HEALTH INFORMATION – NEW POSSIBILITIES

HEALTH INFORMATION – NEW POSSIBILITIES

Tony McSéan
editor

Librarian, British Medical Association,
London, U.K

John van Loo

Librarian, United Medical and Dental School of Guy's
and St Thomas's Hospitals,
London, U.K.

and

Euphemia Coutinho
assistant editor

Administrator, British Medical Association Library,
London, U.K.

SPRINGER-SCIENCE+BUSINESS MEDIA, B.V.

Library of Congress Cataloging-in-Publication Data

Health information, new possibilities / edited by Tony McSeán, John
van Loo, and Euphemia Coutinho.
p. cm.
Includes index.
ISBN 978-0-7923-3584-9 ISBN 978-94-011-0093-9 (eBook)
DOI 10.1007/978-94-011-0093-9
1. Medical libraries--Europe--Congresses. I. McSean, Tony.
II. Van Loo, John. III. Coutinho, Euphemia.
Z675.M4H363 1995
026.61'094--dc20 95-21647

ISBN 978-0-7923-3584-9

Printed on acid-free paper

Contents

2. NETWORKING & RESOURCE SHARING

3. MANAGEMENT & ORGANISATIONAL ISSUES

4. THE LIBRARY IN THE LEARNING ENVIRONMENT

5. DEVELOPING NEW SERVICES & RÔLES

7. INFORMATION IN THE PHARMACEUTICAL INDUSTRY

8. CONSUMER HEALTH INFORMATION

9. PROFESSIONAL ISSUES

10. HISTORY OF MEDICINE

11. POSTER SESSIONS

Introduction

In bringing together and editing these proceedings, we were conscious that we would have to extend ourselves if we were to produce a volume worthy of the conference itself. EAHIL's proud record of successful conferences must be a daunting prospect for any newly-formed organising committee: Brussels in 1986, Bologna in 1988, Montpellier in 1992, all built upon the success of its predecessors and each was an important event in the development of medical and health librarianship within Europe.

The Oslo organising committee, together with their colleagues on the international programme committee, faced a daunting task. A darkening economic climate, a venue far from the European epicentre, Norway's comparatively high cost of living — there were plenty of excuses for retrenchment and conservatism. Instead, through hard work, cooperation and sheer determination, Elisabeth Husem, Arne Jakobsson and their colleagues put together an event which will live in the memory of all of us lucky enough to attend. Perhaps the most notable feature of the conference was that the organisers, through a variety of stratagems, made possible the attendance of large numbers of colleagues from the emerging nations of Central and Eastern Europe, for whom the expense of travel and accommodation might otherwise have been a considerable problem. It is to be hoped that they benefitted from attending, but it is certain that the event was richer, more interesting and more rewarding for their contribution.

In closing this short introduction, we would like to express our thanks to everyone concerned in the compilation and production of these proceedings: to the contributors, almost all of whom responded to our request for a computer-readable version of their papers; to those who helped convert contributors' files from the sometimes surprising formats in which they arrived; to Roselyne Hoet, EAHIL's secretary general for her efforts in marketing this book and ensuring that it got to press at all. Most of all, we must express our appreciation of Euphemia Coutinho of the BMA library, who retyped the papers whose formats defeated us and whose patience overcame computers, laser printers and countless other problems that would have defeated most people.

Finally, we apologise now for any errors not picked up before production, and for the paper that somehow found its way in twice and was not spotted until the indexes had been compiled and camera-ready copy had been printed.

Tony McSeán
John van Loo

CONFERENCE COMMITTEES

LOCAL ORGANIZING COMMITTEE

Elisabeth Husem, Chair
University of Oslo, Department of Psychiatry, Library

Elisabeth Buntz
The National Hospital, Medical Library and Information Centre

Eldbjørg Nåheim Eien
Dikemark Hospital, Medical Library

Tove Gellein
The Norwegian Radium Hospital, Medical Library

Turid Tharaldsen
National Institute of Public Health

PROGRAMME COMMITTEE

Jean-Philippe Accart
Bibliotheque Medical, Centre Hospitalier d'Argenteuil, France

Barbara Aronsson
World Health Organization, Office of Library and Health Literature Services, Switzerland

Suzanne Bakker
Central Medical Library, University of Amsterdam, Netherlands

Elizabeth Buntz
Medical Library and Information Centre, Rikshospitalet, Norway

Arne Jakobsson, Chair
Spri Library, Sweden

Christiane Kay
Medizinische Bibliothek, Zentralkrankenhaus Reinkenheide, Germany

Elisabeth Kjellander
Astra Arcus AB Dokumentation & Bibliotek, Sweden

Ragnhild Lande
University of Trondheim Medical Library, Norway

John Van Loo
Medical Library, United Medical & Dental School, United Kingdom

Deonilla Pizzi
Biblioteca Centrale, Facolta Medicina e Chirurgia, Universita degli Studi di Siena, Italy

Otakar Pinkas
National Medical Library, Czech Republic

Pirjo Rajakiili
Folkhalsoinstitutets bibliotek och informationsservice, Finland

SECTION 1

PLENARY SESSIONS

COMMUNICATION IS A BILATERAL PROCESS

Astrid Nøklebye Heiberg, Psykiatrik Institutt, Universtet Oslo, Blindervn 85, Postboks 85, Vinderen, Oslo, Norway

Health information is important, and we have a lot of new possibilities - without doubt, we all agreee upon that. But then - what do we agree upon? What do we mean by health information, what kind of process is that? What are the possibilities and limitations for giving and receiving information? What do we mean by health, and what do we mean by health information? Who is that information for?

One of the benefits of being a psychiatrist, is that I am entitled to ask questions, not to give answers. Some people - referring to Socrates, say that questions actually may be more useful than answers. So - let us start by scrutinizing our concepts - what is information? No doubt it is a form of communication, one person is in some way conveying her ideas or knowledge or whatever to another person, with the purpose to increase this other person's knowledge or awareness. Let us start with the phenomenon of communication - which we all know is a very difficult task. Certainly all of us have experienced failures here. The typical is within the family:

> "Why did you not arrive at six o'clock?" "But I told you - I should come at eight" "You did not tell me" This also is an excellent starting point for a quarrel. If you want to make that fool proof - just add "always" and "never". "You never tell me", and "You are always late". A more productive way to solve this problem is to say - "You may have said it, but I did not hear it," "I thought I said it - at least I meant to".

This illustrates a very basic condition for communication - which is often forgotten - communication has to come through - it has to be heard, or seen or in some way be received by the sensory system. Many people have dulled senses, especially elderly people, but amazingly also many younger ones, and often they want to hide it. That means that communication has to be clear an preferably unambiguous to avoid misunderstandings. I experienced this the other day, motoring with a new aquaintance. We passed by an area with a lot of moose or elk as we say,- a typical Norwegian countryside with woodland between small villages dominated by the home for the elderly.

I said - "we have to drive carefully because of the elk and deer," she heard me saying "we have to drive carefully because of the elderly," and we had a very confusing discussion about the possible risks for the car and ourselves before the misunderstanding was cleared up.

Misunderstandings show that we have different pictures inside our heads, even if we seemingly have the same experiences. Actually the two of us did not have the same experiences even if we literally were in the same car. I,as the driver, felt the responsibility to follow the signs by the road - warning against elk. She followed the discussion about family that we had just had - a discussion that involved older people. If we could see each others thought bubbles - like in the cartoons, we would probably be amazed at the differences. All information that we get, is linked up to former experiences and adds to or changes the program in our brains. Being with children makes this very evident - all families have cute stories about childrens' misunderstandings, misunderstandings that change the picture the grown-ups try to convey into something which is normally much more dramatic.

My own favourite family story is when our elder daughter at the age of four listened to me telling my husband about a patient we had seen the day before. The patient had been admitted for intoxication after an overdose with tablets called "**insilon**" and I said that considering her difficult life situation she had probably wanted to be taken care of. "Yes"said my daughter. "Yes what" - said I -"what did I say?"
"You said that there was a lady who was very sad, but then she put her mother **in the loo**, and that was what she really wanted"

The moral of these stories is that the different concepts and pictures in our heads are partly derived from earlier experiences, partly from more or less hidden wishes. I got the message of how my daughter felt about her mother.

Because of these internal differences, we can never really know what impact our information will have upon other people. Basically this is the philosophical question posed by Immanuel Kant "Das Ding an sich und das Ding für mich" - we can never know for sure that we share the same ideas.

The next problem is our psychological limitations in receiving information. Our most usual inhibitions is simply being tired. We want to hear - we want to understand, but there is sand in my eyes - so much sand - and they are so heavy - the eyelids are so heavy- I try to keep them up, but they fall - they fall - they fall. I shall stop here, not wanting all of you to fall asleep while I am still the speaker. What I now did, of course, was to use the hypnotic technique of monotonous repetition, keeping the voice even,calm, soothing- we all use that when we try to make babies sleep. Some information is given in the same way, it is given so repetitiously and monotonously that nobody notices any more even if it may be given very correctly, and is meant to be very important and useful. A way to counteract that is to simply try to keep people awake by making them actively associate or participate - or if that is not possible like in big lectures - to stimulate by showing slides and overheads. Some overdo that so that they only use slides, and then the audience is back to more limited stimulation again.

Television highlights some of the problems of communication. It has made visible how limited our capacity for reception is. A basic rule in evening news, is that there shall never be more than one message in one news piece. If a war is terrible and that is the message, you should stick to that, not confuse the picture with varied information about relief work. And if the message is that relief work is fine, you should stick to that, not dwell on the details from the horrors of the war, unless you want to show the contrast. But then the contrast would be repeated. One message at a time. Entertainers break this rule. They introduce new themes all the time, preferably unexpectedly. If you ask the audience afterwards about what he said, they usually can not answer -"but was he funny!"

So far we have dealt with limitations of an involuntary kind, dull senses, differences in experience and knowledge, lack of physiological capacity. But there are more limitations to deal with - those of a psychological nature. Back to television again: we have difficulties in absorbing news from somebody we dislike or who disturbs us in some way. We like the newsreaders because we like them, not because they are good newsreaders. That does not necessarily mean that they are all very good looking - they may be pathetically clumsy, or queer or even ridiculuos - but somehow they appeal to us - otherwise we would not listen.

A friend of mine gave a talk on television - an important political talk, she was a minister. She had been very busy preparing it, so she had not had time to do her hair as she normally did. Next day she met one of her close coworkers in the department and asked how the coworker liked the talk. "Frankly", said the coworker"I had problems listening, I was so distracted by your hair" "My hair" protested the minister " but what about my talk!" "Well" said her colleague "I believe it was all right, but - you must have a haircut" It sounds bizarre - but the story is true. And I have myself made a parliamentarian run back into the cosmetic boot, shortly before the lights went on, when I pointed out to him that his whiskers were unevenly cut.

Sympathy, or lack of sympathy, is mostly unconscious or subconscious. Another subconscious force is resistance against realizing the implications of new knowledge. Often the hopes we have, giving health information, is that it might lead to a change in activity or at least in attitude. The extreme example of this is psychoanalysis, which possibly also might be regarded as a kind of health information. In analysis, the interpretation of resistance to change is fundamental. A friend of mine described it this way : " Here I had been on the sofa for hours and hours, yes actually for several years, telling about my shortcomings and mistakes. Then one day it dawned upon me that it was actually true - that is when I started to change". Open resistance to information will normally have its roots in differences in value systems. We can tell a member of the Jehova witnesses for as long as we wish about the life saving possibilities of a blood transfusion - it is of no interest to him because he is forbidden by his religion to give or receive blood.

In parts of Africa, voluntary organizations have been very active in combatting AIDS by programs for condoms. The information is that the only way of avoiding contamination through sex, is prevention by condoms. But in some of these countries, sex means much more than reaching orgasm. In these countries the value of the woman is determined by her ability to produce sexual wetness. The wetter she is, the higher her value, and the more she is sought by men. A sexually dry woman is looked upon as useless. Then how could a man enjoy her wetness if he is barred from this by a condom? The condom destroys the fundamental pleasure of sexual activity which is so much the proof of his virility and thereby his pride and prestige. What kind of health information reaches them? Let us have an inbetween repetition; if information shall be received, not only given, it has to be

Simple, clear and unambigious
Building upon knowledge about the recipient's knowledge
Activating to be integrated in the recipient's inner pictures
Respectful of the recipient's value systems

With these general rules in mind, we can now turn to health information - is that special in any way? And what new possibilities do we have?

Again, I have no fixed answers,let us look at it together: The recipients are both health workers and patients. The information includes both prevention and cure, knowledge about both normal functions and disorders and disturbances. Traditionally the task of the medical librarian has been to assist the health personell in being updated about the latest development in the often very specialized field that they work in. Gradually now the interest of the public and the patients has come more into focus. The ethical principles of informed consent and autonomy on the part of the patients is being highlighted. This work, information to the patients will probably increasingly be part of the responsibility of the medical librarians. If we look back upon the basic principles for information, we know that we as patients, often are much less receptive than normally because of pain, fear, and maybe influence of drugs. Therefore information to us as patients,must be very clear and simple, and often repeated and discussed. When we use the principle of building upon knowledge, we have to be aware that people normally have very confused ideas about the structures and the function of the body. And even you, when you think about it, how many would be able to make a drawing of how your legs are connected to the rest of the body? Why don't you try it?

Activation of questions and answers can be done by discussion. Here though, I believe that new techonology, allowing the patients to go into programs to seek their own answers, may be some of the very interesting possibilities to develop. Doctors are notoriously not very good informers - for so many years it has been part of the medical culture that patients should not understand what we say. The preference for Latin and Greek in the medical language, is not only that we need a precise tool for interior communications, but also that the patients should be kept out of the discussion. So there is a lot of new interpretation to be done, and who shall be the interpreters? You? Trying to keep to the principle of a limited amount of messages in one lecture, I shall refrain from going more deeply into the very complex questions of how much information shall be given, where is the limit between what is useful for the patients, and what may cause harm through increasing fear and anxiety. Suffice it to say, that there is still a very long way to go before our patients are getting too much information.

My last point is to remind us of the limitation of medical knowledge. Considering the vast influx of articles, this may sound paradoxical. But we should bear in mind that the turn- over of medical truth is shorter than ever -.
Humility is therefore very much needed in our task as health informants. Actually though, my thoughts went a little further than that. An increasing problem is that our patients do not fit very well into our diagnostic categories any more. The diagnosis essential, genuin, idiopathic, which all mean "we do not know", is used more and more frequently. Some start putting a question mark as to whether we are using the right model for thinking, maybe we have the wrong pictures inside our heads? The medical science of today builds upon the model, the inner pictures of natural science. What is in, will come out. What is up, may fall down. Before - now - later. Our thought system are straight lines, our thinking linear, clear, simple. But the queen of natural sciences - physics, is not so clear any more. We now learn about black holes - where nothing comes out - ever. Einstein told us that parallell lines will eventually meet. The concept of interactions is that some activity in one part of the world simultaneously create changes in the balance of systems in the opposite part. Maybe time is not linear, maybe it is circular, repeating itself. I shall stop now - there may be too many questions. Coming together like this in such a big conference gives you the chance to resolve some of these questions. Equally important it gives you the possibility to discuss your role in health information since you are the most important servants of knowledge. I wish you the best of luck.

HEALTH INFORMATICS AND LIBRARIANSHIP

Michael Carmel, South Thames (West) Regional Library Service,Royal Surrey County Hospital, Egerton Road, Guildford, Surrey GU2 5XX, UK

Shared Purpose

The purpose of informatics and library services is to ensure that providers of health care have access to reliable, relevant and up to date information, enabling them to enhance the quality of care. This paper demonstrates the common ground between the two, and the advantages of shared understanding and joint working and draws some conclusions for medical librarians.

The Virtual Library

I am indebted to Lois Ann Colaianni for revisiting the mission statement of health care librarianship (1) provided by George M Gould in 1898 and not significantly improved upon since:

> "I look forward to such an organization of the literary records of medicine that a puzzled worker in any part of the civilized world shall in an hour be able to gain a knowledge pertaining to a subject of the experience of every other man in the world".

This is indeed the virtual library. Today we use electronic networks, storage systems and interfaces to try to come a little closer to the ideal, but the needs of the user remain paramount.

Informatics

The National Library of Medicine offers this working definition in its long range plan (2): "Medical Informatics attempts to provide the theoretical and scientific basis for the application of computer and automated information systems to biomedicine and health affairs. ... (It) is oriented toward the invention and dissemination of powerful information management tools. These include frameworks for organizing and encoding medical knowledge, methods for acquiring and representing judgmental knowledge based on experience, computer networks to permit efficient communications among health personnel, and systems to provide customized advice ..." Informatics has many achievements to its credit in fields as diverse as pathology autoanalysers, CAT scanners, and patient administration systems. Three major areas of work are of intense current interest, and are of direct relevance to the library mission: the management of images, decision support systems, and the electronic patient record.

Image management Medicine has always been the most visual of all the sciences, but never has this been more true than today, with the development of ever more sophisticated ways of peering into as well as at the human body. "Modern medicine has come to depend on the image as the key component for teaching, research and clinical practice. ... Whether we are talking about pathology teaching slides, fluorescent markers in research, or CT scans in clinical practice, the viewing, study and analysis of images has become an all-pervasive part of medicine. Thus in any attempt to improve information management in medicine, the transport and control of image data must be of prime concern." (3) There is a sound logic in using optical discs to store images, computers to organize retrieve them, and networks to transfer them. Many formats are computer generated or enhanced in the first instance, while others have been successfully digitised. The potential gains from computer management include: more efficient organization and retrieval; accessibility at the time of need by use of the network; integration of information from different visual sources; integration with textual and numeric information; security and conservation

3-D browsers, analysis tools and multimedia: It has to be remembered that the primary purpose of images is for immediate clinical use and that optimising that function will always take precedence over management considerations. At the same time there are many gritty problems to be solved along the way, not least those of storage and network capacity and interface design, where the ambitions of the developers always seems to outrun the currently affordable technology.

Decision Support Systems: It is over 20 years since the earliest publicly available diagnostic systems were announced. Yet there are few if any such systems in widespread clinical use today, despite great progress in the underlying knowledge bases, the algorithms and the user interfaces. The use of the terms "expert system" and "artificial intelligence" tend to generate unrealistic hopes and fears, and led to unreasonable disappointment (or relief) when the benefits are found to be limited. Miller and Masarie (4) charge developers, including themselves, with incorporating "an ambitious model for diagnostic decision support that contributed to the current lack of widespread acceptance of diagnostic expert systems." Systems no longer attempt to emulate the decision making skills of an expert, nor do they attempt to provide definitive answers. They offer either: timely reminders for busy clinicians who may have overlooked an important fact or deadline **(alerting systems)**, *or* a method for interrogating a **knowledge base** to retrieve the likely or possible solutions to a given problem (usually diagnostic), ranked by probability. The main obstacles to the use of knowledge base systems in clinical practice, as distinct from education, are familiar to librarians. They include access at the time of use, interface issues, and the difficulties of speedily defining the nature of the problem.

The Electronic Patient Record: There are almost as many synonyms for the electronic patient record as there are definitions. They may be termed: computerised; computer-based; automated; electronic; virtual or online; they may be patient, health or medical records, or even a "patient view". The concept of an electronic record lies in the eye of the beholder. Probably the most successful EPR systems to date are in Europe, among general practitioners in the Netherlands and the United Kingdom. It has to be said however that these are comparatively simple systems involving clear ownership, few users, restricted sources of data, and relatively easily identified patients. Attempts to develop comprehensive hospital record systems reveal great complexity and ambiguity in all these areas. As Dorenfest (5) says: "... the next generation of patient care systems ... will go a long way towards automating all patient care functions with a fully automatic patient record available for all patients ... but today the health care industry is faced with information systems that are far from this vision. .. we must change our approach .. Past difficulties have resulted from oversimplification and improper definition of user requirements."

The common ground: It has been noted that librarianship and informatics share a common purpose, but equally we share many other interests: Monitoring the *quality of information* in the literature, in knowledge bases, and in clinical guidelines int the face of the explosive growth in the literature and research is a central problem in clinical practice, given the need for simple but authoritative answers. The current concern with "knowledge based care" has brought a new urgency to this issue. The *users of systems*, especially clinicians, need encouragement and help to define their needs, which are themselves constantly changing, and training in using existing systems. At the *infrastructure* level there are problems network capacity (especially for image management and transmission), connectivity, and architecture, and software and os compatibility, especially where investment in existing systems cannot be written off. Language is often a major hidden barrier to effective access to information. We need more than one standardized language, because each is based on different usages and a different frame of reference. Yet we also need a common language system for all aspects of health care. Still more important is the need for ***common interfaces*** and work stations which will simplify the procedures for the user without undermining functionality. As Purves (6) says: "It has become apparent that for the future systems to be useful in the consultation they have to be one step ahead of the clinician and present clinically relevant information and decision support at different stages in the consultation process (i.e. differential diagnosis, producing a list or evaluating hypotheses; selecting a course of action; managing continuing problems; and anticipatory care. This requires an effective interface, a knowledge base, decision support software and management guidelines all packaged into a patient orientated workstation." Access to library services should be an integral part of the same package.

IAIMS

Probably no institution or project has done more to bring this about than the IAIMS Program of the National Library of Medicine (USA). The Integrated Advanced Information Management Systems (IAIMS) is a program of the National Library of Medicine which for ten years has been encouraging designers to adopt an integrated approach to information systems, to the benefit of patient care, research, education and administration. Seventeen institutions have received grants, even though it seems not to have achieved its early rather simplistic aims. IAIMS is a highly successful programme in that it has:

(a) influenced the **culture of the institutions** involved and their corporate attitudes to sharing of information, resources and skills;

(b) change of the **cultures of the main professional groups** involved, breaking down tribal barriers;

(c) created a new breed of multiskilled professional, with "mix and match" training at a high level (MSc, PhD) for doctors, librarians and computer specialists;

(d) mapped the main problems of integration in detail;

(e) identified the critical success factors in integration;

(f) created a sufficient range of specific products and services to act as exemplars for future work.

The next great challenge for IAIMS will be to find ways to disseminate the attitudes knowledge and skills which have been acquired or developed in a small number of centres. The process is as important as the product. It will not therefore be possible for other centres to easily "buy-in" to the benefits of IAIMS. This applies even more to other countries and cultures who will have to go through their own learning and development process.

Conclusions

The development of libraries and informatics over the past twenty years shows a great deal of common ground and shared interests, not only in technology, but even more in areas related to the quality of information, its accessibility, interaction with users including marketing and training, organisational issues, and economic issues. There is little interaction between the two in Europe. The interaction which exists in the USA has proved productive for both sides. Interaction is hard work, and requires constant effort and goodwill. Where successful it is almost invariably the result of direct and conscious action by the National Library of Medicine and its development programmes. IAIMS is at the heart of this process. Europe would benefit from a research programme adapting the IAIMS principles to European patterns of health care, research and teaching. The main missing element in Europe is a strong leadership focus equivalent to the NLM. We should try to develop such a focus.

References

1. Colaianni, L "That vision thing" (Janet Doe Lecture) Bull Med Libr Assoc 80 (1) Jan 1992
2. USA. National Library of Medicine. "Long Range Plan". Executive Summary. p31 (extracted)
3. (From) Eaton, EK "IAIMS Grant application on behalf of Tufts University" unpublished report, Boston, 1993.
4. Miller, RA, and Masarie, FE "The demise of the 'Greek Oracle' model for medical diagnostic systems" Meth Inform Med 29, 1990, 1-2
5. Dorenfest, S.I. (1993b) "History, benefits, past problems and future directions in efforts to computerise the patient record" (Abstract of paper) American Medical Informatics Association, 1993 Spring Congress: final program. St Louis, 1993. 56.
6. Purves, I "Implications for family practice record systems in the USA: lessons from the United Kingdom" Abstract in American Medical Informatics Association, 1993 Spring Congress, final program. St Louis, 1993. 54.

UNDERGRADUATE EDUCATION IN HEALTH INFORMATICS

David Bawden, Department of Information Science, City University, London, EC1V 0HB, England

Abstract
This presentation considers the scope of informatics as a discipline, and health (or medical) informatics as an instantiation in one professional domain. Educational approaches to the subject are reviewed, with an emphasis on integrated and information-related approaches. The new BSc degree in Health Informatics at City University is outlined

Informatics
Many, perhaps most, commentators would regard health informatics as, both pragmatically and philosophically, a part of the health-care disciplines. I begin from an opposite perspective, seeing the subject as an instantiation, in one application domain, of the discipline of informatics. Both perspectives are valid. Indeed, this dichotomy, while it may cause some confusion, is a source of creative tension which can stimulate the interdisciplinary interactions valid to the development of subjects such as this. The term "informatics" is one with a long history, but relatively little consensus as to meaning. Originating in Russia during the 1950s, it was adopted in English, German (informatik) and French (informatique). It has often been used as with rough correspondence to term "computer science". However, an alternative meaning has come into widespread usage, to denote a broader discipline, dealing with all aspects of the handling of information and knowledge, and often used synonymously with "information science/s". That is the sense in which I shall use the term.

I regard informatics as a field of study with its focus being the central concept of information, and knowledge. The application of several different forms of knowledge can clearly be seen within the literatures of the informatics disciplines. More formally, we can say that informatics is: *an interdisciplinary field of study, involving several forms of knowledge and associated paradigms, given coherence by the centrality of the concept of information, and underpinning several practical disciplines*. The practical disciplines referred to would be such as: librarianship; records management; software system development; and so on. This approach provides a rationale for a broad-based approach to the application of informatics in particular application areas, such as health-care.

Health Informatics
I should first address a question of terminology: health informatics or medical informatics ? There has been much divergence of opinion as to which is the better term to use. I prefer health informatics, to indicate an inclusive approach, so that informatics is seen as serving *all* of the healthcare professions, not just medicine. There is as much debate about the proper definition of health informatics as about informatics *per se*.

> "Like information science, health informatics has not been defined to the satisfaction of all its proponents. Definitions vary from emphasising the theoretic and scientific basis for the use of automated information systems in biomedicine, to a discipline that includes the fundamentals of medicine, engineering and information science .. Many of the definitions, however, emphasise broad-based information-related issues, and contain the concepts of acquisition, organisation, analysis, evaluation, synthesis, management, communication, and dissemination of information as well as technological literacy." [Lunin and Ball, 1989]

The National Library of Medicine, in its long-range plan for 1986, defined medical informatics as "an interdisciplinary field that combines medical science with several technologies and disciplines in the information and computer sciences. It provides methodologies by which these fields can contribute to better use of the medical knowledge base and ultimately to better medical care". Greenes and Shortliffe (1990) took an even broader view: "the field [is] concerned with the cognition, information processing, and communication tasks of medical practice, education and research, including the information science and technology to support these tasks."

Blois (1984) suggested that "it will be the task of this new discipline {which he termed medical information science] to better understand and define the medical information process .. in order that appropriate activities will be chosen for computerisation" and that progress would not be possible without first "analysing the nature of medical knowledge [as] .. a necessary prerequisite to the proper utilisation of computers in medicine.

These views, and others, emphasise the importance of understanding the nature and application of information and knowledge at a high conceptual level. They stand, however, in distinction to a rather pragmatic "computer skills" approach, which has pervaded much thinking on health informatics training and practice (Ball et al 1989).

Education in Health Informatics

The history of education for health informatics is complex, and includes many different approaches and tactics (Detlefsen 1993, Haynes etal 1989, Ball et al 1989, Mohr 1989). This is both inevitable and appropriate, given the different perspectives which are taken on this area, and the extent and variety of relevant knowledge and skills. There are a number of frameworks for categorising the way in which health informatics is taught. The most obvious is according to the institution and level of teaching, bearing in mind that this may be in-service training (eg Woods and Coggan 1994). In a comprehensive review of the totality of education and training in this area, Haux et al (1992) use a two-dimensional framework of educational level (professional school - polytechnic - university) and nature / orientation (medicine-incorporating-informatics to informatics-incorporating-medicine). The subject may be taught with emphasis on depth, as one component speciality within a disciplinary program: either a health-care discipline (medicine, nursing, etc) or an informatics discipline (computer science, library/information studies, etc). This is the most common means, and the easiest to manage and teach. Thus, informatics modules are generally available as optional or, increasingly, compulsory, elements in medical training, both in the USA and in Europe, and also in training for the other healthcare professions. On the other hand, health information options are now commonplace in library/information training, and health informatics increasingly features in computing and IT courses. Alternatively, with an emphasis on breadth, it may be taught as an integrated speciality, comprising elements of the many relevant disciplines. This challenging approach is, in many ways, to be recommended (Mohr 1989). The best known example is, perhaps, that of the University of Leiden medical curriculum (Tuinstra 1989).

My particular focus here is on undergraduate, first-degree, education, as it is understood in a British context. This make for some difficulties in international comparisons; in the USA, for instance, Masters programmes are a more appropriate comparison, in many ways. Nonetheless, some general points may be made, of which the most important is that this route of education for health informatics has been, and remains, of less significance than that of graduate study. In the graduate route, education in health informatics builds on, and enhances, an initial education either in informatics, or in the health care disciplines. I do wish to suggest that I believe that this concentration on the graduate route is mistaken; on the contrary, my view is that this, in general, the most appropriate way into this field. Nonetheless, there is room for a alternative approaches, of which an initial specialisation in health informatics is one. Undergraduate specialisation implies an integrated approach, rather than one of "grafted on" specialist modules, or somewhat artificial "joint degrees". Further, given the nature of professional education in both Europe and the USA, it implies a course rooted in informatics, rather than one rooted in the health sciences.

Examples of such course are few. Haux et al (1992), speaking of an "information-related approach" refer to "university level .. study of medical informatics .. as an integrated applied subject or as a subsidiary subject within a framework of informatics", an example of the former being the University of Hildersheim and of the latter the Technical University of Munich. The University of Heidelberg offers a 4-year program, leading to a Master's qualification, with joint themes of health sciences and information/computer sciences, plus integrated studies in healthcare systems and applications of informatics. In the USA, BS degrees are generally too limited in scope to offer a significant health informatics component; Stanford offers a Masters in Medical Information Sciences, having as its core subjects medicine, computer science, decision making, medical computer science and health policy / social issues. Perhaps the clearest example is the BSc in Health Information Science at the University of British Columbia in Canada (Protti 1983, Anglin 1989), having as its core subjects computer science, administrative systems, biomedical science and statistics, and economics. In Britain, Manchester University is launching an undergraduate degree in Medical Informatics during 1994.

City University Health Informatics BSc

This degree is planned to build upon City University's twin strengths in Health Sciences and in Informatics. There are already several initiatives in the teaching of health informatics at the University, including a Masters in Medical Informatics, and health informatics modules on Masters degrees in Information Science and in Information Systems and Technology. The course will be informatics-based and integrated. Some students may come straight from school or college course, although we anticipate a particular demand from mature entrants, with non-graduate healthcare experience. The course will have five main themes: healthcare systems; information technology; information systems and services; data, information and knowledge; and organisational, social and ethical issues. The course runs for three years of full-time study, with an optional "sandwich" year of practical experience. For the first two years, students will study informatics modules in common with those on other courses in the departments of Information Science, Computer Science and Business Computing, and will also follow courses in logic and language of healthcare, healthcare systems, and health information and knowledge. General informatics modules, for example computer networks, and systems analysis and design, will be "flavoured" by health care examples. There will be a strong emphasis on communication and interpersonal skills, on information literacy, and on languages; somewhat unusual in British informatics education. In the final year, students will chose from a variety of specialist options, in health informatics and general informatics with a health flavour.

We see the particular challenge of this course as attracting students to a niche subject, and providing a genuinely high quality education, as well as a training for a professional area. In curriculum design terms, the challenge is the integration of a great many diverse subjects, allowing students to obtain a good overall knowledge, while permitting specialisation. We envisage a variety of career paths for graduates of this degree, including clinical informatics, health information systems analysis and design, library/information services, and education. We believe that the course will be a valid complement to graduate study in the area.

References

Anglin CR, Health information sciences at UVic; the student perspective, Methods of Information in Medicine, 1989, 28, 285-291.

Ball MJ et al (1989), Information education and the professions, Journal of the American Society for Information Science, 1989, 40(5), 368-377

Blois M (1984), Information and medicine, Berkeley, University of California, Press.

Detlefsen EG (1993), Library and information science education for the new medical environment and the age of integrated information, Library Trends, 42(2), 342-364.

Greenes RH and Shortliffe EH (1990), Medical informatics: an emerging academic discipline and institutional priority, Journal of the American Medical Association, 263(8), 1114-1120.

Haynes RB et al (1989), A review of medical education and medical informatics, Academic medicine, 64(2), 207-212.

Haux R et al (1992), Recommendations of the German Association for Medical Informatics, Biometry and Epidemiology for Education and Training in Medical Informatics, Methods of Information in Medicine, 31, 60-70.

Lunin LF and Ball MJ (1989), Introduction and Overview, Perspectives on Information Science and Health Information Education, Journal of the American Society for Information Science, 40(5), 365-366.

Mohr JR (1989), Teaching medical informatics: teaching on the seams of disciplines, cultures, traditions, Methods of Information in Medicine, 28(4), 273-280.

Protti DJ (1983), A comparative analysis of the German Informatiker der Medizin Diploma and the Canadian Bachelor of Science in health information science, in Pagès JC et al (eds), Meeting the Challenge: Information Science and Medical Education, Amsterdam, North-Holland.

Tuinstra CL (1989), Integration of medical informatics with other courses in the medical curriculum, Methods of Information in Medicine, 28(4), 243-245.

Woods SE and Coggan JM (1994), Developing a medical informatics education program to support a statewide health information network, Bulletin of the Medical Libraries Association, 82(2), 147-152.

MAKING DECISIONS IN THE YEAR 2000: Realising the Potential of Consumer Health Information Services

Bob Gann, The Help for Health Trust, Highcroft Cottage, Romsey Road, Winchester, SO22 5DH, UK

Abstract

This paper reviews the development of consumer health information (CHI) services in the last decade and looks forward to the major CHI trends in the milennium. It concludes that although there have been major advances, many CHI services are still complacent, passive, static and superficial. There remains a need to embrace advances in quality assurance, health informatics, outcomes and effectiveness if we are to provide the information services to which consumers are entitled in the year 2000.

Introduction

There is no doubt that consumer health information has been one of the last decade's information "megatrends"[1]. During the 1980s and early 1990s increasing attention has been given to the provision of information on health care issues to patients, relatives, carers and the wider public. Over this period, medical libraries have had an increasing inclination and ability to provide information to patients. At the same time, there has been a blossoming in new consumer health information services, combining the subject expertise of the medical library with the accessibility of the public library. And there has been an unprecedented expansion in the amount of published literature on health topics for lay people.

Social and Political Change

There are a number of reasons for the development of consumer health information services in the 1980s and 1990s. One is undoubtedly an increasing consumerism in society generally, which is reflected in our behaviour as patients. People are no longer content to be told what's good for them. They want access to information which enables them to weigh up risks and benefits, and to make informed choices between options in health care[2-3] There now seems to be a political consensus on the need for more information for health care consumers. In 1990 the British Labour Party issued a policy document, *A fresh start for health*[4], which supported the development of a patient population which is "more self confident, more assertive and more knowledgable". This new orthodoxy is most clearly expressed in the UK government's *Patient's Charter*[5] launched by the Secretary of State for Health in 1991. As part of the Charter, the government required all Regional Health Authorities (14 in all) to set up consumer health information services from April 1992. The Department of Health issued Health Service Guidelines HSG(92)21 providing a detailed specification of the services to be provided. RHAs were instructed to set up a freephone service to provide the public with information on local NHS services, waiting times, complaints procedures, Patient's Charter standards, coping with illness and treatment, and maintaining good health. In January 1993 the Secretary Of State for Health launched a single national freephone number for health information throughout the UK. Members of the public can now dial Freephone 66 55 44 and wherever they are in the country they will be automatically routed to their nearest Regional Health Information Service (RHIS). This number was publicised by a major national press advertising campaign. For the first time anywhere in the world, ordinary people can access a national consumer health information service, free of charge with a single telephone call.

This national system is underpinned by a rich network of locally based consumer health information services in a variety of settings: libraries, advice centres, disability centres, health shops, mobiles, hospital information points.[6-7] It is important to remember that consumer health information services were not created, top down, by the Patient's Charter. Some of the most innovative and excellent services have developed, bottom up, from local community initiatives, often on a multi-agency basis. The recent boom in consumer health information services may have a political impetus but it is founded on the vision and local good practice of services since the late 1970s.

Scratching the Surface?

It would be tempting to be complacent about the rapid development and successes in consumer health information over the past few years. We have certainly seen major changes in attitude to the availability of information, political enthusiasm at the highest levels, and, in a time of financial stringency, the availability of new funding for CHI initiatives. But, if we look more carefully, we will see that the potential of consumer health information services has hardly been realised. We are still scratching the surface. Too often CHI services in the UK (and in other countries too) can be: **complacent** : we are content that services are provided at all, not that they are done well; **passive** : we are content for consumers to come to us and we do not exploit new technologies; **static** : our information does not develop rapidly to meet current concerns and is not based on the best current evidence; **superficial** : we provide generalist information which does not answer the questions people really want to know or give them real power in dcision making.

Beyond the Complacent Information Service

In the recent debate on the ordination of women priests in the UK, misogynist commentators have been fond of quoting the English lexicographer Dr Samuel Johnson's opinion of preaching women and acrobatic dogs: "It is not done well, but you are surprised to find it done at all."[8] Until recently this might have been a reasonable summary of opinion on consumer health information services. We were so pleased to see information services being established at all that we were not over concerned about whether they were done well. This may have been acceptable in the early days of an emerging information specialism but it is the sign of maturity in any discipline to be concerned with standards and quality. In other areas of health care and information provision there are clear standards linked to accreditation schemes. Consumers deserve no less. By the year 2000 we must establish a rigorous quality framework for consumer health information, learning from the best European and worldwide practice. It is likely that the National Health Service will move towards a national accreditation scheme for consumer health information services, whereby services which meet quality standards will be entitled to receive calls via the national freephone number and display a nationally - or eventually internationally - recognised "Health Information Service" symbol.

A key aspect of the development of quality services has been the increase in training opportunities for consumer health information staff. Discussions are now under way with appropriate academic institutions and the National Health Service Training Directorate into the establishment of a modular, distance learning diploma in consumer health information. With harmonisation of qualifications we could see a consumer health information qualification recognised throughout the European Union by the year 2000.

Beyond the Passive Information Service

Currently consumer health information services reach a very small section of the population. Work in Wessex and Cambridge is beginning to identify the nature and extent of unmet need for health information. A symposium issue of *Health Libraries Review* devoted to consumer health information reviews work in this area.[9] Individual services are beginning to be responsive to local community needs through a range of initiatives. Helplines are being promoted through talking newspapers for visually handicapped people. Minicom lines are being installed for people with hearing difficulties. Services in areas with large ethnic minority populations are employing outreach workers with relevant language skills or joining tele-interpreting services. Information technologies are certain to be of increasing importance in enabling CHI services to bring information closer to the consumer. We are beginning to see the development of interactive systems designed to involve patients in shared decision making[10] First developed in the USA by the Dartmouth based Foundation for Informed Medical Decision Making and now being piloted in the UK by the Kings Fund Centre[11], these SDPs (shared decision making programs) are based on interactive videodisc technology. The aim is to review the published research on the outcomes of different treatment options (for example surgery or watchful waiting for enlarged prostate) and to present this information in a way which is tailored to the individual patient's history and priorities. By providing information about the risks and benefits of different treatment options, the patient is actively involved in decisions about his or her own care.

Every day thousands of Americans participate in electronic self help groups without leaving their homes. As long ago as 1984 the New Jersey Self Help Clearinghouse was piloting support groups for people with rare conditions over the CompuServe network.[12] A logical extension of the teleconferencing concept, using networks and bulletin boards provides the opportunity for housebound people, those in remote areas, or those with rare conditions to gain new access to mutual support and information.There is now sufficient interest in the application of health informatics for consumers for the first National Conference on Consumer Health Informatics to have been held in Wisconsin in July 1993[13]. The conference reviewed developments in computer and telecommunications applications in the light of the Clinton/Gore administration's commitment to a national information infrastructure.

Beyond the Static Information Service

Ten years ago we were delighted when we heard examples of patients being provided with information about how a particular treatment is carried out and what to expect when you come into hospital. Evidence from a recent UK study by the Audit Commission into communication in hospitals[14] indicates that this is still a major need which is not always being met. But it is also true that when we do provide information it does not always reflect the most up to date evidence on clinical practice. We need to ensure that information to consumers is evidence based and swiftly disseminated. A conference organised by the UK Cochrane Centre and CHIC in November 1993[11] looked at ways of strengthening the links between the research and reviews community and those working to disseminate information to consumers. There is considerable potential for CHI services, self help groups and the media to route to the public information on the effectiveness and outcomes of treatment, which is now being compiled by centres like the NHS Centre for Reviews and Dissemination at York and the UK Cochrane Centre in Oxford. Many treatments which have been carried out for years are now being shown to be of questionable benefit. The new emphasis on systematic reviews of the outcome and effectiveness of treatments has recently led to the value of a number of interventions being challenged. And yet patients are still being asked to consent to treatments (and the general public to fund health care initiatives) without accurate understandable information on their effectiveness. Too often the information we provide to consumers is *process* based rather than *outcome* based. Patient information literature tells patients what happens in a particular procedure; it rarely tells them about its likely effectiveness and the pros and cons of having it done in the first place.

There is evidence of change. In 1992 the US government Agency for Health Care Policy and Research carried out a comprehensive review of pain management and produced a set of clinical practice guidelines for professionals[15] At the same time a consumer booklet *Pain control after surgery: a patient's guide* was produced based on the evidence of the clinical guidelines. Now in the UK the CRD at York and the Cochrane Centre are working to produce consumer versions of reviews of effectiveness of treatment for glue ear and cataracts, and of interventions in pregnancy and childbirth. The pregnancy and childbirth work is being carried out in collaboration with the National Childbirth Trust and the independent Midwives Information and Resource Service (MIDIRS).

Beyond the Superficial Information Service

As I give this paper, back in the UK the government is publishing its first set of NHS Performance Tables. From June 1994, health authorities will be required to publish information for the public on the performance of hospitals. These "league tables" are published in newspapers and available in health service premises, libraries etc. They will for the first time give information about how successful hospitals are in meeting Patient's Charter targets on waiting times for treatment, assessment in accident emergency departments, cancellation of operations, and waits in outpatient departments. The publication of these tables has been criticised as being superficial and misleading. There is something in this, but the fact remains that if this information is collected and available it should be in the public domain. A greater concern should be - does it answer the questions the public want to know? We tell patients how long they will have to wait and what the environment will be like, but very little about whether the treatment will be any good when they do get to see the doctor. As an article in the *New England Journal of Medicine* observed in 1988[16]"Patients are forced to judge medical care on quality of amenities because they rarely have suitable information to base it on anything else".

Patients are led to believe that the health service provides a consistent quality of service. This is clearly not the case. For example research has shown very significant variations in outcome of surgery depending on the choice of surgeon[17]. In 1988 the US Congress published a report on providing information to the public on quality of medical care[18] The report encourages provision of information to consumers on hospital mortality rates, adverse effects of treatments, including hospital acquired infections and disciplinary actions against doctors. We have come a long way in the last ten years in providing the public with information on the health services available to them, on self help organisations, and on everyday self care. If we are fully to realise the potential of health information services for consumers we must now grasp the nettle of providing information about quality and outcomes of treatment. It will not be easy to present this information in an understandable way but that is our challenge as information providers - not a problem for consumers.

Sharing Power in the New Millenium

In recent years there has been a growing body of research evidence on the positive effects of the provision of information to patients. This can extend to improved patient satisfaction, reduction in pain, fewer postoperative complications, shorter hospital stays, reduction in blood pressure, improved self management of conditions including diabetes and kidney disease. In 1991, after reviewing the relationship between communication and health outcomes, an international conference in Toronto issued a consensus statement[19] underlining the effect of information giving. This gave particular emphasis to the benefits of information giving in two key areas: reduction of anxiety and increased compliance with medical instructions. The power of information to produce a happier, more compliant patient population is becoming evident. Many people - including many patients - welcome this. But information should be more than an opium of the people. It should be about answering the difficult questions as well as about giving reassurance. It means raising expectations, challenging professional mystiques and outdated orthodoxies, sharing decision making, and above all sharing power.

References

1. Naisbitt, J. *Megatrends* New York: Warner Books, 1982 identifies self help, information technology and personal networking as "megatrends" of the late Twentieth Century

2. Rees, A. Communication in the physician-patient relationship *Bulletin of the Medical Library Association* 81(1), 1993, 1-9

3. Medical libraries and patient information services: symposium *Bulletin of the Medical Library Association* 82(1), 1994, 43-66

4. *A fresh start for health* Labour Party, 1990

5. *The Patient's Charter* London: HMSO, 1991

6 Gann, R. and Needham, G. *Promoting choice: consumer health information in the 1990s* Winchester: Consumer Health Information Consortium, 1992

7. Gann, R. Consumer health information: the growth of an information specialism *Journal of Documentation* 47(3), 1991, 284-308

8. Boswell, J. *Life of Johnson* 28 July 1763

9. Buckland, S. Unmet need for health information *Health Libraries Review* June 1994 (forthcoming)

10. Kasper, J.F., Mulley, A.G. & Wennberg, J.E. Developing shared decision-making programs to improve quality of health care *QRB* June 1992, 183-90

11. Dunning, M and Needham, G. But will it work, doctor? *Involving users of health services in outcomes research* Milton Keynes: Consumer Health Information Consortium, 1994

12. Madara, E. The self help clearinghouse operation: tapping the potential of I & R services *Information and Referral* 7(1), 1985, 42-58

13. *Consumer Connections: Newsletter of the Consumer and Patient Health Information Section of MLA* 10(3), Winter 1993-94

14. *What seems to be the matter: communication between hospitals and patients* London: Audit Commission, 1994

15. US Department of Health and Human Services. Agency for Health Care Policy and Research *Clinical practice guidelines for acute pain management* Maryland: AHCPR, 1992

16. Elwood, P.M. Outcomes management: a technology of patient experience *New England Journal of Medicine* 318(23), 1988, 1197-1202

17. McArdle, C.S. Impact of variability among surgeons on postoperative morbidity and mortality and ultimate survival. *British Medical Journal* 302, 1991, 1501-5

18. US Congress Office of Technology Assessment. *The quality of medical care: information for consumers* Washington DC: OTA, 1988

19. Simpson, M. et al Doctor-patient communication: the Toronto consensus statement *British Medical Journal* 303, 1991, 1385-7

L'INFORMATION MÉDICALE À LA PORTÉE DE TOUS

Patricia Mesmacque, Brigitte Parraud, Tù-Tâm Nguyen, Médiathèque de la Cité des Sciences et de l'Industrie, 30 ave Corentin Cariou,75930 Paris, Cedex 19, France

La Médiathèque constitue le volet documentaire de l'offre muséologique de la Cité des sciences et de l'industrie. Depuis son ouverture, en mars 1986, elle a pour mission de réunir une collection de vulgarisation scientifique accessible à tous les publics. Dans ce but, a été constitué un fonds multi-niveaux, proposant aussi bien des documents professionnels, que des ouvrages d'initiation. Les collections sont présentées sur 3 étages, la Médiathèque couvrant une surface totale de 12.000 m^2. Le public peut y consulter le catalogue informatisé à l'aide de 70 écrans répartis dans tous les espaces ; ce catalogue est également interrogeable à distance par télématique (Minitel). Le fonds est divisé en grands secteurs thématiques, suivant un plan de classement original qui, volontairement, ne recouvre pas les disciplines scientifiques traditionnelles : ainsi nous trouvons des secteurs comme "Agriculture", "Alimentation", "Travail et Industrie"..., quant à la médecine, elle est représentée par les secteurs "Corps humain", "Ages de la Vie" et "Santé et société". Les livres, les revues, les logiciels éducatifs, les CD-Rom et les audiovisuels sont en libre accès. La majorité des imprimés, ainsi que les cassettes sonores, peuvent être empruntés à domicile. Enfin, le personnel se compose de 150 postes, toutes fonctions confondues, les bibliothécaires représente environ 80% de l'effectif.

Voilà définis, globalement, la mission d'information documentaire de la médiathèque, ainsi que les moyens matériels et humains mis en oeuvre. Le service médecine-santé s'inscrit dans cette démarche, mais présente en plus, la particularité d'être la première bibliothèque de santé ouverte à tous en France. Cette position originale nous a amenés à réfléchir sur trois points. Tout d'abord **notre spécifité documentaire** : quels fonds rassembler, quelles méthodes pour y parvenir ? Ce qui revient à définir les collections. En second lieu **la médiation nécessaire** pour rendre accessible les contenus de ces collections au plus large public, c'est-à-dire redéfinir nos compétences, notre métier. Enfin **une mise en scène globale de la science** dépassant la distinction musée-bibliothèque.

1 - La spécificité documentaire

Lieu d'information médicale unique en France, la Médiathèque offre à tous ses visiteurs l'accès à des ouvrages de vulgarisation comme de référence, ainsi qu'à des documents de niveau professionnel, médical et paramédical : 9000 titres, 20 000 volumes, 370 périodiques, 300 audiovisuels... L'éventail des sujets couverts par notre plan de classement, déborde largement la médecine clinique : ainsi, les documents sur la cosmétologie, le thermalisme, la santé publique ou la psychanalyse, y ont une place de choix et correspondent à une forte demande de la part du public. Même à l'intérieur des domaines plus "classiques" de la médecine, notre repérage doit être large, puisqu'il répond à la volonté de constituer un fonds multi-niveaux, afin de répondre aux besoins d'information de tous les publics. Mais nous sommes tributaires de la production éditoriale française qui est très sectorisée. Ainsi dans les disciplines purement médicales, la production reste le plus souvent d'un niveau très spécialisé. Même s'il paraît de plus en plus d'ouvrages ou de collections de vulgarisation, ils ne couvrent pas encore tout le champs des sujets que nous traitons.

En fait, nous balayons l'ensemble de la production éditoriale, depuis la vulgarisation médicale jusqu'aux ouvrages les plus techniques. Nous sommes aidés dans cette tâche par un dispositif centralisé de demandes de services de presse, en collaboration avec de nombreux éditeurs qui apprécient de pouvoir utiliser la médiathèque comme vitrine pour leurs publications. Il est alors nécessaire de compenser cette ouverture optimale par la recherche de critères rigoureux dans notre politique d'acquisition. Par exemple, l'imagerie médicale est un sujet très développé dans l'édition spécialisée, qui a tendance à publier abondamment des titres spécifiques à chacune des parties du corps humain ; aussi, nous avons volontairement limité notre fonds à l'acquisition des titres les plus généraux, des quelques ouvrages de vulgarisation, et à une revue de référence dans ce domaine. A l'inverse, pour un sujet tel que le sida, il nous a paru important de présenter, dans un lieu neutre, des sources d'information utiles au plus large public. Nous avons donc poussé notre politique d'acquisition vers une plus grande exhaustivité : nous proposons ainsi 200 titres de monographies médicales, romans, témoignages, et bandes dessinées. Afin de compléter cet ensemble nous proposons au public dix revues spécialisées ou d'associations, des films, des didacticiels et des classeurs documentaires.

Nous avons dit que notre acception d'un concept de santé élargi, implique pour nous un problème de couverture documentaire ; aussi, pour combler les lacunes de l'édition, nous avons mis en place un circuit d'exploitation de la littérature non commercialisée. Un premier type de littérature "grise" s'adresse surtout à un public professionnel : ce sont les plaquettes de présentation et rapports d'activités d'entreprises. Cela peut concerner aussi bien les cosmétiques Clarins que l'Institut Pasteur, Sandoz ou Rhône-Poulenc. Ces documents, que l'on trouve rarement en bibliothèque, et jamais dans le commerce, sont utilisés par les lecteurs faisant des études de secteur ou de marché, et par tous ceux qui ont besoin de bien connaître une entreprise, par exemple pour une recherche d'emploi. Un second type de complément documentaire est offert par les brochures d'éducation pour la santé, publiées par divers organismes dans un souci de prévention : Ministère des affaires sociales et de la santé, Comité français d'éducation pour la santé, ou encore des laboratoires pharmaceutiques.

Des dossiers thématiques contenant des brochures d'éducation pour la santé, permettent, dans notre service, de pallier les lacunes éditoriales : c'est le cas, par exemple, du tabagisme. Les brochures de vulgarisation médicale les plus intéressantes sont demandées en grande quantité, puis diffusées gratuitement au public, accompagnées d'une présentation de documents de notre secteur traitant du même sujet. Ainsi, les thèmes de la maltraitance ou de la contraception, présentés ponctuellement de cette façon, ont recueilli un vif succès auprès du public ; celui-ci apprécie ces brochures, qui permettent un accès rapide à une information précise, et lui donnent la possibilité de repartir avec un document synthétique. Bibliothèque de vulgarisation, la Médiathèque de la Cité des Sciences et de l'Industrie reste nécessairement généraliste, et ne saurait être un centre de documentation spécialisé. Nous avons donc recours aux autres partenaires du réseau de santé, vers lesquels nous orientons des demandes que nous ne pouvons prendre en charge jusqu'au bout. Ainsi, une lectrice faisant une étude approfondie sur la grossesse des adolescentes, sera aussi orientée vers le Centre International de l'Enfance, ou l'Institut de l'Enfance et de la Famille. De même, un enseignant souhaitant emprunter des films sur la vie des enfants dans différents pays, sera orienté vers le Centre de documentation de l'UNICEF, car nous ne prêtons pas les audiovisuels de notre fonds qui sont tous transférés sur vidéodisques. Autrement dit, nous pallions les limites de l'offre documentaire ou de service de la médiathèque par le recours aux partenaires du réseau santé. Des outils de repérage d'institutions ou d'associations ont été constitués, sous forme de classeurs d'adresses mis à la disposition du public. Ces classeurs sont régulièrement alimentés par les informations ou les documents que nous récoltons, lors de nos visites de bibliothèques ou de centres de documentation du réseau santé. Après cette rapide esquisse de notre spécificité documentaire, nous allons aborder maintenant le rôle particulier de la médiation dans notre travail.

2 - La méditation nécessaire

Mettre à la libre disposition du public, dans un même lieu, des documents de niveau vulgarisation et de niveau professionnel représente un bouleversement dans le paysage documentaire français. A la médiathèque, la multiplicité des niveaux et des supports, la diversité des visiteurs et des attentes crée la nécessité d'une médiation documentaire qui facilite, en particulier aux non-initiés, l'appropriation du contenu des fonds. En effet, dans la plupart des cas et pour différentes catégories de public comme les scolaires, les amateurs ou les simples curieux, l'intervention active des bibliothécaires permet de renseigner individuellement les lecteurs, ménager une variété d'accès, permettre une diversité d'usages, proposer des réponses plurielles et adaptées, réorienter vers d'autres lieux et ressources en complément. C'est pourquoi des formations à la communication interpersonnelle et à l'accueil du public ont été systématisées pour le personnel.

Cet aspect est particulièrement important dans notre domaine où nous sommes souvent amenés à recevoir des personnes motivées par des questions de santé personnelles ou touchant leur entourage. Disponibilité, écoute, respect de l'anonymat, accompagnement du lecteur dans sa recherche et facilitation de son autonomie doivent être les composantes de notre attitude quand sont abordés des sujets comme la leucémie, le traitement de la maladie de Parkinson... Les exemples sont nombreux et certains ont été repris dans le film que vous avez pu voir. Dans ces situations délicates, la satisfaction du lecteur dépendra étroitement de la mise en oeuvre de compétences multiples : connaissances techniques, savoir-faire documentaire mais aussi, savoir-être relationnel. Il nous paraît également primordial de faire comprendre au public que nous n'avons nullement vocation à nous substituer aux thérapeutes mais que notre apport informatif peut être un élément dynamisant dans la relation médecin-malade qui est fondée sur le principe du consentement éclairé du patient.

C'est dans cet esprit de convivialité que nous avons voulu compléter ce travail de médiation au quotidien par l'organisation d'animations qui aménagent un accès différent à l'information de santé. Les rencontres-débats autour d'un livre ou d'un film réunissent auteurs et lecteurs et font de la Médiathèque un lieu ouvert et neutre où néophytes et professionnels peuvent échanger points de vue, savoirs et expériences à propos de la santé et de la maladie. Lieu de lecture, lieu de parole, mais aussi lieu d'apprentissage, la Médiathèque a inauguré dernièrement une animation d'un genre différent : une démonstration des gestes de premier secours par les pompiers de la Cité des sciences destinée au public adolescent a remporté un vif succès. Nous avons fait une présentation de tous nos manuels et brochures de secourisme à cette occasion et l'après-midi s'est terminée par une séance de consultation des logiciels éducatifs sur le thème "Prévention-sécurité". C'est ainsi que des adolescents peuvent apprendre à s'informer sur un sujet en utilisant différentes ressources documentaires et en découvrant des métiers présents à l'intérieur de la Cité. Cette participation ponctuelle des pompiers aux animations de la Médiathèque, participation qu'il est déjà prévu de renouveler pour l'an prochain, nous a conforté dans notre recherche de synergie avec l'ensemble des acteurs de la Cité des sciences pour une mise en scène globale de la science.

3 - La mise en scène globale de la science

Elle doit intégrer l'espace muséologique et l'espace documentaire. De façon générale, nous nous sommes toujours attachés à faire écho aux productions de la Cité. Les thèmes abordés par les expositions temporaires nous donnent l'occasion de mettre en valeur les documents de notre fonds qui peuvent aider les visiteurs sensibilisés par l'exposition "à en savoir plus...". Ainsi, des expositions comme celles du "Sang des hommes", "La Fabrique de la pensée", "Les Cinq sens" destinée aux enfants ont crée l'occasion d'éditer des sélections bibliographiques et de faire des présentations d'ouvrages à la Médiathèque. Sur le site même de l'exposition, des documents sont proposés, simplement mis sous vitrine ou organisés en véritable salle de documentation. C'était le cas lors de l'exposition "La Douleur" qui avait délibérément pris le parti de la complémentarité entre démarche muséologique de sensibilisation et approche documentaire.

L'exposition consacrée aux "Métiers de l'hôpital" a fait réaliser de très utiles dossiers documentaires mis en consultation sur le lieu de l'exposition. Nombreux sont les visiteurs qui sont venus à la Médiathèque pour pouvoir les emprunter, découvrant alors toutes les ressources de la section médecine-santé. Les renvois d'un espace à l'autre ont un résultat positif mais encore insuffisant. Car notre voeu est d'aller vers une véritable intégration musée-bibliothèque offrant à chacun la possibilité de choisir ses chemins de la connaissance et de reconstruire sa propre unité du savoir. Un tel projet doit s'appuyer sur les deux volets muséologique et documentaire de la vulgarisation.

Conclusion

Bibliothèque multimédia, la Médiathèque apporte des éléments de réponse à propos des questions vives et en controverse. Elle propose le moyen de s'informer de manière contradictoire en présentant les positions en présence (débats sur l'éthique biomédicale, les médecines différentes). Avec la pérennité de ses collections elle constitue un centre de ressources de référence qui permet d'approfondir ce que les médias ne font qu'effleurer. En donnant la priorité à la médiation humaine elle propose au simple profane de s'initier aux concepts de base et aux savoir-faire, et aux professionnels de s'autoformer et de poursuivre leur formation. Nécessité de la médiation documentaire, volonté d'améliorer le dialogue soigné - soignant autour de l'utilisation d'un même fonds documentaire et de son animation... Nous aimerions que ces quelques réflexions nées de notre jeune expérience de 8 ans puissent créer l'occasion d'échanges entre nous et, pourquoi pas, aboutir à la création d'un code de déontologie propre aux bibliothécaires ?

LOOKING TOWARD THE FUTURE WHILE WORKING IN THE PRESENT[1]

Lois Ann Colaianni, Associate Director, National Library of Medicine, Bethesda MD 20894, USA

It is my pleasure to attend this, the Fourth European Conference of Medical and Health Libraries. I can clearly remember the excitement and anticipation as the first conference opened in Brussels in 1986, and the vigor of the second conference in Bologna two years later. The European Association for Health Information and Libraries started as an idea but came into being through the efforts of a small number of European health sciences librarians. EAHIL can be viewed as a significant step toward the global organization of health sciences librarianship. Other steps are also being taken. In 1992 the first Regional Congress on Health Information Sciences for Latin America and the Caribbean was held in Brazil, and the fourth Congress of the Association for Health Information and Libraries in Africa was held just two months ago. The development of these regional and national health sciences library associations comes during times of great change. Have you thought about the changes that are occurring in your lives and your libraries and information centers? If your experiences are like the majority of health sciences librarians I encounter, you must learn many new skills in order to be successful professionally and provide up-to-date services in your libraries. Colleagues in other libraries in your country and in other countries are also confronted with major changes and the rapidity with which they are occurring. Professionally we face challenges and all around the world, events seem very unsettling. It is times such as these when some of the people looking at half a glass of water see it as half empty; others as half full. I hope that you are all persons who see the glass as half full.

Times characterized by great challenges such as these also present great opportunities. Our success as a profession depends on our ability today to plan strategically for the future. We must look forward while working in the present. On Saturday, Rachael Anderson will discuss some of these opportunities in the context of new or expanding roles for health sciences librarians. This morning I will address these opportunities in the context of a global vision of health sciences librarianship. I will mention two trends in the world that affect this vision and then suggest some specific ways health sciences librarians could begin to pursue such a global vision.

The first trend, facilitated by modern communications, is the increasing international cooperation in health promotion and disease prevention and biomedical research. This is prompted by the unnecessary deaths of millions of children from preventable diseases; the HIV/AIDS epidemic; the rise in incidence of tuberculosis and malaria; and the "brown plague", tobacco smoking, to name a few. In 1977 the World Health Assembly resolved that "the main social target of governments and WHO in the coming decades should be the attainment by all citizens of the world by the year 2000 of a level of health that will permit them to lead a socially and economically productive life"[2]. Similar resolutions have been enacted all over the globe. Cooperative efforts in biomedical research, public health programs and epidemiologic studies, disaster relief, and drug development are well documented in the literature. Results in health services research are being shared internationally as nations examine each other's health care delivery systems for better ways of providing quality health care to everyone at an affordable price. International cooperation in health care and research is a world-wide trend.

John Naisbitt in his new publication *Global Paradox* provides some thought-provoking insights into my second trend. He describes the developing global village, but he says that although people want to come together to trade much more freely, they want to be independent politically and culturally. He sees the global paradox as powered by the explosive developments in telecommunications, encouraging strategic alliances, creating global networks, and empowering everyone. Everyone can have the power of a personal computer and through a modem or local area network connect

---

[1] A shortened version of the paper presented at the conference.

[2] World Health Organization. *Global Strategy for Health for All by the Year 2000*. Geneva, Switzerland: World Health Organization;1981.

to everyone else, thus "the bigger the world economy, the more powerful its smallest players"[3]. The challenge he sees for a successful global future is balancing the tribal concerns with its issues relating to culture, ethnicity, or religion, with the universal or more global concerns. We have a global village drawn together by communication, travel, and common interests in the economy and health but divided by the needs for independence and the increasing power of the smallest unit, a tribe or indeed, an individual. Success in this world, he says, requires strategic alliances. Naisbitt identifies the trend of empowered small players establishing powerful alliances in the world economy.

What are the implications for our profession? Globally, our profession provides information necessary for health care and biomedical research and yet individually we are part of different political, cultural, religious, and ethnic groups. What advantages might strategic alliances have for our future? What if we removed some boundaries in our thinking? Health sciences librarians might use strategic alliances to form a virtual international health information center.

Consider some of the requirements for a virtual health information center. Electronic networks exist and are spreading throughout the world. In addition to the electronic networks health information resources exist for many subject areas and others can be developed. Many health information resources such as MEDLINE and AIDSLINE from the National Library of Medicine, ISI's Science Citation Index and EMBASE have been created as international resources. There are regional resources such as LILACS and national resources such as SPRILINE and SWEMED. We already have significant portions of the communication network, the connections, and biomedical and health information resources for a virtual information center, but how would we function in such a center? Networking permits individuals almost unlimited access to all the people who are on the network. Some months ago a graduate student in northern India needed a couple of articles to complete his dissertation and sent me an Internet message requesting copies of them. If a virtual health information center existed how would I be expected to respond? Should I fill the request bypassing information resources in India? Should I refer him to the National Medical Library in India, the International MEDLARS Center in New Delhi, or the library in his institution? Would there be a directory of libraries so that I would know what services his library provided or what serial titles they held? If there is an infrastructure, will it be developed by associations of health information professionals such as EAHIL and the Medical Library Association in the U.S.; or national medical libraries such as NLM and the Karolinska Institute Library in Stockholm; or will the structure be composed of informal relationships between individual colleagues?

On what value system would a structure be based? Are the values that underlie the activities of the 4,000 libraries in the National Network of Libraries of Medicine in the U.S. the same as those in other parts of the world? Will librarians across the globe with network access agree to standards of practice? Even if some of us agree to cooperate and share resources, how will we communicate, not technically but in choosing the words we use and our style of writing? Lee Sproull and Sara Kiesler have spent more than ten years studying communities of people using electronic mail. In their book *Connections* they discuss how electronic interactions differ significantly from face-to-face exchanges and actually change the way work is conducted. They found that people were less constrained in the electronic environment, expressing extreme positions more freely, a phenomenon called "flaming". Do people communicating outside their own environment or at a distance devote less time to the social niceties? Sproull and Kiesler also found that communication even in organizations that have open access was not an easy task. The cues that most of us are accustomed to in face-to-face communications are absent. Gone are heads nodding in agreement or puzzled expressions when the message is not clear. They observed that groups of three persons took approximately four times as long to reach a decision electronically as they did in face-to-face situations. How much cooperation are we willing to foster to perform our library tasks? Electronic networks remove the necessity for individuals working on the same intellectual task to be in physical proximity. A cataloger at NLM could contact a cataloger in Germany for name authority information about a German author. Will colleagues respond with an authoritative answer to a message.."Does anyone know...?"

At this meeting sessions are addressing our roles and services, designing a library, pharmaceutical publications, marketing the medical school library, psychiatric reforms in Nordic countries, managing change, DRUGLINE, problem-

---

[3] Naisbitt J. Global paradox: the bigger the world economy , the more powerful its smaller players. New York, Morrow; 1994. p 50.

based medical curricula, and many, many more topics. As you listen to these presentations think about how handling the information from these sessions in the networked environment. What if there were international discussion groups on problem-based curricula and mental health issues and a bulletin board where a notice describing DRUGLINE's contents and access mode could be posted for the entire world to read when they had a need for this information?

Each of us is appropriately focused on our roles in our own library or information center and the environment of the city, state, and country in which our library exists. As increasing numbers of health professionals are directly empowered through electronic connections, some librarians are concerned about what the future role of our profession will be. One future direction for us is to build the health information resources we create into a virtual international health information center. In order to do that we must think beyond ourselves, our libraries, our countries, and our regions. We must have the vision of an international profession and develop the infrastructure through which we can cooperate. Electronic networks offer unlimited opportunities for achieving significant objectives that improve the services in our libraries. Networks also offer the possibility of health information for all in the next century; a possibility limited only by our vision and our efforts.

Well, it's only an idea, as EAHIL was a decade ago.

THE FUTURE OF INFORMATION PROVISION: Managing the Process of Change

John Cox, Managing Director, Carfax Publishing Company,PO Box 25, Abingdon, Oxon, OX14 3UE

An analysis of how the market for individual research papers has developed, why document delivery is now being treated as a matter of importance both by publishers and librarians and how such developments may reach new markets for rsearch literature. It concludes with some observations on future developments. For the past 40 years, the volume of scientific and medical research information has grown at an astonishing rate. It has been distributed largely in the form of those printed volumes we call journals. There has always been a marginal activity, which we now call document delivery, in supplying copies of individual articles to customers who cannot find the journal issue they need in their own library. The British Library Document Supply Centre, and other national and regional libraries, have been supplying copies of documents in this way for 30 years. As long as it did not really affect the economic basis of journal publishing, document delivery was not seen as an issue of importance. However, since the mid-1980s the world of scientific and medical journals has increasingly been beset by change and uncertainty. It has become more difficult to maintain collections in the face of static budgets, the exponential growth in information, and price increases that regularly exceed the prevailing inflation rate. Journal subscriptions have been cancelled at an increasing rate over the past five years. Librarians are searching for ways of deploying their resources more evenly to meet their patrons requirements more effectively.

This crisis has been felt most keenly in academic libraries. The following facts serve to illustrate the situation:

a The proportion of the university library materials budget devoted to serials is now 70 percent. It is much higher in the case of collections of mainly scientific and medical material.

b. Collections of monographs and conference proceedings have been seriously eroded.

c. Library expenditure, as a proportion of overall university expenditure, has declined. As an example, in the UK it has declined from 4 percent in 1980 to 3 percent in 1990.

d. Inter-library loan traffic has increased dramatically. Most of this traffic is in the form of individual articles photocopied by one library and supplied to another, without attracting any form of payment to the publisher.

So we have an economic crisis in which our customers are seeking alternatives. And what makes recent developments in document delivery so potent is the convergence of that economic need with technological opportunity. The availability of indexing and searching tools on CD-ROM and on-line has brought increased awareness of, and ability to find, a complete range of the literature for any particular requirement. Document delivery provides researchers and practitioners access to the literature in their fields, even though their own library's holdings have been eroded. Modern telecommunications and computer technology clearly provide us with the opportunity to store and transfer information speedily and inexpensively. As a result, inter-library loan traffic has grown to an estimated 20 million documents circulated worldwide. And a new generation of document delivery services has been launched. The "new generation" document delivery services have two components: a current awareness service based on journal table of contents, and a speedy document delivery mechanism that will deliver, usually by fax, the article required in no more than 24 hours. This immediacy has transformed what was traffic between libraries into a growing commercial activity. A large number of players have already taken up their positions:

a. National libraries (BLDSC, CISTI, INIST etc) have been delivering documents for many years, but are now using new technologies to upgrade their services.

b. Library utilities like the Research Libraries Group and OCLC.

c. Abstracting and indexing services like ISI.

d. Secondary publishers like UMI.

e. Subscription agents like EBSCO and B. H. Blackwell.

Moreover, telecommunications companies like AT&T and Mercury are expressly targeting the medical and scientific communities with research information services. I would like to use UnCover to illustrate what is happening. UnCover was established by CARL as an on-line current awareness service, based on 10,000 journals table of contents, in 1988. In September 1991, UnCover unveiled its article delivery service, allowing libraries or individuals to order through the network a faxed version of the original document. In March 1993 Blackwell and CARL created a joint venture and established UnCover as a separate company. UnCover plans to enhance the existing service from its current 15,000 titles to around 25,000. This will make it the most comprehensive article database in the world, addressing the needs of users in North America, Asia, the Pacific, and Europe in equal measure.

UnCover is committed to the observance of publishers' copyright, and he maintenance of publishing as an integral part of the scholarly and medical research process. When you look at an UnCover display, the order screen indicates two prices for document supply. The first is a fixed service charge for UnCover. The second is a variable publisher fee, determined by the publisher, and taken from the publisher direct or from the Copyright Clearance Centre. UnCover has made great efforts to develop close relationships with the major medical and scientific journal publishers. It already has a system of direct licences with those publishers, which grant UnCover the right to store articles electronically and therefore cut the delivery time to less than one hour. While 10 percent of UnCover's article database is stored as full text electronically, those articles account for 17 percent of the articles requested by customers. As market demand increases, we aim eventually to deliver such articles wholly electronically to the personal computer on the customer's desk.

The market that lies ahead of us will be complex and varied. Supplying individual articles creates the opportunity to reach individuals directly as well as supplementing inter-library loan. Above all, it can create new revenue streams that are denied to the traditional scientific and medical journal with its low circulation and high subscription price:

1. None of the 20 million inter-library loan documents attract copyright payments for the intellectual property owner. If only 10 percent of this traffic is time sensitive, and could be captured by a 24 hour service, some 2 million documents, at a copyright fee of, say $5 per item, ie. $10 million, could be captured for publishers. In reality, the potential is much larger. Efficient commercial suppliers like UnCover can sell a document for less than $20, including the copyright fee. At the same time, traditional inter-library loan transactions probably cost $25 or more simply to process. The "new generation" document delivery companies can bring service benefits to the library as well as lower costs, and create a revenue stream that will underpin the research publishing process.

2. Document delivery may also bypass the library and reach the individual practitioner or researcher directly. A significant part of UnCover's turnover is generated by individuals who pay by credit card. Whether they are using personal or corporate cards does not matter in the sense that this traffic is not using library funds. Appropriate pricing and slick and speedy service will help to realise this potential.

The future systems of supply for medical and research information will largely be dictated by developments in the mass market, and in business to business communication. There are some trends which we need to watch most carefully:

1. Personal computers will continue to drop in price while their processing and storage capacity increases. The new generation of multi-media PCs will become commonplace.

2. We will see an ever closer integration of different types of telecommunications technology. Traditional telephone companies are working with and purchasing cellular companies and technologies: AT&T and Macaw Cellular is

an example. Global satellite television may facilitate the provision of scientific, medical and technical information.

3. Software for the universal communication of documents that preserve the original content, structure, look and feel will improve. Adobe Acrobat is the first, and is based on Postscript, which is already a de facto international standard in electronic typesetting.

Collaboration between organisations in different but complementary fields is accelerating. Let me give you two examples:

1. RED SAGE is a collaborating venture between the University of California at San Francisco, AT&T Bell Laboratories and Springer Verlag: a library, a telecommunications and software utility, and a publisher.

2. The British Library and Mercury Enterprises have announced a joint venture in which a CD-ROM based current awareness service, and a two hour fax or image transmission based document delivery service will be developed, covering journal articles, conference proceedings, patents and grey literature.

These ventures exploit the need that telecommunications companies have for 'content', that publishers have for new methods of reaching their market, and that libraries have for access to information they can no longer afford to own. In the longer term, the truly electronic journal, that uses the power and storage capacity of modern technology, must develop. We will see an increase in compound documents with audio and video. This creates new barriers to open and effective interchange. Multi-media documents require huge storage and delivery capacities, and will stretch existing networks to their limits. The document will inevitably move beyond merely being a derivative of the printed article. The pace at which this happens depends on the user's requirements, and his or her perception of the value and status to be attributed to non-print media. The peer reviewed article is still the authoritative report on a piece of research, and is the mechanism by which such research may be judged and may be developed further. In the electronic environment, there is no reason why the process of peer review and quality control should not continue to apply. But authors and readers still defer to the traditional printed journal as the benchmark of scientific and medical research.

The journal publishing industry is facing a dramatic change in the way in which its product is created, delivered and used. Many journal publishers already use sophisticated electronic techniques to accomplish the technical processes of design, illustration, text editing and presentation. The electronic infrastructure is already being created where a journal publisher will, in future, publish material in many forms: in the traditional printed volume form, or on CD-ROM, or on-line, or electronically on demand. But all of this will continue to involve investment. As the copyright owner, the publisher is entitled to control the exploitation and use of his property, but he should be responsive to legitimate market demand, and in particular to the demand of both libraries and individuals for access to the material in a variety of formats, very often through agencies such as document delivery companies operating under a direct licence. It is clear that the economic basis of research publishing will be assured only if all these outputs create revenue for the publisher.

Librarians will also have to change. The very word librarian implies the management, ownership and control of book collections. But what medical practitioners and researchers need today is a range of information resources, with the librarian as the navigator, providing access to whatever his patron requires. If librarians do not grasp the initiative, and actively deliver such services to their patrons, rather than making them passively available, they will be bypassed by those patrons who, with modern technology, can access information sources directly. I foresee a future in which an individual, be he a doctor, researcher or student, will be able to dial into a variety of information sources, and have the material he requires delivered electronically to the personal computer on his desk. The technology already exists. The user is going to be better served than he ever has been in the past. It is for those of us who serve who need to be innovative and flexible; the market will then choose between us.

THE FUTURE OF MEDICAL JOURNALS: An Editor's View

Magne Nylenna, Editor, The Journal of the Norwegian Medical Association,Fjellveien 5, N-1324 Lysaker, Norway

The future of medical journals may be more influenced by political and cultural trends than by technological developments in medicine and the media industry. Medical journals will probably become more reader-oriented and general. The difference between data bases, ideally constructed to produce explicit answers to explicit questions, and medical journals, constructed for general updating and debate and presented to their readers on regular intervals, will become more visible. Editors of medical journals should be prepared for a continuous fight for editorial freedom and integrity.

What is A Medical Journal?

Journals are not the same as data bases, although both may store and present identical information. While data bases serve mainly as sources of specific information, ideally constructed to produce explicit answers to explicit questions, medical journals present unasked for, even unexpected and sometimes surprising information to their readers. To clinicians, and perhaps even to scientists, there are at least two ways of reading. One way is the search for a solution of a defined problem. You have a question, and you look for an answer. This is a way of reading very familiar to librarians, and data bases are an excellent solution. The other way of reading is to be currently open to new impulses and to learn of advances in medicine and health care. You do not really know exactly what you are looking for, but by browsing and through serendipity you may come over something interesting and useful, just as you do when you read the daily newspapers. For this purpose, medical journals, and in particular general medical journals, are perfect. By scanning tables of contents and browsing through abstracts the reader is updated on a broad range of topics. Journals also serve as fora for debate, and as market places for ideas, creativity and personal standpoints. Scientific quality is ensured through a system of peer review. However, medical journals are not simply passive vehicles of information. All editors influence the way that science appears in their journals through their editorial policy, their decisions as to which papers are accepted or rejected, their choice of editorials, their priorities as regards news and book reviews, and the lay out and appearance of the journal. It should be emphasised that the difference between journals and data bases holds good irrespective of production format, whether this be paper or electronic media.

Medical journals have always been linked to the social issues of their day, and editorial philosophies have been changed with changes in society and science (1,2). Changes in the medical journals' contents, appearance and organisation reflect changes in society: Over time, journals have become more democratic and user-oriented. Systems of peer review and quality assessment have been improved. Ethics and political issues have been awarded more attention. The speed of publication has increased, reflecting the higher tempo in all fields of society and the demand for rapid access to medical information. Production routines have changed along with technological developments, and the economics and business aspects of the production have become steadily more important.

Global Lifestyles and Cultural Nationalism

Futurology is a challenging and risky discipline. Everyone who tells fortunes should keep in mind the huge number of errors made by prophets over the years (3). A well known technique in futurology is *trend extrapolation*, which means projecting into the future what has recently been taking place. This may be better than using a crystle ball, and is perhaps useful over a short period, but it is not a very reliable method in the long term. Extrapolations can perhaps be made on the basis of trends in science, technology and economics, but religious, social and political changes are not easy to predict in this way. Few people could have predicted the recent political changes in Eastern Europe and South-Africa by trend extrapolation.

John Naisbitt has become famous for his Megatrends which are based not only on trend extrapolation, but on several techniques, including so-called genius forecasting, which means making judgements about the future by extraordinarily well informed and competent persons. According to Naisbett, one of the megatrends of the 1980s that is relevant to us should be the shift from the industrial society to the information society. We have all experienced the truth of this prediction. A megatrend of the 1990s which I believe to be of importance for the future of medical journals is what

Naisbett & Aburdene have called *Global lifestyles and cultural nationalism* (4). It could be called a paradox, and it is certainly somewhat confusing that two seemingly contradictory trends run together.

The increasing internationalism is obvious to all of us. Trade, travel and television produce a global lifestyle. Wherever we live on earth we can listen to the same American rock music through our Sony walkmans, dress in Levis or United Colors of Benetton, eat McDonald burgers, watch CNN news and drive a Toyota car. Though this is mainly an economic and consumer-based development, it has several cultural implications. One of them is the proliferation of the English language. Language is a corner-stone of culture. English is now becoming what has been called the world's first truly universal language. The language of the information age is English, and there are now more than 1 billion English speakers in the world. English has become the language of science in general and of medicine in particular. Today more than 80% of all scientific papers are published first in English, and the majority of scientific periodicals are in English. On the other hand, there is simultaneously an increasing awareness of the threats implied by this "one universal language" . People in many parts of the world insist on keeping traditional languages and cultures alive. This is what Naisbett & Aburdene call a trend toward cultural nationalism, a trend against uniformity and a desire to assert the uniqueness of one's culture and language. This consciousness of culture and language is highly visible in Europe of today. In France it leads to a strong negative attitude to English, and even regulations against the use of it. In Belgium it leads to high tension between different parts of the same country. In Wales, Catalonia and Lappland it leads minorities to a fight for their cultural identities.

This trend of cultural nationalism is also reflected in an increasing interest in ethnic food and art, an enormous patriotism in sports, and perhaps even in a religious revival. If an outside culture gains too much influence in a country or community this may bring about strong reactions. Unfortunately, under certain circumstances, this cultural nationalism can turn into political nationalism, become a threat to peace and, as we all know, even lead to war. Tragic examples of this exist in Europe today. It is not by mere chance that all the national medical journals in Scandinavia have columns for language and national medical terminology. The pressure not only to publish or perish, but to publish in English or perish leads to reactions in many smaller countries and cultures. This sort of cultural nationalism is not limited to smaller countries and cultures. When some major American medical journals retreat from the true international system of physical and technical units, SI-units, and insist on so-called conventional units (5), this can be viewed as an example of just the same thing. Though general trends in society and culture are relevant for the future of medical journals, developments in medicine and in the media industry are of special interest.

Medicine and the Medical Profession

There has been an explosive development in medicine during the last few decades. Before antibiotics were discovered in the late 1930s doctors had few really effective weapons in the fight against disease and illness. The techological developments since World War II have given medicine new power. Key words are transplantations, new, more effective drugs, and genetic engineering. In spite of this "the medical world is in a sorry state", as The Economist put it in a survey of the future of medicine a few months ago (6). Neither patients nor doctors regard technological progresses as the most typical and visible part of medicine today. Patients' expectations have increased even more rapidly than the medical developments, and doctors and hospitals all over the world complain that they cannot satisfy what has become an ulimited demand for medical care. Patients and doctors alike are frustrated, the doctors' authority is diminishing, and the doctor-patient relationship suffers. In addition politicians and the public feel uneasy about the increasing costs of health care in most countries.

The medical profession is in trouble, and the future does not look as bright as it did a few years ago. Discussions about the future of medicine are not dominated by the scientific developments that can be expected from the new biology, but by economics, lack of resources and a possible reorganisastion of the health care system (3). Add to this medicine's responsibilities for overpopulation, the destruction of the environment and a number of other threats to mankind, and the crystle ball becomes rather dark. Biotechnology and molecular biology will undoubtedly have increasing impact on clinical medicine, but the future of medicine may be dominated by more political issues. Medicine's dilemma of being both a business and a profession will become more apparent. Already today we can see an increase in papers on ethics, economics and legal matters in medical journals, and possibly this is just the kind of trend that may be extrapolated.

Media and Information Technology

Medical journals stand with one leg in the medical and scientific community and one leg in the world of media and information technology. The developments in this field have probably been, and will be in the future, as great as in the field of medicine. The mass of information is rapidly increasing, and most of us have become "information addicts" in one way or another. People have been complaining about the information overload for the last 500 years, and you may have noticed that the ones who complain most are the ones who have produced most information themselves. Up to now, however, it seems as if the means of coping have increased faster than the mass of information. Doctors spend 2 - 4 hours per week on medical articles and journals (7), and their main problem is to decide what to read. Doctors' reading habits have not yet been sufficiently investigated, and the medical journal of tomorrow will have to pay more attention to its readers' needs and demands.

Naturally electronic publication is a challenge to medical journals, as it is to all other sorts of media. Two decades ago it was predicted that, within a few years, the electronic journal would supersede the traditional paper journal(8). This has not been the result so far, and I do not believe it will happen even during the next two decades. As regards the information revolution, health care is still in the dark, and there is no doubt that there will be great changes in the way information is distributed and stored over the next decades. Electronic media will increase and the next generation of doctors will have quite another relationship with screens and terminals. Even so, I believe that paper journals will still survive and play an important role along with tomorrow's electronic professional information systems, just as daily newspapers do in today's era of radio and television. Up till now, no new medium has ever killed an old one. But medical journals for sure will have to adjust to a new situation. Publishing, like medicine, is both a business and a profession. As with medicine, the business part has become more important and visible over the last years. The rising costs of subscriptions to journals are a cause of concern both to librarians and editors. Merging of publishing houses, stronger demands for efficiency in production, and more focus on profits are typical trends.

For editors the economic pressure may represent a threat to editorial freedom. Editorial integrity implies freedom to put the interest of the readers first, and an editor, even of a medical journal, must always keep the ideal purpose of the press and the principles of editorial freedom in mind. This goes beyond political pressure and goverment interference. Editors must have full authority to determine the editorial content of the journal, and neither owners nor advertisers should be allowed to influence editorial decisions. An increasing number of journals and the development of electronic media with almost unlimited capacity are no guarantee for quality assurance and editorial integrity. Remember that free float of information is not necessarily a float of free information.

Conclusions

I expect the following trends in medical journals during the next two decades:

- greater diversity between journals, which means a more pluralistic market
- more reader-oriented journals, meeting the needs and demands of their readers
- more general journals, in the way that more ethics, health politics and material of general interest will appear even in specialist journals
- a more visible difference between journals and data bases, electronic media even more suitable for data bases than for journals
- a continuous fight for editorial freedom and integrity

References

1. Lock S. As things really were? In Lock s, ed. The future of medical journals. London: BMJ, 1991:21-35.
2. Fletcher RH, Fletcher SW. Medical journals and society: threats and responsibilities. J Int Med 1992;232:215-21.
3. Smith R. Through the crystle ball darkly: medical journals and the future. In Lock S, ed. The future of medical journals. London: BMJ, 1991:187-210.
4. Naisbitt J, Aburdene P. Megatrends 2000. London: Pan Books, 1990.
5. Nylenna M, Smith R. Americans retreat on SI units. BMJ 1992;305:268.
6. Wyke A. The future of medicine. The Economist March 19, 1994 (suppl).
7. Nylenna M. Norske legers lesevaner [Norwegian doctors' reading habits]. Nord Med 1991;106:53-4.
8. Long M. The future: electronic publishing. In Hall GM. How to write a paper. London: BMJ, 1994:107-12.

THE NATIONAL MEDICAL LIBRARY (NML), PRAGUE ON ITS WAY TO INTERNET

Otakar Pinkas, Národní lékařská knihovna, Sokolská 31, Prague, Czech Republic

Abstract
An outline of major changes in the Czech health care system and in the network of Czech medical libraries is presented. Recent developments of the Czech educational and scientific network (CESNET) are described. Arguments are brought out stressing the necessity of the National medical library, Prague to become an active member of large information networks including Internet.

1. Introduction
Transition of our country to free market economy has been connected with radical transformation of the Czech health care system. Owing to this situation our Library as well as other Czech medical libraries and information centres has to cope with a number of serious problems. The objective of this paper is to outline the most principal changes, to present principal ways of solution and to sketch out our aims ensuing from the existence of rapidly developing information networks providing new perspectives in both national and international scientific communication.

2. Changes in the Czech Health Service System and Medical Librarianship
Among the most profound changes associated with the transformation of the Czech health service system the following ones should be mentioned:

- the new health service system includes both public and private services,
- the patient has his or her choice concerning the physician and the health establishment,
- the newly built insurance system is the main source of financial provision of medical services,
- transformation of the district public health centres into independent administration subjects was accomplished in 1992,
- transformation of some medium and major hospitals has been in progress since 1993,
- some 33,000 health care workers have moved into the private sector,
- research activities have been reduced and grant system has been introduced,
- health care funding is supported by sponsors, foundations etc.

The library and information network undergoes a corresponding conceptual transformation. In the sphere of medicine and public health the network comprised some 300 units in 1992. The funding of some 150 libraries in the so-called regional and district public health centres through the Ministry of Health came to an end in 1993; nowadays they are financed solely by local authorities. The remaining 150 medical libraries and information centres are still parts of organizations under the state (government) authority and as such they are financed by the Ministry of Health. The privatization of public health centres resulted in 1993 in the decrease of the number of information users; this trend has been evident also in this year. Local community authorities do not usually allocate adequate means to maintain medical libraries and consequently some of them have ceased their existence. A new scheme of financing public information services should be applied in the nearest future. Means from the state budget will be allocated mainly to libraries providing first-rate services to the broadest public. Employment of the grant system for the needs of medical libraries is also envisaged. The decrease of the number of users and the decline of the number of medical libraries in the Czech Republic have a naturally significant impact on the contents and range of present-day NML's activities.

3. Using CESNET
At present, CESNET (Czech Educational and Scientific Network) comprises all 15 academic centres in the Czech Republic, with Prague - Brno connection as its axis. On international level the central node in Prague communicates with partners through Bonn and Vienna. Implementation of optical cables based metropolitan networks is under way

in Prague and Brno. CESNET is being financed by the Ministry of Education so that all schools and academic institutions can use it freely. On the other hand, organizations under the authority of the Ministry of Health (among them NML) have to pay all necessary expenses. Information services provided by CESNET:

- addressing services,
- ftp archives searching on CESNET, ftp anonymous servers,
- surveys of ftp archives mirroring,
- gopher, library catalogues and bibliographic databases,
- conference forums - listserv, other servers, news,
- computational servers.

Since July 1993 NML has been exploiting switched line connection with 2,400 b/sec transmission speed with Internet IBM node computer in Prague. We have been using KERMIT protocol for E-mail and discussion groups. We participate in the international librarian forum Comenius (in English). Functions of integrated library systems are being tested by access to OPACs of foreign and Czech libraries. To a lesser extent we have been experimenting with file transfer. Effectivity and speed of communication have increased substantially since SLIP (Serial Line Internet Protocol) implementation in February 1994 but problems concerning transfer of files with Czech diacritics pertain. Besides being very expensive, communication lines in our country still do not work well and reliably. A monthly charge of some 40 USD is being paid for using communication services and a monthly charge of cca 450 USD is planned for operating a leased line connection with 9,600 b/sec transmission speed. Although all seven medical faculties and both pharmaceutical faculties have already joined CESNET, this unique communication means is still being employed only by some academic libraries.

4. New Objectives of NML and the Modern Information Technology

Besides producing significant bibliographic data bases, the NML provides a broad range of library and information services to physicians through the country. It takes gradual steps to become an active member of CESNET, a specialized nation-wide library network CASLIN (Czech and Slovak Library Information Network) and Internet. Another strategical point of interest is the production of printed outputs, diskettes and CD-ROMs; these products are still more and more available, less expensive and very widely used. NML's permanent aim is economical use of resources and economic effectivity. Nearly all our services and products are charged to the users but fees are very low and generally acceptable. This represents also the way to raise the prestige of the librarian's work and to diminish inadequate exploitation of resources.

We aim at improving quality and timeness of our information. Micro CD/ISIS, widely used in our libraries, lacks data entry support allowing validation of data and usage of authority files. Transition to the usage of more complex library software systems is nowadays a general tendency in all major Czech medical libraries. MeSH thesaurus which has been up to now used only for the indexing of the medical national bibliography is being applied since 1994 also in our cataloguing practice. Our records conform to the UNIMARC format and the English language will be used not only for title translation but also in the user's interface in order to make access to our products more "foreign user-friendly". NML has developed and continues to improve seven external databases, besides them it maintains several internal databases. All databases are made available for relatively modest fees.

The most significant among them is the Czech and Slovak national medical bibliography (CS NMB). With its backfiles since 1978 it contains over 160,000 indexed citations; some 10,000 citations are added each year. It is available as a monthly publication on diskettes and now also on CD-ROM. It may be accessed online, too. The union catalogue of foreign medical periodicals (UC FMP) with some 5,000 entries since 1976 is available on diskettes or in printed form; directory of participating libraries (LOC) is also available both on diskettes or in printed form. Another of our electronic products, the Czech version of MeSH, has found its use in several libraries. In this year it is being implemented into integrated library software packages of medical faculties. Since 1991 we have been monitoring health information in daily and weekly press (HDP). The size of the HDP database is equal to 30,000 bibliographic records. Not only these but also other NML databases will be made available through our server in CESNET. By fixing our own prices we shall be able to determine indirectly the extent of databases usage. The first NML CD-ROM with four databases in hypertext is scheduled for release in October 1994. It will consist of following databases: CS NMB, UC FMP with LOC, HDP. At present, cca 40 personal computers however, not interconnected, are at our disposal. A LAN project on the basis of a RISC server and UNIX operating system has been worked out in February 1994. Our LAN shall be connected via leased telephone line with CESNET and full connectivity in relation to other networks shall be provided. In the first project phase 32 workstations shall be included in LAN. Requests for proposals of an integrated library system were submitted to 4 foreign vendors in May 1994. In June 1994 the Unix DEC 3000 model 300X AXP with 64 MB of internal memory, with 3 GB of disk memory and other peripheral equipment was ordered.

5. Conclusion

NML is striving to meet information needs of its end-users in the new health care system and continues its cooperation with library partners in Czech and Slovak Republic. It aims at improving the level of its services and products, it tries to apply new ways of managing and even marketing in its practice with the objective to provide services for acceptable prices to all clients. It tries to become an active member of CESNET and at the same time to make its products currently available in printed form, on diskettes and on CD-ROM. Our information strategy is based on adherence to international standards and recommendations and on successive introduction of English. These steps as well as new ways of communication via Internet present main pre-requisit for gradual incorporation of NML into the European medical library community.

References

1. Analýza současného stavu a cílové záměry transformace zdravotnictví v České republice. Zdravotnické noviny, 43, 1994, č. 18, s. 3 - 10.
2. Seminář rozvojových projektů CESNET. Praha 23.2.1994. Praha, České vysoké učení technické 1994, 46 s.
3. VACHEK, P.: Informace pro nové uživatele sítě Internet. Verze 3. Praha, ČVUT 1992. 8 s.
4. SVOBODA, M.: Česká a slovenská knihovní informační síť CASLIN. Vznik, principy a předpoklady realizace. i'93, 35, 1993, č. 6, s. 150 - 161.

PROFIL D'UN SPECIALISTE DE L'INFORMATION: Le Documentaliste Hospitalier

Jean-Philippe ACCART, Centre Hospitalier d'Argenteuil, rue du Lt-Col. Prudhon 69, F95107 Argenteuil, France

Résumé
La documentation au sein de l'hôpital est en plein essor. De plus en plus technique et spécialisée, celle-ci doit faire appel à des professionnels de la documentation. La législation actuelle au sein de la fonction publique hospitalière ne reconnait pas la spécificité de cette fonction. Cet article se veut un reflet des préoccupations actuelles des bibliothécaires et documentalistes hospitaliers : c'est à la fois une réflexion sur un statut propre et également un descriptif d'actions individuelles et collectives autour de ce thème.

Depuis les trente dernières années, la fonction de documentaliste a beaucoup évolué. La gestion des documents est devenu primordiale dans un monde où l'information est prépondérante, et pour cela, les hôpitaux n'y échappent pas; la fonction de documentaliste a donc pris tout son sens, son caractère utile et indispensable n'est plus à démontrer à l'heure actuelle. De plus en plus spécialisé et spécifique, ce métier nécessite un niveau d'études supérieures correspondant à un BAC + 3 ou 4. De nombreuses formations existent : Institut National de la Documentation et des Techniques (INTD), Ecole de Bibliothécaires-Documentalistes de l'Institut Catholique de Paris (EBD), Institut d'Etudes Politiques (IEP), Institut Universitaire de Technologie (IUT), etc... On dénombre à l'heure actuelle 65 formations diplômantes accessibles en formation initiale ou continue.

Richesse et diversité de la documentation hospitalière
Depuis le début des années 1980, plusieurs facteurs ont fait évoluer le domaine de la documentation hospitalière, et parmi ceux-ci, l'arrivée des nouvelles technologies, l'avancée du professionnalisme, la gestion de données en nombre croissant, la mise en place de réseaux locaux, ainsi que la diversité des utilisateurs potentiels.

Les hôpitaux publics français se divisent en 3 catégories d'établissements :

* la première catégorie concerne le centre hospitalier régional (CHR) et le centre hospitalier universitaire (CHU) qui assurent des activités de soins, d'enseignement et de recherche dans des domaines très spécialisés.
* la deuxième catégorie concerne le centre hospitalier (CH) ayant une fonction d'hôpital de secteur,
* et enfin le centre hospitalier spécialisé (psychiatrie, pédiatrie)

Ces hôpitaux sont gérés par un conseil d'administration présidé par le Président du Conseil Général si l'hôpital est départemental, ou le Maire de la ville si l'hôpital est municipal.

Tous ces hôpitaux réagissent différemment par rapport à la gestion de leur documentation, qu'elle soit médicale, paramédicale, administrative ou technique. On assiste depuis ces dernières années à un intérêt croissant des équipes de direction et du corps médical pour la documentation au sein de l'hôpital. Aussi fait-on appel de plus en plus à des professionnels.

Le but de cet article est de faire le point sur cette actualité en évoquant plusieurs aspects particuliers :

1) un essai de définition du métier de documentaliste hospitalier : ses spécificités, son champ de compétences et d'action au sein de l'hôpital.

2) les nombreux éléments de réponse apportées "sur le terrain" par les équipes de direction, le corps médical, les documentalistes, l'Ecole Nationale de la Santé Publique (ENSP) de Rennes, ainsi que la mise en place de plusieurs associations professionnelles (ou mouvements associatifs) proches des besoins des professionnels .

Le métier de documentaliste hospitalier : essai de définition
Le Rôle des institutions

- La Direction des Hôpitaux, au Ministère de la Santé, s'est intéressée au développement des bibliothèques médicales et a incité chaque hôpital à créer sa propre bibliothèque.
- Une enquête de la Conférence des Présidents de C.M.E. (Commission Médicale d'Etablissement) en 1989 a synthétisé les réponses et a présenté des résultats très inégaux, mais qui, tous, reflétaient un réel besoin.
- Les directeurs généraux des Centres Hospitaliers Universitaires ont également pris, en 1991, cette question à coeur.

Ainsi, les professionnels recrutés dans les hôpitaux publics pour prendre en charge des structures telles que bibliothèques médicales, paramédicales, administratives, centres de documentation etc doivent-ils correspondre de plus en plus à des profils déjà existants et définis. Au sein des hôpitaux , on trouve : *des archivistes, des bibliothécaires, et des documentalistes.* Aujourd'hui, on parle des "métiers de l'information" et plus généralement des " spécialistes de l'information".

Le Statut de la profession
A l'heure actuelle, le statut de documentaliste hospitalier est inexistant, car la fonction publique hospitalière ne reconnait pas la spécificité de la fonction de documentaliste. Cela crée des situations statutaires très différentes selon les établissements hospitaliers qui possèdent des bibliothèques ou des centres de documentation. Les personnes qui s'en occupent sont : agent de bureau, secrétaire, secrétaire médicale, infirmière, adjoint des cadres, chef de bureau, titulaire, contractuel, catégorie B ou A selon les cas, ... Tous les cas de figures sont donc représentés. La plupart du temps, l'évolution de la carrière est assez lente. Cette situation pose également le problème de la reconnaissance du métier au sein de l'hôpital lui-même : il y a souvent confusion des titres et des compétences... Le rôle et la fonction du documentaliste restent donc à déterminer.

L'existence d'un statut est très importante, car il définit la situation de la profession dans son ensemble et permet d'y attirer et d'y conserver les personnes ayant le profil requis. En son absence, on voit les situations individuelles réglées de façon aléatoire et bien entendu repoussées vers le bas de l'échelle socioprofessionnelle, et ce d'autant que la profession ne constitue pas un groupe de pression suffisant. C'est le cas pour les documentalistes hospitaliers, bien que de plus en plus d'hôpitaux fassent appel à eux. A titre indicatif, on peut dire que le nombre de documentalistes en France est évalué à 20 ou 30 000. De plus, 1000 diplômes de documentation sont délivrés chaque année.

Le métier de documentaliste hospitalier : éléments de réponse

Quelques éléments de réponse nous sont cependant donnés qui font augurer d'un avenir meilleur pour la profession.

Premier élément: La "Nomenclature des emplois-types de l'hôpital" de l'Ecole Nationale de la Santé Publique de Rennes Sous forme de fiches, cette nomenclature dessine les grandes lignes de la fonction et dégage des traits principaux. Ainsi selon la fiche consacrée au métier de documentaliste, celui-ci est responsable du centre de documentation de l'établissement ; il dispose d'un budget dont il assure la gestion. Technicité, information, communication prédominent parmi les qualités requises :

- la technicité. Il gère et réceptionne les abonnements, dépouille, transmet les informations aux services intéressés. Il a accès à des banques de données et procède à des recherches documentaires. Il veille à la conservation des documents et effectue leur classement et leur archivage.
- l'information. Il analyse les informations et les transmet aux services concernés.
- la communication. Sa fonction le met en relation avec tous les services de l'hôpital. Il communique avec d'autres centres de documentation ou bibliothèques.

Son esprit d'analyse et de synthèse doit lui permettre d'apprécier l'importance des informations dont il a connaissance et leur usage. Il représente pour tous les services de l'établissement un gain de temps en facilitant l'accès à l'information et apporte une amélioration qualitative de l'information utile.

Deuxième élément: au sein même des hôpitaux

* la préoccupation croissante ***des équipes de Direction*** au sein des hôpitaux pour une mise en place effective de bibliothèques hospitalières s'adressant à toutes les catégories professionnelles de l'hôpital : les personnels médicaux, paramédicaux, administratifs, techniques .
* le Corps médical, de par la nécessité d'être au fait des dernières connaissances scientifiques et médicales, est un élément moteur de la documentation à l'hôpital. Les structures documentaires qui se sont développées à son intention sont en général organisées et ne demandent qu'à croître.

* la volonté ***des documentalistes*** d'être reconnus au sein de l'hôpital en tant que professionnel à part entière : bibliothécaire - documentaliste hospitalier ou médical. La nécessité d'un statut spécifique est avancé.

Troisième élément: l'émergence de mouvements associatifs divers. L'Association des Documentalistes-Bibliothécaires Hospitaliers (ADBH) créée en 1985 à Lyon : depuis 1972, des rencontres informelles avaient lieu entre documentalistes des écoles paramédicales privées et publiques de la région lyonnaise. Echange d'informations, réflexion sur un statut spécifique, relations avec des documentalistes de Montpellier marquent ces années. Un groupe de travail élabore un projet de statut, et c'est en 1985, afin de donner plus de crédibilité à celui-ci, que l'ADBH est créée (J.O. du 15 mai 1985). En moins de 10 mois, le petit groupe de 5 personnes réussit à rassembler 70 documentalistes représentant plus de 40 départements : les 2/3 exercent dans des centres de formation, les autres à l'hôpital. Cette association poursuit ses activités à l'heure actuelle. Le réseau des documentalistes des Centres Hospitaliers Spécialisés (CHS) : ce groupe a démarré en 1984 avec 9 documentalistes. Actuellement, 32 documentalistes (publics ou privés) se sont regroupés, issus des bibliothèques médicales et des centres de documentation paramédicaux et administratifs. Une rencontre annuelle de deux journées a lieu . Ce qui a déjà été réalisé: un catalogue collectif des périodiques reçus dans chaque centre de documentation avec l'état des collections; un catalogue des ouvrages anciens de psychiatrie; un catalogue collectif des thèses et mémoires; une liste de mots-clés un catalogue collectif de documents audio-visuels.

Le prêt entre bibliothèques et l'échange de bulletins documentaires ainsi que le choix commun d'un logiciel documentaire (TETO) sont à signaler.

* un second réseau est celui notamment appuyé par Mr Alain HALBOUT, président du Centre National de l'Equipement Hospitalier (CNEH), et par la Conférence des Directeurs Généraux de CHU : plusieurs réunions se sont déjà tenues à Paris afin de réfléchir sur les problèmes de la profession. Cette réflexion a porté sur le fait que les établissements hospitaliers ont un besoin sans cesse croissant d'informations rapides nécessaires à la prise de décision. Or l'apport de ces informations ressort de compétences spécifiques, d'un métier. Une approche sur un statut spécifique a été entreprise ainsi que la mise en chantier d'un annuaire professionnel. A l'heure actuelle, 130 personnes participent à l'animation du réseau. Un Bureau et une Présidente ont été élu en mars 1994.

* il existe également le groupe sectoriel "Médecine, pharmacie, biologie" au sein de l'**Association des Documentalistes Bibliothécaires Spécialisés** (ADBS). Un sous-groupe "Santé Publique" a été mis en place récemment, ainsi qu'un groupe "Fonction publique", qui inclut les hospitaliers.

Conclusion

Dans l'état actuel des choses, le statut du documentaliste à l'hôpital demande à être clairement mis à plat. Souhaitons que grâce aux différentes initiatives et propositions faites dans ce domaine soit de façon individuelle, soit collective, on aboutisse à un règlement de cette situation pour le moins ambigüe. La mise en place d'un tel statut n'est envisageable que si dans chaque hôpital certaines conditions sont remplies:

- le recrutement d'un professionnel bibliothécaire-documentaliste et d'un(e) aide-documentaliste,
- la volonté du Corps Médical et de la Direction de mettre en place ce service avec :
- un budget propre
- un noyau actif d'hospitaliers intéressés au développement du service : médecins, paramédicaux, administratifs
- des moyens informatiques : traitement de texte, accès aux banques de données, logiciel de gestion documentaire, CD ROM, moyens vidéo...
- une offre de stages, de formations, et la possibilité d'adhérer aux associations professionnelles, de participer à des congrès professionnels
- la mise en place d'un réseau documentaire : liens fréquents avec d'autres centres de documentation hospitaliers, visites, échanges de documents (photocopies, tirés à part) et d'informations.
- un plan de développement à long terme pour la documentation à l'hôpital

En effet, les activités d'information sont en plein essor et leur utilité sociale de plus en plus importante et reconnue. Une carrière dans cette profession apparait aujourd'hui comme prometteuse, passionnante en raison de ses finalités, de ses modalités et de son évolution technique. Elle apporte une discipline, un art de travailler et de se comporter, un renouvellement de ses connaissances personnelles qui seront toujours un atout irremplaçable.

Références

Divers

(1) Résultats de l'enquête de la Conférence Nationale des Présidents de C.M.E des Hôpitaux Généraux. 1990.

(2) Comptes rendus des réunions des documentalistes hospitaliers au Centre National de l'Equipement Hospitalier-PARIS

Articles

(3) "Une Gestion des ressources documentaires innovantes" / Francoise BLONDEL et al,... in GESTIONS HOSPITALIERES , no 311, décembre 1991,p. 914-917

(4) "La Mise en place d'un centre de documentation pluridisiplinaire et informatisé au Centre Hospitalier d'Argenteuil / J.P. ACCART, in TECHNIQUES HOSPITALIERES, no 556, janvier 1992, p.48-51

(5) "Documentaliste à l'hôpital: des compétences et un métier" /J.P. ACCART, in TECHNOLOGIES ET SANTE, no 9, janvier-mars 1992, p.31-35

Ouvrages

(6) Les Métiers de la documentation /APEC, 1989

(7) Nomenclature des emplois-type de l'hôpital / Ecole Nationale de la Santé Publique, Rennes, 1990

(7) Sciences et techniques de l'information et de la documentation / C GUINCHAT, M. MENOU.- Paris : UNESCO, 1990.- p.509-527

SECTION 2

NETWORKING & RESOURCE SHARING

DEVELOPING A REGIONAL MODEL FOR SHARING LIBRARY RESOURCES WITH PARTICULAR REFERENCE TO THE HEALTH INFORMATION NEEDS OF RURAL COMMUNITIES

Stephen Pritchard, University of Wales College of Medicine, Heath Park, Cardiff CF4 4XN, UK.

Abstract

Information technology increasingly enables information sources to be accessed remotely without regard to geographic barriers. Regional library services to health care teams are now able to supplement library centred information delivery with a range of traditional and technologically based services delivered directly to the workplace and to the consumer. Clinical decision making in rural practices can benefit from improved access to the knowledge base of medicine. The application of these principles to a developing regional library system for health is described and possible future developments are outlined.

Introduction

It has been claimed (1) that no library owns more than 6% of the world's knowledge and yet, until recently the opportunities for individuals to use even a fraction of this information were dependent on the ease and convenience with which they were able to travel to an extensive and well- resourced library. Despite the availability of mediated online literature searching and postal interlibrary loans the depth and range of information sources offered to students, researchers and practitioners was related directly to the size of accessible libraries. Health care generally and medicine, particularly, have a long history of the establishment of regional systems to spread the benefits of library use more equitably (2). Where libraries are supported by public funds it can be argued that tax-payers in locations remote from significant collections of material have not been receiving value for money. Of at least equal importance with financial accountability is growing evidence (3) (4) (5) that access to timely and relevant information by physicians improves patient care by, for example, reducing: mortality, length of hospital stay; rates of hospital acquired infection; numbers of tests or procedures. The increasing ability of appropriate information technolgy to provide direct access to significant information sources beyond the library walls and in a user-friendly way enables the potential for health gain to be delivered to practitioners and, hence, to patients regardless of geographic location. At the same time opportunities for sharing library resources, for example by networking library automation systems or specialist databases, are further enhanced.

The earliest account traced in MEDLINE of the application of automated information services for rural health care is now almost twenty - five years old (6) and, indeed, precedes the appearance in the database of the word "telemedicine" (7) to describe the broader concept of using remote telecommunication for health care delivery. Since then recognition of the need to support rural medicine has spread globally with published reports describing projects from Alabama (8) to Australia (9) and from Norway (10) to Nambia (11). In certain instances the needs of rural communities may even be said to be moving to centre stage. A service devoted to rural medicine is now available on the Internet (12). One of three key recommendations in a recent American report states "Library and information services should be extended through outreach to underserved health care providers in urban and rural areas" (13). Similarly the recently published "Library and Information Plan for Wales" cautions " In a world where ... information deprivation will lead almost inevitably to a depressed quality of life it may no longer be possible to justify significantly inferior rural access to library and information services."(14)

Traditional Solutions

In a number of respects Wales, politically and administratively a part of the United Kingdom, parallels the geography and demography of a number of other European regions. It is a small country, occupying an area of approximately 21000 square kilometres with over 60% of the population of 2.9 million living in the industrial/post-industrial south on just 17% of the land surface. At least one person in three, therefore, lives in the large,relatively thinly populated, rural hinterland with few significant urban centres and poor transport links. The predominately upland landforms mean that journey times, particularly on a north-south axis are long. Indeed on a time map south Wales is further from north Wales than London is from New York.

Health care is served largely by approximately 45 small libraries, many with a history of poor resourcing and part-time staffing. In spite of this provision large areas of the country are remote from any library at all - in mid and west Wales, particularly, many practitioners are over ninety minutes by car from their nearest library and which may be able only to offer a rather restricted range of information sources. Like a number of other areas within the UK and Europe Wales has developed a regional medical library service based largely on traditional techniques to attempt to spread the benefits of information access more fairly. Over the last twenty years this traditional model has evolved to include core library and information services delivered from libraries in local hospitals and postgraduate medical education centres with secondline support from a larger library with "regional" responsibilities. Typically the local libraries have adopted a multidisciplinary role - to medicine, nursing, the basic sciences and the professions allied to medicine - offering collections of books, journals and non-print media, loans renewals and reservations, interlibrary loans, reference and enquiry services, formal or informal reader instruction. More recent developments have included standalone installations of core databases on CD-ROM. This provision at local level has been supplemented by support services from a larger library with a partial role as a regional back-up centre. In Wales this role has been played by the University of Wales College of Medicine which has designed a series of extension services in association with the local medical libraries. Services available through this scheme currently comprise an umbrella of professional support including: document delivery on demand (journal articles and books) via mail or fax as appropriate; information services including access to a wider range of standalone and networked CD databases as well as online sources; negotiation of regional discounts for multiple subscriptions - particularly to CD services; assistance with staff appointments, training and development. Another aspect of cooperation within Wales has been the professional support and development activities of the Association of Welsh Health Librarians including a voluntarily compiled and updated union list of periodicals held by health libraries in the region which is the basis for an active self-help interlibrary loan scheme.

The Needs of Rural Health Care

While this traditional two tier model has been succesful in Wales and elsewhere in providing medical and other health practitioners on site or in close proximity with access to timely and relevant information it has been less successful in meeting the needs of health care teams serving rural communities. Research findings in this area may be summed-up in a study of the information requirements of health care providers in rural Hawaii "All interviewees expressed the need for improved access to health-related information." (15). Typically rural practitioners see the traditional model as failing to address their needs in a number of ways. It takes no account of the phenomenon of "distance decay" in which the degree of take-up of any service is inversely proportional to the distance the consumer has to travel. In the case of health care libraries the problem will be compounded if the nearest, accessible library is poorly funded or open for restricted or unsuitable hours. Many of the perceived problems centre on the twin obstacles of time and isolation. Rural workers are conscious that time invested in travelling to libraries is not always justified by the benefits and resources offered. The traditional model's reliance on hard copy sources is seen as inappropriate for the needs of practitioners in isolated locations. A more subtle response sometimes expressed is resistance to the concept of "outreach" solutions which may be seen as grace and favour disbursements from the privileged centre to the disadvantaged margins. An effective service to rural communities must confer ownership by recognising that expertise and benefits will accrue at both ends of the link. A related concern is that traditional regional services fail to focus specifically on rural health problems - for example, farming and forestry accidents and injuries, agicultural toxicology, mental health problems of isolated communities. In addition there is a strong perception that library and information services to rural areas must be capable of enablingaccess to the knowledge base of medicine to directly influence health and treatment outcomes.

There are a number of specific problems to be overcome in providing effective and efficient library and information services for rural health care teams. Information must be available electronically - paper based solutions are increasingly viewed in rural areas as an ineffective response. Assistance may be needed in identifying, acquiring and supporting the appropriate hardware. Crucially there will have to be easy, work place and local access to cheap and reliable telecommunication systems. Rural practitioners are acutely aware of a multiplying plethora of information sources to which they might gain access. They are equally aware that they require support in discovering exactly what these services offer, what information is contained, what hardware, software, telecommunications and passwords are required to gain access and, of course, how to search effectively the sources chosen and how to obtain and use the results. A great deal of the expressed needs also revolves around the issues of initial training and subsequent support.

An Emerging Model

Recent developments make it possible to identify the elements of an emerging, technology-based, model of library and information services offering the potential of improved support to health care in rural areas. This model retains all the relevant aspects of traditional regional systems, and takes account also of practice based collections of books and journals, but focuses increasingly on the ability of appropriate information technology to deliver access to the medical knowledge base beyond the library walls. This model may be said to be deconstructing not only the traditional library but also geographic obstacles by emphasising service delivery regardless of the locations of library, information source and user. It is also clear that this approach has potential advantages for urban conurbations with their problems of traffic congestion and parking restrictions.

Although in its early stages a number of requirements are already clear. The emerging model must be based on a sound needs assessment in collaboration with those it is intended to serve. Cheap and reliable telecommunications - regionally, nationally and internationally - are essential backed up by investment in appropriate hardware and software. There are undoubtedly good grounds for work place or practice based standalone installations of one or two core and heavily used databases on CD but this will be supplemented by easy access to regional and specialist databases. It is crucial that a mix of whatever appropriate technologies are available is employed. For example, access may be provided to a number of different networks for different purposes. Similarly satellite communications whether for education or document delivery will be utilised where possible. It will be necessary to devise programmes of user instruction that can be delivered locally and meet the needs of rural users. A complementary requirement is for a fast, responsive help "hot line" whether by telephone, fax or email. Regular reviews of performance, progress and strategy will be essential to ensure that service responds to changing needs and developments. Above all the processes and technology must be as transparent as possible to the users and function, therefore, entirely as an enabling tool.

A Pilot Model in Wales

Using a number of the elements identified above an experiment is currently in progress to establish a pilot service between the university medical school library, the local hospital library and a remote rural medical practice in mid-Wales. A needs assessment of both practioner and community requirements is being carried out as part of a dissertation project by a postgraduate LIS student. The question of telecommunications is being addressed in a number of ways. BT's ISDN lines capable of carrying text, graphics and sound have been installed and these will be supplemented by links to a local county community information service employing touch screen technology as well as to the national academic network and the Internet. Cooperation with this county data network, which is in the process of extension into other parts of Wales, offers the exciting prospect of information delivery and access directly at local community level for use by patients as well as health care providers. With financial support from the Dean of Postgraduate and Continuing Medical Education the practice has been equipped with a CD workstation and a first year's subscription to MEDLINE. In addition equipment has been installed providing remote links to the local hospital library as well as to the university medical library.

Sources available remotely at the university will include, in the first instance, access to the automated library system as part of a scheme to extend the benefits of sophisticated automation at a cost within the reach of smaller libraries and units. Consequently the OPAC is in the embryonic stage of development towards a national union catalogue of health related materials. The university's networked range of databases on CD will also be searchable thus supplementing MEDLINE provision locally with access to nursing, social sciences and general science sources. It is hoped that database access will be supported by facilitating cooperative document delivery from the resources of medical libraries throughout the region. Future developments are planned to provide access to specialist databases for rural health covering issues of regional interest as well as international perspectives via the Internet.

A number of issues remain to be resolved in particular the crucial ones of training and support. It is recognised that these are not only staff intensive in the first instance but must be capable of development in reponse to changing user needs and changing solutions against a rapidly evolving technological background. Above all this support must be delivered to the user in their own locality. It is believed that networked training packages may be valuable here.

The Future

There is in existence already an informal network of medical practitioners throughout Europe and the United States active in the field of health care for rural communities. In addition to self-help, support, exchange of information, ideas and experience members of the group organise an annual conference. A number of the members are very conscious of the potential for improved clinical and health care decisions-making offered by faster, easier access to up to date, relevant and timely information. Is there a role for a similar network of librarians with an interest in this area? In association with health care workers such a grouping would be in a position to monitor and, perhaps, influence developments, in particular the paramount requirement for full text clinical information, not just bibliographical data, to be searchable and retrievable remotely in electronic format. Similarly a network of this sort would provide a broad-based forum for cooperation with the medical and health care professions to ensure that the emerging model of technology based regional systems paying particular attention to the needs of rural health would be firmly integrated with the accelerating field of telemedicine in which technology is used to provide fast, responsive diagnosis and treatment at a distance. In this way cost effective and efficient access to the total relevant knowledge base of medicine would contribute to improved outcomes for health care in communities remote from traditional library services.

References

(1) LAW D Address to the UK Library Association Medical, Health and Welfare Group Conference 1993

(2) TABOR RB Libraries for health: the Wessex experience; a collection of experiences contributed by the staff of the Wessex Regional Library and Information Service 1967 - 1977. Southampton, Wessex Regional Library and Information Service 1978

(3) MARSHALL JG The impact of the hospital library on clinical decision making: the Rochester study. Bulletin of the Medical Library Association 1992; 80 (2): 169-178

(4) HEPWORTH J Personal communication of research in progress

(5) KLEIN MS et al Effect of online literature searching on length of stay and patient care costs. Academic Medicine 1994; 69 (6): 489-495

(6) MILLER OW et al Assessing the potential of automated health care in a rural area. Biomedical Sciences Instrumentation 1971; 8: 19-32

(7)GRAVENSTEIN JS et al Laser mediated telemedicine in anesthesia. Anestesia and Analgesia 1974; 53 (4): 605-609

(8) BATTISTELLA MS et al Medical information for Alabama rural physicians. Alabama Medicine 1990; 59 (8): 21-24

(9) HUMPHREY JS etal Evaluating the importance of information sources for preventive health care in rural Australia. Australian Journal of Public Health 1993; 17 (2): 149-157

(10) RINDE E etal Telemedicine in rural Norway. World Health Forum 1993; 14 (1): 71-77

(11) LISSE EW An overview of networking for physicians and problems of network consulting in remote areas. Annals of the new York Academy of Sciences 1992; 670: 19-28

(12) MARSHALL UNIVERSITY SCHOOL OF MEDICINE Ruralnet gopher (Gopher to ruralnet.mu.wvnet.edu)

(13) MEDICAL LIBRARY ASSOCIATION & ASSOCIATION OF ACADEMIC HEALTH SCIENCES LIBRARY DIRECTORS Health care reform and the health sciences librarian: excellence in health through access to information. MLA etc 1994 (?)

(14) CYMRU LiP WALES MANAGEMENT GROUP Library and information plan for Wales (British Library R&DD report 6109) CLWMG 1993

(15) LUNDEEN GW & TENOPIR C Information needs of rural health care practitioners in Hawaii. Bulletin of the Medical Library Association 1994; 82 (2): 197-205

THE INTERNATIONAL TORTURE DOCUMENTATION NETWORK (ITDN)

Svend Bitsch Christensen, International Rehabilitation Council for Torture Victims, Borgergade 13, PO Box 2107, DK-2107, Copenhagen K, Denmark

Abstract
Over the last decade, more than 50 rehabilitation centres for torture survivors have been established around the world. Some of these centres have recognized that a documentation centre, similar to the one at IRCT in Copenhagen, should be part of their structure. Based on an increasing demand for information from abroad, IRCT has decided to contribute to the establishment of new documentation centres around the world.

Introduction
Already one year before a WHO working group in 1986 recommended the establishment of clearing houses for scientific literature on organized violence, the Rehabilitation and Research Centre for Torture Victims (RCT) had started collecting literature on torture, the effects of torture, and on the rehabilitation of torture survivors (1). In October 1987 RCT opened its International Documentation Centre with a collection which at that time comprised 1,500 books, articles, manuscripts, conference papers, etc. At the end of 1993 it comprised about 14,000 items, including newspaper cuttings, slides, and videos.

The collection of the Documentation Centre focuses primarily on the medical aspects of torture. However, it also comprises relevant studies on medical ethics, post-traumatic stress disorder, cross-cultural psychiatry, disaster psychiatry, concentration camp survivors, humanitarian and international human rights law, etc., as well as documents from the Council of Europe's Committee for the Prevention of Torture and the United Nations Committee Against Torture. The material is mainly written in English, Danish, Spanish, German, and French, but literature in Russian, Arabic, Urdu, Farsi, Turkish, Nepalese, Filipino, Japanese, and Korean is also represented.

The Documentation Centre takes an active part in HURIDOCS, the Human Rights Information and Documentation System Network, which is a global network comprising about 200 human rights organizations and institutions (Inter-governmental and Non-governmental). HURIDOCS has developed several standard formats for the registration of information on human rights. The formats are guidelines for the recording and exchange of data and are based on AACR2. The standard formats take into account manual and computerized routines and procedures in a documentation centre (2). In 1992 the Documentation Centre joined the International Refugee Documentation Network (IRDN), which is a network within HURIDOCS open to organizations and individuals who work in refugee-related fields of research, information, etc.

Since its start, the Documentation Centre has been a member of the Danish Research Library Association and the European Association for Health Information and Libraries. Staff members have been active in relevant professional groups in the field of medical information. The material in the Documentation Centre is registered according to the HURIDOCS standard formats for bibliographic material in a local database with UNESCO's CDS/ISIS database programme. The RCT collection is open to organizations, institutions, and individuals working with the treatment of torture victims or somehow participating in the work against torture. Services offered include searches in the local database, and lending and photocopying services.

New Perspectives
Over the last decade, more than 50 rehabilitation centres for torture victims have been established around the world. Some of these centres have recognized that a documentation centre, similar to the one at RCT in Copenhagen, should be part of their structure. Based on an increasing demand for information from abroad RCT has decided to contribute to the establishment of new documentation centres around the world. The first such documentation centres were established in 1991 at the Rehabilitation and Health Aid Centre for Torture Victims (RAHAT) in Islamabad, Pakistan, and in Centro Educazione ai Diritti Humani (CEDU) in Bologna, Italy. In 1992 the Behandlungszentrum für Folteropfer e.V. in Berlin, Germany, and the Children's Rehabilitation Centre in Manila, the Philippines, started documentation

centres. When starting the cooperation, data was transmitted from RCT's bibliographic database to the databases of the newly established documentation centres. These data then formed the basis for the recording of literature in the new documentation centres (shared cataloguing). With the establishment of the centres in Islamabad, Bologna, Berlin, and Manila, the first steps were taken towards the creation of a proper network of torture documentation centres.

Training

The establishment of new documentation centres involves training. Three international teaching seminars for librarians and documentalists were offered at the IRCT in January and November 1993 and in May 1994 with 50 participants from 31 different countries (3). The seminars were held in cooperation with the Royal School of Librarianship, the Danish Refugee Council, and the Danish Centre for Human Rights. The subjects taught ranged from the development of libraries, HURIDOCS Standard Formats, the CDS/ISIS database software, to introduction of E-mail and workshops on networking and division of labour. As a result of the seminars, it has been decided to formalize close cooperation between the rehabilitation centres in the area covered by the IRCT Documentation Centre. This has taken place with the creation of the International Torture Documentation Network (ITDN).

Networking

Networking is something that cannot be forced upon someone and only come into being when it is realized that a common need exists. This means that the relationship between the participants, the conditions for participation, and the benefits that one gets from networking should be clear. One has to consider the structure of the network, i.e. should it be formal or informal, centralized or decentralized, bilateral or multilateral? Trust should be established among participants and the roles clearly defined. Benefits of networking, such as contact with other people working within the same area, solidarity, avoidance of duplication of work, and waste of resources, should be recognized. When working with documentation on human rights and torture, experience has shown that no single library or documentation centre will be able to cover all aspects of a these topics. In other words, there is a great need for co-operation among organizations working with rehabilitation of torture survivors and victims of other forms of organized violence. In the day-to-day work all participants will profit from a network. It will become easier to exchange and obtain information from each other, which is of great importance for the overall work for the participating organizations.

Building Up the Network

It was agreed that, when starting a new documentation centre, data from the RCT bibliographic database would be transferred to the database of the new centres, as was done when the first centres were set up. At present this data amounts to 5,300 records in HURIDOCS standard formats. Centres that are not yet computerized would receive printouts from the database on a regular basis. A necessary condition for the functioning of the network was compatibility of information systems, i.e. a mutual language, thesaurus, and standards for recording of literature. Requirements also included the use of software that produces compatible files and the use of specific media to transfer data, i.e. diskettes, filing cards or electronic mail.

For several reasons the CDS/ISIS software has been proposed as the most appropriate programme for international co-operation, even though there are faster and more sophisticated database programmes than CDS/ISIS. One reason, not the least important, was that the programme is free of charge for non-commercial enterprises and has a worldwide distribution. Another was that the programme has user interfaces in English, French, and Spanish. The programme runs under DOS on IBM-compatible computers. It also provides on-line help and menus for data entry, search, printing of cards and accession lists, import/export facilities, and possibilities for programming in PASCAL. Finally, the programme has a thesaurus-programme which makes it possible to use the same index terms. When the new centres begin to register documents, their records could be exchanged between the centres on a regular basis. A common database with all data from all the participants will also be considered in order to offer online access to organizations and institutions that do not have their own documentation units.

Division of Labour

Decisions with regard to a division of labour among the different centres have not yet been made. One might consider the allocation of certain responsibilities to individual centres, e.g. the collection of literature in a specific language, on specific geographical areas, on specific groups of torture victims (women, children, adolescents), or about specific aspects of torture problems (the transition from dictatorships to democracy, doctors' participation in torture, the problem of non-prosecution of torturers). A very natural contribution to the network will also be the recording of articles in journals that are published by the organizations participating in the network.

Conclusion

In the future it is of high importance that a policy is laid down as to the way of cooperating and how often exchange of data should take place. It is the intention that the work inside the network should be on an international and global plan. This means that strengths and weaknesses must be considered regarding economic abilities, trained personnel, etc. After the establishment of new documentation centres on all five continents a strengthening, as regards geography, languages, and contents, of the registration of knowledge about torture will be in focus.

References and Notes:

1. Geuns H van, ed. Health hazards of organized violence. Rijswijk: Ministry of Welfare, Health, and Cultural Affairs, 1987.
2. Noval AM ...[et al.] HURIDOCS Standard Formats for the recording and exchange of bibliographic information concerning human rights. Oslo: HURIDOCS, 1993.
3. AFRICA: Cameroon, Ghana, South Africa, Zimbabwe. AMERICAS: Argentina, Canada, Chile, Guatemala, United States, Uruguay. ASIA: Bangladesh, Burma, Egypt, Israel, Nepal, Pakistan, Palestine, The Philippines, Sri Lanka. EUROPE: Albania, Austria, Croatia, Estonia, France, Germany, Greece, Latvia, Lithuania, Russia, Sweden, Turkey.

SHARING LIBRARY RESOURCES

Márta Virágos ,Central Kenézy Library, Medical University of Debrecen, 4012 Debrecen, PF. 31, Hungary

This paper offers a discussion of new tendencies of library network on a regional and national level, respectively. The concept of resource sharing, with particular attention to co-operative acquisition and cataloguing, is examined in relationship to library networks

.

Before talking about the topic specified in the title of my paper I will offer a brief outline of the situation of libraries of academic institutions in Hungary. At present, the system of higher education in Hungary, according to internationally accepted typology is a single public system on two levels: university and college. Almost all of the academic institutions are controlled by the state. In Hungary, the classic university structure was suspended in 1945, mainly for political reasons, and the respective university schools were separated from one another . The formerly integrated library collections were likewise separated and because of insufficient funding, the currently available resources are becoming increasingly less adequate and more obsolete.

With the new Act of Higher Education the university system is facing a radical restructuring which will result in a doubled intake within five years and lead to substantially new methods of teaching and learning. The reform of higher education involves both the actual contents of curriculum development and structural organisation of university education, with a substantial increase in student enrolment, which, in turn, makes the updating of institutional infrastructure, including the operation and services of university libraries, an issue of top priority. Libraries which provide essential access to reading material and information are crucial components of higher education and their efficient and cost-effective development will produce benefits to the whole university community. University administration lays special emphasis on the automation and development of library networks. The main goal is to be completely accessible to all, in offices, laboratories, classrooms, and public clusters through the university network system.

Current efforts to generate a library network in Hungary are taking place on two levels: regional and national.

1. Regional: Higher education in Debrecen dates back to 1538, the foundation of the Reformed Theological College. With the addition of new departments and faculties (arts, humanities , medicine, law and sciences) the classical university structure functioned till 1949 when that self-contained University was divided, with the School of Law actually discontinued and the others organizedd into separate institutions subordinated to different government authorities. For the past decades Debrecen has grown to become one of the biggest cultural and educational centres of the country, with new institutions of higher education. The administrators of the disintegrated universities never ceased to be desirous of a newly integrated University. The first important step toward reunification was made in 1991, when the UNIVERSITY of DEBRECEN was formally re-established, first as an initially loose association of the University of Agriculture, the University of Medicine, the Academy of Theology of the Reformed Church, Lajos Kossuth University of Arts and Sciences and the Institute of Nuclear Research of the Hungarian Academy.

The major objectives of the founding institutions can be summarised as follows:

(1) Improvement of the quality of university training by transforming the University into one of European standards in the sense of quality and availability; creating a broader spectrum of undergraduate and postgraduate courses, which would provide degrees accepted internationally;

(2) Improvement of scientific research work by building up a joint information network, laying the foundation of computerised bibliographics and library documentation, encouraging joint research projects.

The Kenézy Library is a key participant in the Universitas Project, and its main goal is the implementation of an integrated library automation network among all the major academic institutions of the city of Debrecen. There is a union card catalogue that has been built for decades as part of the traditional co-operation of these libraries. The participating main libraries function as network centres for the smaller libraries working as institutes, departments, seminars and clinics. Both the centres and the branch libraries are situated far away from one-another. Network centres assume the tasks of ordering periodicals and the acquisition and cataloguing of foreign books for the whole of their respective network constituents. Owing to a World Bank grant, the participating libraries have been able to purchase and install a state-of-the-art local area network and requisite software to computerise their operations and make available a Public Access On-line Catalogue for efficient access and resource sharing.

The aims of the application of the integrated library system are the following:

*to make the processing and availability of all materials possible that serve as the bases of instruction and research at the university;
*to offer possibilities for the unified handling of the databases of co-operating libraries, and the accessibility of one another's databases with proper authorisation;
*to be capable of providing and receiving information for and from domestic and foreign networks respectively.

The Carlyle Voyager integrated library software and the uniform Sun hardware, both acquired in 1993, are capable of incorporating textual, sound, and pictorial information into the data base.

2. National network. A complementary collaborative effort is currently under way to obtain the necessary financial and technical resources to link the four medical university libraries of Hungary in a nation-wide network. In Hungary the four medical universities are regionally well distributed, the one in Budapest being the biggest. The overall student population numbers about 11,000 with faculty and teaching staff of about 3,500. The major medical libraries in the country are university libraries, which offer their services to hospital patrons as well. For the purposes of a better utilisation of the domestically available resources, the university libraries for the past decade have co-operated in some areas, e.g. in co-ordinated acquisition policies and started to implement the integrated library system leading to the creation of resource sharing catalogues and data bases. They prepared a joint proposal within the framework of the "Catching up with Europe" scheme and a detailed action plan comprising the subsequent phases from planning through development, implementation and continuos monitoring.

The respective fields of activities include

*preparation of standardized recommendations for the co-ordinated development of LANs, WANs and data bases in the university libraries concerned;
*implementation of the local area network system where it is needed;
*implementation of the automated library system; and
*implementation of a multi media centre in each of the participating libraries.

The network will provide the following new services for the benefit of the whole university community of each partner but in a wider sense the information given by the system will be accessible to every academic institution:
- electronic mailing facilities;
- appropriate access to all computerised bibliographies and library documentation;
- access to collections of periodicals and books in full-text format;
- shared, multi-user, simultaneous access to on-line catalogues.

The exponential growth of information sources has created a major problem for libraries. The information needed to support education, research and patient care is becoming more complex and unmanageable.

Increasingly, CD-ROMs are proving to be critical resources for libraries, offering new and less expensive opportunities for computer-assisted searching of important files. The CD-ROM option, just coming to our library in 1988, had the potention to bring the data base itself into the library and allow users to access it directly in the university LAN system. A library consortium of three universities of Debrecen, the University of Miskolc and Safarik University, Kosice (Slovakia) elaborated a proposal for a resource sharing CD-ROM network. This Central-European project aims to upgrade the level of information availability for teachers and students with substantial improvements in the acquisition of CD-ROM databases and establish an interconnection of library services between the partner institutions by creating a wide-area network. The network has to maintain maximum hardware and software flexibility which would allow the WAN to involve a generalized reference service system involving additional shared data base applications.

The networking system comprises two network file servers with 21 CD-ROM drives, as well as 18 gygabytes of magnetic storage, Novell networking software, and management softwares. The network is fully integrated with the University's campus network, enabling access from more than 1,000 workstations.

Conclusion

In the library the program will place more emphasis on information access and dissemination through the application of new technologies. On the institutional level the system will offer -mutual use of distributed databases built by member libraries, -faster network links to encourage users to increase the volume of the information transmitted. Libraries are and will remain central to the management of scholarly communication for the foreseeable future. And the implementation of electronic information technology makes it possible to envision radically different ways of organizing collections and services which the library has traditionally provided.

A EUROPEAN CLEARING HOUSE ON HEALTH SYSTEMS REFORMS: the New Possibilities of A Europe Wide Approach to Information Exchange

Lorraine M Bate, Nuffield Institute for Health, Leeds University, 71 Clarendon Road, Leeds LS2 9PL, UK.

In this paper I shall be describing the EC Clearing House on Health Systems Reforms, the context of current European health care reform in which the Clearing House came about and the information support and analytical and evaluative work planned.

A recent study on the future of European health care by Andersen Consulting is an interesting review of health system developments in 10 European countries. I quote from their conclusion:

> The key theme of European health care in the future will be change, change for the role of governments from direct provider to enabler, and supported change for hospitals from reactive provider to productive competitor. Doctors will be an integral part of the change process. Patients will demand and drive this change. [1]

Not only is change the theme for the future, it is the theme today in European health care. Almost every country in Europe is either in the midst of reforming its health care system or is contemplating reform. Appearing almost as a motif in all European health care reform is the idea of moving toward primary health care with less reliance on secondary hospital care. The introduction of `approved' drug lists is also frequently reported in an attempt to reduce the national drugs bill. And competition is promoted as a means of ensuring greater efficiency and higher quality of care. The total free market approach of United States health care is not favoured, however, as in the Netherlands where the original recommendations of the Dekker Commission, based on the US model, were abandoned. Perhaps sometimes our governments do learn from the mistakes of others. I quote from an article which appeared in the UK Health Service Journal at the conclusion of a series of articles on European health care. The author is American:

> The US is a more plausible source of health policy ideas, of which we have a huge supply, than health policies, of which (pick your description) we have either none or only bad ones. If this series has encouraged readers to look at European experiences instead of US theories, it will have done enough.[2]

European health care reform is happening at the same time as the much debated Treaty on European Union (the Maastrict Treaty for those who need to be reminded) ricochets through national governing bodies. The Treaty includes a new Article on Public Health, Article 129. In the article it is accepted that the health of people in Europe depends on much more than the provision of health care and health services. There is an emphasis on the need to cooperate and coordinate activities between member states to combat the major causes of diseases. Article 129 covers public health activities at Community level and their relationship to work in member states, and gives a legal basis for a planned framework for action in the area of public health, of course always in the context of the principle of subsidiarity.

Further to this awareness continues to grow about the importance of information in health care decision making. In the European Commission's Specific Research and Development programme in the field of biomedicine and health under the third framework programme, otherwise known as BIOMED, there is a greater recognition of the role of the EC in the development of information relevant to the Community's health needs. An editorial in the journal The Lancet in January this year pointed to the important role both the European Union and the World Health Organization have to play in improving systems for data collection and transmission.[3] For example, The European Nervous System is an EU initiative intended to facilitate rapid transfer across Europe of computerised information. The initiative includes a project on health which also involves the World Health Organization.

As each country sets about the process of change much information is generated about the development of health care system reforms. In order to learn from the experiences of others we need to collect that information, make it available to others and use it in comparative analysis of the emerging research findings within countries. It is with this in mind that the Nuffield Institute for Health at the University of Leeds has been awarded funding by the European Commission Biomed programme to establish a European Clearing House on Health Systems Reforms. The Clearing House is funded as a concerted action research project. Concerted actions are designed to fund not the research but the costs of bringing the multinational teams together. The idea behind concerted actions is that they constitute not a block of activity with a known end but an enabling activity to encourage new methods of research and new directions of research. These new methods and directions are made possible by the growing banks of information developed as a result of the programme participants' frequent exchanges of information.

As a concerted action research project the European Clearing House on Health Systems Reforms will have the following objectives:

1. To establish a central repository for published and unpublished information about the introduction and development of health care systems reforms in EC member states and in COST countries (those members of the framework for Cooperation in Science and Technology who are not also members of the EC).

2. To establish a European-wide network of health service researchers and policy analysts concerned with health systems reform

3. To provide a forum for the exchange of information and experiences of health services researchers

4. To establish a critical appraisal function to evaluate health service research

5. To develop health service research questions

The Clearing House will produce a twice yearly newsletter and a series of articles and papers emerging from international meetings and workshops.

Collected data will be held in the Information Resource Centre (IRC) of the Nuffield Institute for Health. The IRC is one of the UK's largest libraries specialising in health and social care management and offers information services outside the Institute through the Health Management Information Service, or HELMIS. The Information Resource Centre has been involved in a number of information projects; currently we have staff working on a community care innovative practices database, a register of quality in health care training and sources of information, and a health outcomes clearing house which has also recently been awarded funding under the EC concerted action programme. The database of information for the European Clearing House on Health Systems Reforms will be developed using BRS Search information retrieval software and housed on a University of Leeds platform. Information Resource Centre databases are accessible through JANET, the Joint Academic Network in the UK and internationally through INTERNET. The IRC also becomes a World Health Organization Documentation Centre in 1994. As well as the dissemination activities the IRC will undertake on behalf of WHO European Region the IRC's designation as a Documentation Centre will ensure WHO information on national health systems is available to the Clearing House.

What other databases are available which will be of use to the project?

MEDLINE contains some non-English language material. Health Planning and Administration, the database produced jointly by the National Library of Medicine and the American Hospital Association, is the better database for health systems information but has a smaller proportion of non-English language material than MEDLINE.

The National Library of Medicine has also recently launched its HSTAR database online. This is a health services research database with references to government reports, books, book chapters, meeting abstracts and newspaper articles as well as material from MEDLINE and several other NLM databases. This is a particularly interesting development but again its usefulness in the European health care context is limited.

HECLINET, the database of the Health Care Literature Network is the product of a consortium of the Hospital Institutes of Austria, Denmark, Germany, Sweden and Switzerland. The headquarters of the project is in Berlin and the database is available on the German host DIMDI. 60% of entries are in the German language.

URBADISC is the European CD-Rom database of urban planning and policy, consisting of the UK Urbaline, the French Urbanet and the Spanish Urbaterr databases. Although not specific to health care some aspects of health policy are covered on the URBADISC database.

One source of information of direct relevance to the Clearing House project is the database on health care reforms being developed by WHO European Region for the EURO Health project As part of the development the project has produced the country profiles HITS (Health care in transition overviews) and ROVERS (Reform overviews) with which some readers may be familiar. The Clearing House and WHO EURO will be discussing joint developments. One of the problems of collecting European information is of course the differences in language. MEDLINE assigns English language keyterms to non-English language abstracts. HECLINET assigns abstracts with German and English keyterms with a German to English thesaurus. URBADISC indexing is in French and English using a two-way thesaurus.

So a variety of approaches have been adopted for accessing the content of multilingual databases. I have no solutions, unfortunately. Within the limits of the Clearing House project we do not have the funds to develop multilingual thesauri. It is probable that the material we receive will be translated into English. So I mention these problems of multilingual databases not to offer solutions but to highlight the issues. The participant countries of the project, at least in the first year, are the UK, the Netherlands, Finland and Spain. The idea is that each project participant will represent a group of countries. The Department of Public Health at the University of Helsinki, for example, will monitor policy and planning activities of governments and health authorities in Denmark, Finland, Norway and Sweden as well as health care research and development in those countries. The centre will scan government and health authority plans and reports, professional journals and reports about planning, implementation and evaluation of organisation change and funding arrangements in health and social services. Cooperation will be sought with government agencies, national associations of health authorities as well as hospital institutes in the different countries. The Centre will abstract, translate and submit documents of interest to the Clearing House and will promote the work of the Clearing House in the Nordic countries. Interest in the project has also been expressed by France, Germany, Italy and Sweden. The Clearing House aims to have six participant nations by the end of the first year of the project.
So, I have described the European Clearing House for Health Systems Reforms, its aims and objectives. I have said a little of existing information sources and of the problems in dealing with multilingual material. But the emphasis today is on dissemination of information that is in a form most likely to be acted upon. Much has been written on the problems of disseminating information on current best clinical practice to practitioners, for example. Sometimes even when the information is available, it is not acted upon. Thus we have the variations in clinical practice that we have in the different regions of the UK, for example. In the United States the process of disseminating information so that it is acted upon by practitioners is termed `diffusion'. An area of particular interest in the UK currently is the process of subjecting original research to meta analysis, or review, and disseminating the resulting overviews. A similar approach will be adopted in the European Clearing House on Health Systems Reforms. Published and unpublished literature will be critically appraised and cross national themes and trends drawn out.

Information which has been subjected to review is viewed as of greater value than the primary information. It is no longer sufficient to create a database of primary information, to supply searches of that information and leave it at that. I believe the information profession - our profession - should recognise this. Indeed this may be the future information professional - someone with a greater understanding of the information they are working with and the importance of dissemination in a way which will have maximum impact. I may be accused of arguing that information professionals should in fact be researchers. But no, I am saying that we should have a better understanding of information and how it is used. This will aid interaction between information professionals and those who use the information we provide.

In conclusion, one conclusion I have come to is that national concerns about the Maastricht Treaty aside, there is considerable advantage in having a large organization like the European Commission behind health initiatives. The United States may not have got its health care structure in any sort of reasonable order, but nation-wide initiatives in dissemination of health care research findings by the Agency for Health Care Policy and Research show an understanding of the difficulties in ensuring information take-up amongst health care practitioners. Both the Agency and the US National Institutes of Health are government funded. One interesting idea which emerges out of a recent EC evaluation of its biomedical and health research programme is the suggestion that we may be moving towards a European

Community form of National Institute of Health. As a health information professional I find this of greater interest than arguments for and against a single currency.

References

[1] Andersen Consulting and Burson-Marsteller The future of European health care Arthur Andersen, 1993 p.vi
[2] White J Market choices Health Service Journal 8 April 1993 p 23
[3] Health issues for Europe (editorial) Lancet 29 January 1994 pp 245-246

A LOW COST UNION CATALOGUE: the School of Medicine of Turin (Italy) experience

Valentina Comba, Anna Maria Giordano, Uberto Moreggia, Paola Petroni & Paola Santimaria,
Biblioteca Centralizzata di Medicina e Chirurgia, University of Turin, Italia

Abstract.
The project for a new School of Medicine of Turin union catalogue is presented; the costs, the time of work are evaluated, the software choice discussed. The practical choices related to the kind of organization are pointed out: the network approach allowed the librarians to exchange information and professional knowledge, to share experiences and to be more involved in the project.

Introduction.
The need of an updated union catalogue of the Department libraries in the School of Medicine was clearly perceived by users and librarians. Until last year the union catalogue was a printed alphabetical list, published in 1982, with some partial (handwritten !) updates; the printout was only available in some libraries. The swift evolution of the access to biomedical information, from the online searches to the spread of CD-ROMs, has demonstrated the limits of the old union catalogue and the library services related to it. The goal of our project is to produce a new, updated union catalogue wich overcomes the lack of formal organization among libraries: the most important aspect of the project is to involve collegues and librarians in a special effort leading to upgrade the professional level of the service.

The School of Medicine of Turin Department Libraries
The Biblioteca Centralizzata di Medicina, established in 1985, is the main point of reference for the School of Medicine regarding reference services, online research and CD-ROM instruction, but it is only one of the 31 (thirtyone) Department libraries scattered in the teaching hospitals of the city and the surrounding area. Even though the teaching and research activities are organized within the framework of the Faculty of Medicine, no formal and centralized structure is devoted to libraries, which are considered a local service for the Department; with the exception of the Biblioteca Centralizzata, the services are one-person-libraries and very often administrative staff look after the small number of subscribed journals . The libraries may be divided into four groups: the group A of 6 libraries (which includes the Biblioteca Centralizzata) with at least one librarian and a local journal catalogue; the group B of 9 libraries with at least one librarian but no journal catalogue; the group C of 10 libraries with only secretarial staff assistance;
the group D of 6 libraries and no staff at all.

The Project
A network approach: The bureaucratic model of organization was considered useless for the project; in the past years no change was introduced and the old union catalogue was the symbol of the lack of cooperation under a hyerarchical structure; most of the personnel is part of a Department, whose Head is a Professor with very little interest in library service management; the Director (a librarian) of the Biblioteca Centralizzata cannot interfere in the Departments' organization. We tried not to worry about the formal context, but rather involve the colleagues in a cooperative work with a network approach (1). The main aspect of this proposal consists establishing more informal rather than formal relations, and communication among all the people involved, in order to stress the practical aspects of the project and minimize the structure and the formal responsibilities. This model should imply that there is not a "head" of the project but that everyone would interact informally; through informal communication there should be not only practical work to be discussed and carried out, but also trasmission of professional knowledge and practical skills. As the situation revealled very different levels of organization in the libraries considered, we chose to use a basic organization of framework: the Biblioteca Centralizzata is the main point of reference, and some colleagues of the group A libraries are the reference persons for the group B and C libraries. Group D libraries have not been included in the project presented in this paper. As this was our first attempt, no exact timing of the Project was established, except for a maximum length of one year, because the journal titles changes. All efforts were made to simplify and make cooperation easier, with the minimum of expense for each participant.

Methods: software, format and database input. Before the beginning of the project a quite extensive survey was carried out in order to find a software for a personal computer specially designed to produce a union catalogue of journals, with a print output program for all the database and each participating library. We found that there was no software for this task but some library softwares on the Italian market were able to produce a similar result: TINLIB and CDS-ISIS. We decided to use TINLIB not only because the Biblioteca Centralizzata already possessed it, but also because it implied nearly no external computer technical support. We decided to use the UNI 6392 standard, which comes from ISO 3297, as suggested by the Guidelines for the Compilation of Union Catalogues of Serials (2). Moreover the Italian Union Catalogue of Serials by CNR-ISRDS is now moving towards updating the program which will allow our union catalogue to be easily merged in the national database.

The second step consisted in the evaluation of serial databases in order to download the maximum number of the records in the desired format. The ISDS CD-ROM (International Serial Data System) was considered, but we clearly needed a subset of biomedical journals records. We chose to use the data of a biomedical-pharmaceutical union catalogue, with the format UNI 6392, of 4.300 titles: more than 50% were used for the final version of our union catalogue. The following steps for the database input were carried out as follows: merging of the GIDIF,RBM Catalogue (3) records on a text file, through WORD 5.1 Version in TINLIB, merging of Dbase databases (version III and IV) through Paradox (version 3 Special Edition) and WORD into TINLIB, and input of records from paper catalogues into TINLIB.

The Department libraries were asked to write (or to input a Dbase file) a record composed of: **Title, ISSN, Holdings** (with year, and volume number), **Location** (library code). The third step therefore implied some kind of training of the personnel working in the Department libraries; four colleagues were responsible for groups of libraries, helping people to list their journals and check their holdings. All the lists (on paper or on diskette) were collected by the Biblioteca Centralizzata where the librarians performed the following stages of the work.

Input the Database: add the records from Dbase through the cited path to TINLIB, input the records from the paper into TINLIB, check the record matched with existing description in the GIDIF,RBM catalogue.

Check: - catalogue the new records, using the photocopies of title page and the following reference tools:

* List of serials indexed for online users / National Library of Medicine, 1993
* CASSI: Chemical Abstracts Service Source Index / Americal Chemical Society, 1980
* The Serials Directory : an International Reference book. - 6. ed. - Ebsco, 1992
* Ulrich's International Periodicals Directory. - 25. ed. - Bowker, 1987
* Répertoire des périodiques biomédicaux dans le bibliothéques de Suisse. 5.ed. - Académie suisse des Sciences Médicales, 1990
* Catalogo collettivo nazionale delle pubblicazioni periodiche / Consiglio Nazionale delle Ricerche, 1990

checking of the duplicate records in order to find any mistakes in title and holdings description (the number of the volumes were quite useful for this task); printing of a list for each library to be checked by the colleagues; input the changes from those lists and carry overall check of the database.

Print: all the databases were downloaded in WORD for the draft printout. At this stage we needed a print programme in order to obtain the correct order of the data in the record (different from the one which appears on the TINLIB screen), to have a readable layout of the page: these requirements were reached with some macro on WORD, specially written for our catalogue. Despite these routines, some data had to be added or deleted record by record.
- at the end of this phase, the union catalog listed 3.700 titles from 25 libraries, whose address, time of opening and name of the librarian were printed on the first pages and on a bookmark.

Discussion and Conclusions

The choice of the software was also influenced by the lack of organization of many of the libraries: in fact only few of them have a personal computer; therefore the printout was essential. The total cost of our catalogue has been calculated in 18.740.000 Italian lires: this sum includes 890 library staff hours, expertises, printing material. We wish to point out that we had no sponsorship, and most of the software and travel expenses were paid by the Biblioteca Centralizzata; only the printing expenses were shared by the libraries. We also gathered information about the cost of other solutions:

* Genova Medical Libraries Union Catalogue : they had a 15 million lires sponsorship and paid a temporary staff member to collect the data from the libraries (total cost of more than 20 million lires) (this amount was estimate as before)
* Consultancy Agency: the cost for similar service done by a private agency is about 37 million lires only for the bibliographic check and input of the data; if the cost of collecting the holdings data from the libraries is added, it can reach 60 million lires.

The second point is related to the network approach: we certainly employed more time than a private agency, and the project realization was made more difficult because of the day by day library work; we also had no computer technical support, but reached our final product trying different solutions with an unavoidable loss of time. We think, however, that all the time devoted to training colleagues, discussing the results, evaluating the impact of the catalogue on the service has been very useful . In fact we forecast some important changes which will imply a more intensive usage of the catalogue and an increase of the document delivery service:

* in few months a Local Area Network will serve the whole of the main Hospital and the catalogue will be online for 25 libraries
* an upgrading of the TINLIB software on a UNIX computer will allow access to the union catalog on Internet
* the Medical Libraries in Italy are launching a document delivery project (MDD) which implies more efficient service, even for the Department Libraries
* the merging of our union catalogue into the National Catalogue of the CNR-ISRDS will involve the cooperation of this group of libraries at a national level.

These changes need to be accepted and developed by librarians of a good professional level and ready to work in a network which is not only a technological reality, but has a social and human dimension.

Acknowledgments
We wish to thank IF, the Italian Vendor of TINLIB, for sponsoring our participation in the conference.

References and Notes
1. Cfr. Morgan, Gareth. Images : le metafore dell' organizzazione. Milano : Franco Angeli, 1991 (orig.tit. : Morgan, G. .Images of Organization. - Beverly Hills : Sage, 1986)
2. Guidelines for the compilation of union catalogues of serials. - Paris : Unesco : IFLA, 1982.
3. GIDIF,RBM : Gruppo Italiano Documentalisti Industria Farmaceutica e Istituti di Ricerca Biomedica.

EVALUATING GLOBAL INFORMATION ACCESS AND REQUIREMENTS OF COOPERATIVE RESEARCH CENTRES IN AUSTRALIA

Josephine M Marshall and **Lisa M Belkin**. The Walter and Eliza Hall Institute of Medical Research Post Office RMH 3050 Australia. CSIRO Division of Biomolecular Engineering 343 Royal Parade Parkville 3052 Australia.

Background

In 1990 the Australian Commonwealth Government launched the Cooperative Research Centres Program.This radical step in science funding was in recognition of the importance of cooperative ventures between business enterprise and scientific research.Centres are set up within existing organizations. The government contributes 135 million Australian dollars per year to the centres. Participating organizations contribute cash or kind towards 50% of running costs. Centres must be made up of varying types of participants including Universities, private research establishments, Government institutes and business partners. Centres are selected by a lengthy competitive process. At present there are 51 centres covering areas including environment, agriculture, manufacturing and medicine. There are seven centres focusing on Medical Science and Technology in areas ranging from Vaccine Technology to Cochlear Implant, Speech and Hearing. All the centres have been set up to take discoveries to the market place. Centres are located all over the continent of Australia.

Study

As librarians working in two different organizations which are centre participants the authors were concerned that no formal research had been undertaken to assess present information services and needs of professionals working within the centres. We were aware, only too well, by personal experience that no efforts had been made at a formal level to expand current library infrastructure to meet new demands. Libraries were being under utilized in some instances and some participating institutions had no formal library service and no professional library staff thus leading to uneven distribution of quality service within centres. Whilst material resources and staffing for laboratories was increased within centres no additional finding support was forthcoming for libraries. We also knew that the Internet and its vast resources was being underutilised through lack of promotion and understanding.

We realized that the only way to approach these concerns was to undertake a formal research project. We had extensive discussions with scientists involved and noted that our concerns were well supported at an anecdotal level. We also had discussions with the Government administering body, The Office of the Chief Scientist of Australia who was also supportive. We then undertook a detailed literature survey of government papers and articles relating to science and technology in Australia. Over the past 30 years numerous studies of capabilities, trends, strengths, weaknesses and international comparisons of Australian science have been done. Only two reports have assessed, let alone mentioned the adequacy and importance of the library and information services in relation to research. In 1973 the STISEC report on Scientific and Technological Information Services in Australia concluded that although information access and delivery were critical for effective research services were inadequate in Australia.[1] In 1987 a small sample of scientists surveyed by the Australian Department of Science concluded that although supply and demand were basically fulfilling their functions there were several gaps in services. They highlighted the low use of patents as an information source, the widely expressed need for guidance to information and in particular the need for institutions to recognize the essential nature of their information services by allocating a higher proportion of their budgets to library services.[2] In government reports leading to the formation of the Cooperative Research Centres Program no mention was made of information, either infrastructure or importance in relation to research. We then decided on our target group, the seven medical Cooperative Research Centres (CRC's). As these are spread across the continent we decided it would be practical to proceed in stages, commencing with our own state, Victoria. At the time of this presentation only one centre has been fully surveyed owing to time constraints. We hope to complete the seven by the end of 1994 year and present a final report at the International Congress of Medical Libraries in Washington in 1995.

Methodology

A written survey was then developed and tested on research staff within our institutions. The survey was designed to take approximately five minutes to complete, in order to gain the cooperation of busy research scientists. Surveys were then distributed by mail to individual participants in the Centre for Cellular Growth Factors. This is one of the centres which our respective employer organisations are involved in and is made up of five partners- The Walter and Eliza Hall Institute of Medical Research, a private research organisation, the largest medical research institute in Australia, The CSIRO Division of Biomolecular Engineering, a government research institute, The Ludwig Institute for Cancer Research Melbourne, a private hospital based institute, The Biomolecular Research Institute, a state government institute and the AMRAD Corporation a commercial research and development company. This centre is a typical example of the type of collaboration involved in the centres program. Survey forms were sent out to the one hundred and for staff in early May 1994 with a response deadline of ten days. The response rate of 42% covered a wide cross section of different categories of library and information users amongst the participants including postdoctoral scientists, technicians, postgraduate students, clinicians, business management and administration.

Results

For the purposes of the survey information was defined as "resources accessed for research and development purposes".

Question: Where do you obtain information? The first three preferences indicated that the on site library is considered most important. Conferences, meetings and personal communications were second most important as an information source. Responses to this question are consistent with findings of surveys of health professionals in the United States of America in recent years.[3,4,5] It is interesting to note the comparatively low rating of computerised sources. We assume that medical researchers in this study are still relying on printed material as a primary source rather than databases.

Question: How important are the following resources to your research? The study reported on the importance placed on various resources. As predicted journal articles were the most important. Books, conference proceedings and preprints were surprisingly high as a preferred source this may be in part due to the technical staff relying heavily on books for laboratory methods and study. Computerised sources were surprisingly low. The low recognition of patents as an information source indicates use has not increased since the 1987 government report.

Question: Can you obtain journal articles within 24 hours? The answer to this question resulted in a positive 89% yes. This is encouraging and suggests that most libraries involved in the study are providing a fast document delivery service to their clients. Librarians are responsive to the urgent needs of the scientists. The level of those obtaining articles outside libraries is low.

Question: Do you use computers for research information? This question relating to the use of computers for research information showed some interesting results. Initially the results look unfavouable for librarians however we know that the high percentage of those users doing their own searching, in this survey 80%, shows how in particular librarians have led the change. By taking the initiative the library is to a high degree driving the use of computers as a research information tool. Amongst those using using computers Medline is the database of choice closely followed by Current Currents. The combination of these two databases means that these researchers have a good coverage of up to date information available to them. Use of other databases is low.

Question: Are you using AARNet/Internet? A vital question included on the survey was the use of the Internet through AARNetits Australian access point. In the May 1994 issue of "The Scientist" a series of articles on the Internet and its capabilities states that " The Internet is one of the most absolutely critical tools for modern biology. It is in fact changing fundamental aspects of the way scientists work."[6] As alternatives for accessing data bases increases and effective software tools are developed to provide linking of various types of data to answer increasingly complex questions we must conclude that a 52% usage rate amongst respondents is not a good response, particularly when we look at the services used by that group of respondents. A number of our respondents answered "no" initially to this question and then changed their response to "yes" when they realised electronic mail was a component. Of the 48% who are not using the network the figures prove a general ignorance of the capabilities as we suspected prior to the survey. The "no access" figure (14%) is of particular concern. If science is to be practiced in Australia at the same level as in the United States for example and effective collaboration is to be achieved even amongst participants in these centres widespread access to the Internet is integral. This shows a desperate need for promotion and education. Librarians must decide who takes on this role, themselves or computer staff. This could be an ideal opportunity for librarians.

Question: Do you learn about new information developments? 61% of respondents indicated they do learn about new developments. However the very low figure obtaining this information from library tutorials (20%) again demonstrates a need for more promotion, communication and education between librarians and user groups.

Question: How do you envisage accessing information resources in the future? This was the final question on the survey. The answer proved some encouragement for librarians rather disillusioned by previous answers. 45% wanted to continue with their own searching however 52% would like to use a combination of their own and specialist/librarian skills.

Conclusions

Findings based on the study of the first of the seven Medical Research Centers are interesting. Findings such as the fact that journal articles are considered the most critical in the eye of users and the high rating of personal communications, conferences and also books suggests a heavy dependence on traditional sources of information. The speed with which journal articles can be obtained for users shows that librarians involved are very responsive to the fast delivery of information requirements. The increasing use of computers for research information and the high incidence of end user searching show that some librarians are responding well to state of the art technology for their users and can be seen to be in fact driving the use of CD-ROM and networked information databases for searching. From comments at the end of the survey and from ananysis of results there is an obvious urgent need for more education, both in informing of users of new information resources as they become available and in particular Internet and resources. This gives librarians a unique opportunity to take the lead in education for scientists information needs.The gaps in information services noted in Australia in the 1970's and 1980's appear to be growing wider. The low use of patent literature as a valuable source of information highlighted in the 1987 survey has not improved in this survey group.

This survey confirmed our initial concerns regarding information access and delivery to medical research scientists in CRC's. The Director of the Centre for Cellular Growth Factors wrote in support of our project "this is obviously a very important area given the expanding information overload experienced by scientists." We feel encouraged by these initial results to continue on with the project and to follow up with results and recommendations later in the year. Following the final report we hope we can go some way into assisting Australian medical researchers optimise information services and networks to enable a more effective contribution to be made to the development of internationally competitive research based industries and impact upon global health and well being.

Bibliography

1. The STISEC Report Volume 1-scientific and technological infromation services in Australia. Canberra:National Library of Australia 1973:vii.
2. Australia. Department of Science.Scientific and technological information:its use and suppy in Australia. Executive summary. Canberra:Department of Science,1987:S10.
3. Curtis KL, et al. Information seeking behavior: a survey of health sciences faculty,use of indexes and databases. Bull Med Libr Assoc 1993;81:383-92
4. Hurd JM, et al. Information seeking behaviour of faculty: use of indexes and abstracts by scientists and engineers. Am Soc Info Sci Proc1992;29:136-43
5. Grefsheim S, et al. Biotechnology awareness study, Part 1:where scientists get their information. Bull Med Libr Assoc 1991;79:36-44.
6. Hoke F, Scientists predict Internet will revolutionize research. The Scientist 1994; 8:1,8-9.

THE HIDDEN COSTS OF NETWORKING

Margaret Haines, King's Fund Centre, 126 Albert Street, London NW1 7NF, England

There is a tendency today within our profession to equate networking with electronic networking. However, we must remember that networking is still used, especially by other professions, to mean co-operation and this paper will be using this definition ie, the reciprocally beneficial sharing of resources, developed or pre-existing, by two or more bodies[1]

Why do libraries co-operate? Alan MacDougall suggests that "*One of the fundamental tenets of co-operation 'maximising the resource base' is not only believed to be advantageous but positively attainable. Concepts of brotherly and sisterly love, or at least partnership abound. Co-operation then, in the library and information world, is seen as an obvious and guaranteed path to an excellent library service. Or is it? At the other end of the spectrum the unconverted or unbeliever claim to see the false god who deceives. The supposed gift bestowed by co-operation can only be seen, at best, as illusory, or at worst, a counter-productive sham.*"[3] Michael Willis also questioned the motivation behind co-operation when he described it as: "*one of the seven deadly sins of librarianship, resembling a fruitful marriage rather less than a series of casual affairs - absorbing a lot of time and energy and providing pleasure for the participants at the expense of the interests of the family back home.*"[2] Are all librarians this cynical? Based on the experiences of the King's Fund Centre Library, this paper will explore some of the reasons for co-operation, discuss hidden costs and critical success factors, and comment on whether the cynicism of Willis and MacDougall[3] is justified.

Some reasons offered for co-operation include: saving money through sharing resources (staff, storage, materials) with other libraries; improved access to resources and services beyond the means of one library; a positive response to political pressure for more efficient use of resources; the opportunity to demonstrate the use of new technologies; enhanced status and perhaps increased influence within the professional community; and finally, a sense of contributing to the community and displaying professional values. Kennett Dowlin says "*It is hard to quantify but ours is a networking profession. We see co-operation as one of our most important shared values.*"[4] It appears that many libraries still share this value as co-operation does not seem to be on the wane. Wilson and Marsterson describe three categories of co-operation[5]:

Exchange: of material, information, users, records, staff, etc

Coalition: the shared development of service tools/resources (software, staff, buildings, equipment), research, training or publishing activities.

Entrepreneurial: a two-way interaction with one partner gaining a service and the other gaining some financial remuneration for this service.

Within our own sector, we can find many examples of all these types. The National Network of Libraries of Medicine in the USA, initially focused on the *exchange* of resources through interlibrary loan activities and training programmes but later developed a more *entrepreneurial* outreach service to end users.[6] A key lesson espoused by this network is that success depends on meeting the needs of users as well as library staff. In the UK, regional Health Information Plans or HIPs provide an enabling and facilitating framework for planned co-operation and co-ordination of health information services.[7] HIPs are based on the principle of *coalition* amongst many partners including non-library organisations from the health sector. A key lesson from HIPs is the importance of finding funding for the planning stage of co-operation. n Canada, the Health Sciences Information Consortium, a local co-operative of 38 libraries affiliated with the University of Toronto also focuses on *exchange* of materials through interlibrary loans but promotes a `single point of contact' rather than a distributed or decentralised approach as the key success factor.[8] Participants in these networks and others mention a number of factors which can influence the success of the network. Some of the `tactical' factors include:

Funding: what funding is required for co-operation and can all partners contribute to this funding given the short-term nature of some library funding;

Ownership: who has the responsibility for monitoring quality and for management of joint ventures and what is the legal position vis-a-vis revenue and debts;

Communications: how complex is the communications chain, and how can `Chinese whispers' be avoided if there is no central communications source.

Other issues can best be described as more political, eg:

Hidden agendas: do partners' local interests (concepts, timescales, priorities) conflict with the general interests of the network?;

Environment: are there new pressures as a result of government elections such as a push towards competitive tendering which may affect the partnership?

Status: will the personalities of the institutional representatives and the reputations of the partners get in the way of co-operation?

Against this background, I will describe the various co-operatives in which King's Fund Centre Library participates and share some of our conclusions regarding the hidden costs of networking.

The King's Fund Centre Library is a public reference library specialising in health care management. In 1990, this library was facing a number of service-related crises precipitated by budget cuts, increased information demands from users due to the NHS reforms, and an inefficient manual technical processing system. A strategy was developed to improve services for users which included a commitment to co-operation with other libraries in order to: reduce technical service costs, share the burden of enquiries, and provide access to materials not within the remit of the library. In addition, the library's long-term vision was to contribute to a national health information plan based on co-operation between all major information providers and it was hoped that the library's own co-operative ventures might provide one model for this plan. Since 1991, the library has participated in four networks. The first was an international, `exchange' network of 25 WHO documentation centres organised by the WHO Regional Office for Europe in Copenhagen. We receive WHO-EURO publications free but must publicise and disseminate these within the UK. This network has helped us to develop our public health collection for the benefit of our users; however, we have found that our higher profile within Europe has resulted in many additional enquiries from European visitors and libraries.

In 1992, we formed the Healthcare Management Information Consortium with the Department of Health and the Nuffield Institute for Health Libraries. Despite our different parents (a charity, a government department and a university institute), we all act as quasi-national resource centres for healthcare management information. Our aims included the exchange of bibliographic records, co-operative acquisitions, consultancy, participation in international projects, and lobbying for a national health information strategy. We have made more headway in international and special projects than we have in sharing records and collections. This has been partly due to local pressures such as re-organisation of one partner and market testing of another, but there have also been legal problems due to our very different parent organisations. Other inhibitors include lack of time and money for the planning of co-operation and lack of senior management support and junior staff involvement. It still feels that all the responsibility is resting on the three library directors. Our third network has only one other partner - the Health Education Authority. As we now use the same collection management system, UNICORN, we decided to capitalise on a system module which creates electronic links between our online public access catalogues thus permitting our users to search each other's library databases. With funding from the HEA, in 1993 we hired a project manager to oversee collaboration and to produce UNICORN training programmes and manuals for staff at both sites and to develop further links between our speciality databases on health and race. Despite some technical and communication problems, we have made great progress which we attribute to having sufficient funding for project management, and to having agreed terms of reference, priorities and timescales.

In 1994, we joined the European Foundation Centre's Orpheus Network which documents and provides information services on foundations and corporate funding throughout Europe. It is decentralised with each member maintaining a national dossier of foundations with the EFC convening the network as well as maintaining a dossier of cross-frontier funders. This network is providing us, with access to new resources but it is also proving to be very expensive in terms of travel to network meetings.

After four years, what benefits have we seen from networking? We expected and gained increased access to resources. We expected and gained a higher profile nationally and internationally. We expected and to a limited extent, progressed towards our vision of a national health information strategy. However, we expected cost savings and reduced enquiries but achieved neither. We did not expect co-operation spin-offs such as consultancy opportunities, greater access to senior government officials, and professional development opportunities such as presentations and articles. (Must admit that I was the main beneficiary of the unexpected benefits and when reading Willis' quotation about `providing pleasure for the participants', I felt distinctly guilty.) We were prepared to see some costs of co-operation and the costs of publicity, equipment and communications were about what we expected. However, travel costs were higher than expected and I seriously underestimated the amount time I spent on network activities. There were also many unexpected costs such as the legal bill for investigating the status of HMIC, the cost of sub-contracting the preparation of an HMIC consultancy proposal because we were all too busy. In addition, there were hidden but serious costs such as the increased number of enquiries and visitors resulting from our WHO network activities and the fact that time spent away at network planning meetings was time "at the expense of the interests of the family back home" to quote Willis again.

In conclusion, were our networks worth the cost and trouble and would I do it again? The short answer is a cautious yes, but I would not go into any future cooperative ventures without truing to separate personal benefits from institutional benefits as honestly as possible and asking myself the following questions:

1) Will it improve service, save money, eliminate barriers to information or provide something we could not get through our own action?
2) Do our potential partners share a common purpose or subject with us, and do we know their reputations and their personalities well enough?
3) How easy is it to participate and can we guarantee to fulfil our obligations to the network and can our partners and what will happen if we don't?
4) Where do our local priorities fit with network priorities and have we senior managements support for network priorities?

My experience and that of others suggests that the cynicism about the benefits of co-operation can be addressed by ensuring the presence of critical success factors. These included clarity about terms of reference, priorities, timescales and distribution of responsibilities; documented commitment in the form of contracts or legal agreements; staff involvement and support as well as senior management support; time and money for planning; one point of contact within each network partner; built-in mechanisms for feedback and review; and network objectives which are focussed on better services for clients.

References

1. Edmonds, Diana J. Current library cooperation and coordination. (Office of Arts & Libraries, Library & Information Series 15) London: HMSO, 1986.
2. MacDougall, Alan, Cooperation: a conceptual framework for librarians. In: Handbook of library cooperation, Eds Alan MacDougall & Roy Pryterch. Aldershot: Gower, 1992.
3. Willis, Michael. Lust or "cooperation". LA Record, Apr 1990, 92(4): 292.
4. Dowlin, Kenneth. In: Managing the economics of owning, leasing & contracting out information services. Eds Anne Woodsworth & James F Williams II. Aldershot: Ashgate, 1993.
5. Wilson, T D & Marterson, W A. Local library cooperation: final report on a project funded by the Department of Education & Science. Sheffield, Univ Sheffield School of Librarianship & Information Science, 1974.
6. Weise, F O. Developments in health science libraries since 1974. Library Trends, Summer 1993, 42(1): 5-24
7. Childs, S. Health information in the North. Newcastle: Information North, 1993.
8. Leishman, J. The health science information consortium. Bibliotheca Medica Canadiana, 1991, 13(2):96-9.

Section 3

Management & Organisational Issues

MAINTAINING QUALITY: the Accreditation Experience

Anne FitzGerald, Forest Healthcare Trust,Whipps Cross Hospital, Whipps Cross Road, London E11 1NR, UK

This paper describes the North Thames (East) accreditation process and considers its impact on the Library at Whipps Cross Hospital. It concludes that accreditation is a valuable way of not only maintaining quality but promoting it.

Accreditation may be described as "a structured method for measuring quality".[1] It is a relatively new tool in Hospital Libraries in the U.K. with only a small number of regions currently using it. In March 1993 North Thames (East) Region Unit Librarians were made formally aware that their services would be accredited. Prior to this it was the type and quantity of services that were systematically monitored rather than their quality. What I propose to discuss is: how the process of accreditation actually works in North Thames (East); the impact accreditation on the unit library that I manage at Whipps Cross Hospital, with specific reference to communication; some of the positive benefits to be gained from the process, and finally some of the problems of accreditation.

North Thames (East) Regional Health Authority funds thirty one Libraries to provide a service to those in postgraduate medicine. The Whipps Cross, unit Library which is situated in the Medical Education Centre, receives the predominant part of its funding from Region. The Regional Librarian has been instrumental in organising and setting in motion the process of accreditation This began with the setting of minimum standards of provision. These are based on the Committee of Postgraduate Deans (COPMED) and the NHS Regional Librarians' standards [2] they owe much to the original work of John Lancaster, Librarian of the University of Wales College of Medicine. The North Thames (East) standards have been carefully defined and set out in a document which takes the form of a questionnaire [3]. This has to be filled out in advance of an accreditation visit by the Regional team.

The Regional team consists of the Regional Librarian, a medical practitioner, and a senior librarian from a unit library in North Thames (East). All members of the team are given a copy of the completed accreditation checklist / questionnaire in advance of their actual visit. The visit itself is structured by the accreditation document with the visiting team having a formal opportunity to ask the librarian about the specific points that have been highlighted. This "interview" is followed by a tour around the library including ample time for browsing and more informal questions. The visit takes about a day. Following it a report is prepared and the Library is given one of three levels of accreditation: level one - where all levels in the accreditation statement can be applied to the unit library; level two - where the essential elements of the accreditation statement can be applied to the unit library and where there is evidence of continuing progress towards level one status; and level three - where the essential elements of the accreditation statement can be applied to the unit library when formal co-operative arrangements with larger library services are included and where there is evidence of continuing progress towards level two status. The "essential" elements of the accreditation document are indicated by an asterisk. In all there are eight major areas considered in the accreditation document. They are: library philosophy and management; accommodation and equipment; the library collection; library finance; staffing; basic services; inter-library co-operation, and information technology. Under these broad headings 79 individual points are covered.

When I first saw the accreditation document I was somewhat daunted by its range and attention to detail but I came to regard it as a very useful quality checklist. As a newly appointed manager it was just what I needed. I agree with Lascelles who says with regard to quality 'Just deciding where to begin is so difficult that many never get off the starting block.' He goes on to say 'The condition is so common that it even has a name "Total Quality Paralysis"'[4]. Knowing that I would have about six months from the time I received the document to the time my service would be accredited I had to prioritise, taking note of not only what could be done but what should be done. There were simple tasks that could be quite easily performed like improving internal signing and updating the library guide. Other issues needed more long term attention. The quality of communication was the largest single issue that needed to be addressed. When I came into post, there were no formal communication channels but an opportunity was created to form better links when I was invited to attend the Medical Academic Committee. With the accreditation document to hand I spoke at my first meeting about the need for formal consultation with my users particularly on issues of policy. It was agreed that the academic committee would provide such a forum.

I also knew that I needed to have broader consultation with my users. This seemed particularly evident in the area of stock selection. I wanted to ensure that the collection was both timely and relevant. A new journals holdings list was compiled and all departments were sent a copy with a covering letter. The letter advised of the imminent 10-20% journal price rise and asked recipients to prioritise the journals in their discipline. The response rate was 76%. This reflected the value placed on journal subscriptions. As a result of this survey I was able to cancel two subscriptions and replace them with two notable new ones. I was also given a clear idea of which journals were the most highly rated.

In addition to this I wrote to departments about the current book stock. Each consultant was sent a printout of the current holdings in his/her speciality and a list of the texts suggested by Hague & Jackson [5]. They were asked to prioritise for purchase. Using the list gave the exercise some focus and once again the response was high at 70.5% As far as possible I followed up purchase suggestions using the suggestions made. Good communication obviously needs to extend to staff too. In preparation for accreditation I was prompted to: set up weekly staff meeting; prepare a full induction programme for a new member of staff; rewrite the staff procedures manual, and consider the issue of staff appraisal. I think that given the time constraints I was under before my new staff member was appointed I might not have prepared an induction programme. It was, however, worthwhile because it did give her a wider feel for the organisation. Staff appraisal was only introduced in April 1994 but it has already had an impact on individual staff awareness.

Continuing on the theme of communication I would like to discuss user education. I have always tried to ensure that users are aware of all the facilities and services available. This has tended to be on a rather "ad hoc" basis. Earlier this year I was able to make education more organised by writing a letter inviting all the "firms"/ medical teams in the hospital to short firm specific library induction session. This brought a small but significant response from five of them. The major lure was our new CD-ROM windows version of Medline from 1966 to date. Even consultants who had worked on the main site for several years wanted to come. It certainly appears that those firms having formal induction sessions have subsequently tended to exploit the full range of services available.

I have only touched on some of the issues that the North Thames (East) accreditation process made me address. It certainly was a useful focus which not only made me aware of areas where quality needed to be maintained but also those where standards needed to be raised. It is, however, a fledgling tool and as such has some problems associated with it. Some librarians are very apprehensive about accreditation. Others are critical of the document and of the results. There are those who see it as a developmental opportunity whilst others see it merely as a scoring system which offers them nothing tangible. Another problem with accreditation can be finding the time to do it. For the visiting team there is nearly two days work, and for the unit librarian there is the hard work involved in assessing his or her service effectively.

At present the North Thames (East) document lacks any accompanying guidelines. The Regional Librarian did, however, set up two working parties on writing aims and objectives and quality control. Both produced useful papers. The Regional Librarian is also available for consultation about specific points. Indeed he came to Whipps Cross for an informal pre accreditation visit. South Western Region has produced a "Toolkit" [6] which accompanies their own document. This I found very useful starting point but there are gaps in its coverage because the process of accreditation is new there too. Those responsible for it and those involved in it need to build on their experiences. This is the plan in North Thames (East) where it is hoped to make examples of good practice available to unit Librarians. With fuller backup material the accreditaion document will not only make demands and set standards but show how improvements can be made. Essentially, the introduction of the accreditation process has proved what a powerfully persuasive tool it can be. By its nature accreditation is on-going - helping to identify and set in motion many new service targets. Although the process is still in its infancy it has proved itself to be a valuable catalyst for change. For me the major benefit of accreditation is that it supports unit librarians in the task of maintaining and improving quality. Finally, constructive use of comprehensive checklist document can also help to prevent "Total Quality Paralysis". There can certainly be no excuse for "remaining on the starting block" [4].

References

1. EAGLETON, K.E. Quality Assurance in Canadian Hospital Libraries- the challenge of the eighties. Health Libraries Review 1988 5(3) pp.145-9
2. COPMED in consultation with NHS RLG Accreditation of Unit Libraries in support of Postgraduate Medical and Dental Education London 1992. (Available from the NHS Regional Librarians Group)
3. NORTH EAST THAMES REGIONAL LIBRARY SERVICE Accreditation of Unit Libraries London 1993. (Available from John Hewlett, Regional Librarian, North Thames (East)
4. LASCELLES, D.M. DALE, B.G. A review of the issues involved in quality improvement International Journal of Quality and Reliability Management 1988 5 May pp.76-94 quoted in FOREMAN, L. (ed) Developing Quality in Libraries London 1992
5. HAGUE, H. JACKSON, M. Core collection Medical Books and Journals 1992 Medical Information Working Party, London 1992
6. TRINDER, V.(ed) SWEHSLINC Accreditation Toolkit (national edition) South West England Service Libraries in Co-operation) 1993 (Available from Valerie Trinder SWEHSLinc)

THE MANAGEMENT OF INTEGRATED INFORMATION SYSTEMS AND THE ROLE OF LIBRARIANS

Jean G. Shaw, University of Leicester, Clinical Sciences Library, Leicester Royal Infirmary, PO Box 65, Leicester LE2 7LX, UK

Abstract

The characteristics of an integrated information system are defined and examples of the management issues, which may be encountered, are given. The management structures found in the Integrated Advanced Information Management Systems, funded by the National Library of Medicine in the U.S.A., are examined and the implications discussed. Integrated information systems are dynamic and librarians are urged to use their skills both in their implementation and their exploitation.

Access to information is made possible by technology, but to make access easy and hence useful rather than time-consuming we need integrated information systems. My purpose here is to examine examples of integrated information systems, look at ways in which they have been implemented and comment upon some of the implications for our profession as managers of information. Integrated information systems are as important to industry and commerce as they are to health services and education. Technology is enabling us to revolutionize information flow, but if we are to avoid information overload, librarians and information managers need to have an understanding of the nature of integrated information systems.

There is probably no one universally accepted definition of an integrated information system, but there are some definitions which I think are particularly helpful. These come from a recent survey of commercial organizations and other large organizations, such as the National Health Service, in the U.K. (Brittain 1992) "A single source of data, which can be shared across applications... and allow the fulfilment of organizational goals and objectives." "The inputting and storage of data relevant to the functions/departments of the company, so that there is no duplication or replication of input and that access is available to all who need it." "Providing a window on the world for the user with invisible technology." "The tools [computer systems] are glued together so that the user does not see the joins". In summary, they avoid the duplication or replication of tasks; they make information easily accessible to those that want it, and they can give rise to new services.

That we can contemplate such a concept is due to computer and network technology. In 1982 Nolan proposed six stages in the evolution of computerized data handling. In the final stage the concept of shared data and data as an important resource comes to maturity - an integrated information system. In the following examples of integrated systems, there are some which have taken place at a comparatively modest level and others (mainly from America) which involve the whole institution. Many of you will be familiar with integrated library systems. The key component of the system is generally the catalogue record. It is this record which is "attached" to the borrower's file, when the item is borrowed from the library. There is no separate file for circulation as there used to be in older automated but unintegrated, systems. The order record, once on file, will be upgraded not recreated. Interlibrary loans are typed directly into the system by the reader. The same mechanism generates reminders for both interlibrary loans and the local lending system. These are all features of an integrated system. Information is not copied from one piece of paper to another. The menus for the different functions use the same format, so that once learnt it is easy for the staff and users to manipulate. And it can create features that are of real benefit to the user. Perhaps the most dramatic in this instance is that users can see from the catalogue, whether the books they want are on the shelves or not. So here we have a system in which the data is input only once, it is shared amongst the applications and the sum of the whole is greater than its constituent parts. Note also that it is an dynamic system. If booksellers' and publishers' computerized systems comply with the same recognized standards, there could be integration with libraries acquisitions systems.

From a management point of view there are a number of issues concerned with the implementation of an integrated system. At whatever level it is initiated an integrated information system is based on the concept of shared data. To implement it effectively and efficiently old practices may have to be abandoned. This is not always easy for librarians or library assistants to accept. Some may well have to come to terms with a deskilling of their operations. These are human issues which management may well have to face and plan for if the morale and committment of the work force is to be maintained. For instance one of the main obstacles in setting up an integrated Health Intelligence function in a District Health Authority in the U.K., was not technological, but human (Gregory-Royce 1993). Information activities, previously carried out by a number of departments needed to be brought together, but the consequent loss of control and autonomy was, not unnaturally resisted. Without support from themost senior level of management such projects may be rendered ineffective if other senior staff regard them as being opposed to their interests.

Integration creates a much greater awareness of the importance of an integrated approach to long term strategic planning. Even on the scale of a single library, the necessity for closer co-operation and the pursuit of shared values for the enterprise appears to be a corollary of operating an integrated system. The degree to which problems will be met, are likely to vary. Personal as well as organizational factors are involved. But if top management is to show sustained committment any integrated information project must be central to the aims and priorities of the parent body . This is a point made by many writers on information policy (eg. Orna 1990), and has been said one way or another in all the examples used in this article. Much of the pioneering work on integrated information systems in the medical field has taken place in the U.S.A, where the National Library of Medicine funded and supported a number of Integrated Academic Information Management Systems (IAIMS). Though an early emphasis on the library's role in generating an integrated information system has given way to a wider, institutional commitment, libraries still play a significant role, though in some projects it is tangential rather than central (Lorenzi 1992; Fuller 1992).

One of the interesting results of the IAIMS projects was that no one model for integration emerged. Successful projects addressed the aims and objectives of their institution, but medical schools are complex. The institutional emphasis may be on clinical or basic research; the degree of involvement of the teaching hospital or parent university may differ. Such differences may be carried over into the form of the integrated information projects themselves and so be reflected to some degree in their management structures. At Columbia (Roderer et al. 1992) the emphasis was on easy access to numerous information sources for as many people as possible. Control of the network gave sufficient leverage to the IAIMS project leadership to foster co-operation, since co-ordination rather than authority over the disparate and dispersed information resources was the preferred organizational model. Five new units were set up to promote this end.

1. Centre for medical informatics - new
   Multidisciplinary with strong personnel links to the hospital
   Research in the IAIMS context

2. Administration for the Health Sciences Division - new
   Liaison with the University administration

3. Core Resources -technology group -new

4. Hospital Department of Clinical Information Services -new
   Considerable overlap with 1. Clinical information

5 Joint Security Task Force - new
   All three organizations represented (Hospital, Medical School and Columbia University)

6. Scholarly information systems
   Managed by the existing University Health Sciences Library

The precise way in which these teams interact is not specified, but Roderer et al. (1992) emphasize the overlap in personnel between groups and the importance of the links. In their words the IAIMS leadership is an "information architect" rather than a "Czar".A similar sort of structure in which there is no very definite hierachy amongst the teams can be demonstrated in the Médiathèque initiative at the psychiatric hospital in Neuilly sur Marne, France (Charpentier

1994) This exemplifies the importance of the human element rather than technology. The hospital had been concerned at the lack of contact and information flow between the different hospital professions. So at Neuilly sur Marne the aims were achieved by the physical integration into one area of several small libraries and other conventional information sources, along with with facilities which foster contact between personnel (both staff and patients), such as the cafeteria, hairdressing, banking and kiosks. This project not only provided a place where all might meet informally, but in setting up the multidisciplinary teams to design and implement the project they made some headway towards the very goal that they wished to achieve.

At Georgetown (Broering & Bagdoyan 1992), and indeed in many of the other IAIMS projects, the management structure is more hierachical, but is again largely dependent on teams . The Georgetown project is directed by a key individual, the Librarian, though in other IAIMS projects this responsibility is shared by a multidisciplinary team There are two subgroups, one for technical support and the other for training and education, which is mainly the responsibility of library staff. Though this is the core of the IAIMS management structure it is embedded in that of the institution. Regular meetings are held with high level executives in the Medical School. There are meetings with key people both inside and outside of the institution, and periodic reviews of the process involve still more people in providing feedback.

If there are any lessons to be inferred from the examples above the most obvious must surely be the committment and total support of the top management of the parent body. In the American examples the degree of organizational change is considerable. The creation of management structures which require the active participation of senior personnel cannot be lightly undertaken and feedback procedures encroach on the time which might otherwise have been devoted to research or other duties. Multidisciplinary teamwork is one of the common features in the IAIMS and the other projects described here no matter what the aim or the formal management structure adopted. Team building and its associated management techniques is therefore crucial to the success of a project. Matrix management, in which project teams are formed, disbanded when no longer needed, and reformed to undertake the next objective, was the management strategy adopted at the University of Washington (Fuller 1992). All this is a more fluid structure than we find in traditional library management, but Fuller points out that the people who are best at planning a project are not necessarily those who are best at carrying it out or managing it when it reaches it conclusion. If librarians are to work effectively in multidisciplinary teams, we may need to adopt a more assertive attitude. To often we see ourselves as the passive providers of services rather than as an active colleague with special skills in information systems and management, which are badly needed if the vast amounts of information that become available are to be retrievable.

Successful integration of information is dynamic. We need to ensure that information projects are compatible with one another; that they adhere to recognized international standards. Only in this way will it be possible for one initiative to join up with another thereby making ever increasingly powerful information systems. Intrapreneurship, innovation within an organization to achieve goals, has been demonstrated in a library environment at the University of Miami School of Medicine (Lemkau et al. 1991) The integration of the computer and audiovisual services with the library led to the creation of collaborative projects such as the marketing of video systems and a networked slide making service. The library played an important role in both of these projects, which first became self-financing and then profit making. Thus new services can be created which benefit both the creators and the users.

The integration of information systems will have far reaching effects on the whole of the information industry and librarians are not alone in having to come to terms with it. Publishers and subscription agents will also need to redefine their role as integrated systems and electronic publication blur the boundaries. Will they, rather than our libraries, take on the document supply service? Maybe. We already have competitors. In the future there may be less stock to manage and a greater emphasis on retrieving, managing and making available new sources of information. Old skills such as indexing, classifying and cataloguing will be applied in a new medium. We may find ourselves more involved in educational roles, but I hope that librarians will continue to exercise their knowledge and skills in working with other professions, so that the benefits of integrated information systems can be exploited to the benefit of all.

References

Brittain M ed. 1992 Integrated information systems. London: Taylor Graham. (British Library Research and Development Reports, 6054.)

Broering NC & Bagdoyan HE 1992 The impact of IAIMS at Georgetown: strategies and outcomes. Bull Med Libr Assoc 80(3):263-275).

Carpentier SM 1994 De la bibliothèque á la médiothèque au C.H. Maison Blanche. Newl Eur Health Libr no. 26, Jan, 9-10.

Fuller SS 1992 Planning the future: IAIMS planning premises at the University of Washington. Bull Med Libr Assoc 80(3):288-293.

Gregory-Royce R 1993 Creating a health intelligence function. IFM Healthcare Newsl 4(4):2-6.

Lemkau HL, Burrows S, Stolz F 1991 Bull Med Libr Assoc 79(3):271-275.

Lorenzi NM 1992 Introduction: integrated academic information management systems (IAIMS). Bull Med Libr Assoc 80(3):241-243.

Nolan RL 1982 Managing the data resouce function. 2nd ed. St.Paul (Minn): West Publishing.

Orna E 1990 Practical information policies: how to manage information flow in organizations. London: Gower.

Roderer NK, Long AC, Clayton PD 1992 IAIMS at Columbia - Prebyterian Medical Center: accomplishments and challenges. Bull Med Libr Assoc 80 (3):253-262.

MARKETING MEDICAL SCHOOL LIBRARIES

Beatrice M. Doran, Royal College of Surgeons in Ireland Mercer Street Lower, Dublin 2, Ireland

Abstract
Medical School Libraries have to compete with other resources in their institutions for decreasing funds. It is therefore vital (if they wish to survive in the present economic climate) for them to market their services. An effective marketing plan will give the medical school high visibility and illustrate the Library's essential role as a support service to the teaching and research carried out in the Medical School. Various marketing devices open to Medical School Libraries are discussed with examples from the Library of the Royal College of Surgeons in Ireland.

Introduction
To survive in the present economic climate of reduced funding, rising costs of materials and staff shortages medical school libraries need to improve their situation by promoting themselves with the same marketing and advertising techniques used by successful businesses [(1)]. Medical school libraries, like other academic libraries, have to compete with other resources in their colleges and universities for decreasing funds. For this reason, it is important for medical school libraries to pay great attention to marketing their services. We must ensure that the administrators, academic staff, governing bodies and alumni, as well as our students recognise the Library's value to the parent institution. We need to have an effective marketing plan which will give us high visibility, and illustrate our importance as a support service to the teaching and research carried out in the medical school. If we do this, our libraries will become a selling point for the medical school in promoting the school to potential students, and also to major donors to the institution.

What exactly is marketing? According to the Chartered Institute of Marketing in the United Kingdom: *Marketing is the management process responsible for identifying, anticipating and satisfying customer requirements* ***profitably.*** In most organisations marketing is now a strategic management process. It seeks to integrate advertising, selling, pricing, new service developments etc. with the needs of customers in order to achieve long term customer satisfaction. An important part of any marketing strategy is the marketing mix [(2-3)]. This is normally recognised as being the four Ps - **Product, Price, Promotion, Place**. I now want to look at each of these in the context of medical school libraries. The core **product** offered by the medical school library or indeed any library is its basic library service, the provision of books, journals and other multi media products to support the teaching and research carried out in the medical school. More and more libraries are beginning to emphasise the value-added services they provide. These are particularly important in medicine with the urgency of our clients information needs and the complexity of the subject matter. Members of the health care professions, therefore, place particular emphasis on the value-added services that a quality medical library can provide. Such services include tailor made bibliographies, packages of information in the form of articles and news extracts, online searches and document delivery. Providing these services is, in a way, simply marketing our resources. We must also ensure that news of new products and services reach not only our regular library users, but that news of new products and services also attract new customers.

The question of **price** is probably the most difficult aspect in the marketing context. The price that we charge for our services will obviously have an influence on the revenue we generate. Our regular users expect our basic services to be free. But we should charge for our value-added services. In the present financial climate we need to maximise the revenue which can be generated through charging for specific library services. We should also be trying to extend further income generating activities in our libraries by packaging and charging external readers for information. In the context of the marketing mix **promotion** plays an important part. We need to create and develop an awareness of our library services and the services we offer our customers. Publish or perish may be the academic cry. Promote or perish could be ours [(4)]. There are three obviously promotional methods that we can make use of : the published word, personal contact, and atmospherics - that is the way the library is planned and designed for use. We must advertise our services regularly, indulge in personal selling, publicity and sales promotion [(5)]. We need to produce attractive leaflets describing the services on offer. In fact, everything which we send out to our customers should be an advertisement for our services. Do we use graphic designers to help us put across our message to our users and potential users? Do we advertise on campus wide networks?

Never forget the importance of the part played by the library staff in the promotion of the library services. Your manner whether in person in dealing with library users or on the telephone will affect the use of your library. Smiling at customers will help you establish personal relationships with them. No one likes to be greeted with a sour face if they come to the library issue desk. Did you know that smiling on the telephone changes the tone of your voice and makes you appear more friendly [(6)]. Most libraries have readers cards with their name on it - library staff should be encouraged to address readers by their name. It makes a great difference not only to promoting the library and its services but also in making our customers feel important - it shows we care enough about them to ascertain or remember their names. Think of the clubs you are members of and how nice it is to be greeted by name!

Word of mouth is by far the best way of attracting new users of our services. People who receive a poor service in the library are more likely to tell ten people about it. If they receive a good service it is likely that they will only tell one person about it! We should be constantly endeavouring to improve the quality of our library services and facilities by creating an atmosphere in which quality becomes the most important concept. Internal customer care means looking after your own staff. A successful marketing programme begins with the library's own staff. A monthly staff bulletin can be an important adjunct to library public relations [(7)]. High quality library service begins in the minds of the library management team. As managers, we have to create and enhance a culture of service, communicate quality standards and find the necessary resources to help solve problems and remove any obstacles to the quality of our staffs job performance. Your staff need to know that you care about them before they will consider caring for your customers. Find someone doing something right and praise them for it! Try and support your staff in their work, and let them know that they are a valuable source of information and ideas on the Library and its services. We should do everything in our power to encourage our staff to work as a team [(8)].

Place within the marketing mix refers to the location in which library services are offered. The right information to the right people at the right time must be our aim. For our users to be satisfied customers, services must be made available when and where the user can use them most effectively. Place also incorporates all the distribution channels - e-mail, fax, the postal service etc. - whatever means you use to get the information to the person who wants it [(5)]. In the context of place, new libraries provide excellent opportunities to attract new users and they can act as a showcase for collections and services. Students use libraries as a place to study but they also use libraries as a place to meet other students. Many a romance has started in the Library! Libraries, then, are social centres for our student population. The physical structures furnishings and atmospheres should all be considered an integral part of marketing the services provided by the library. If, like us, you are fortunate enough to have one of the most modern medical school libraries in Europe, the attractive environment is in itself a marketing device in that it is a physical symbol of the medical school's commitment to learning and research.

The 1990's are generally acknowledged to belong to the customer. We live in an era when quality management and indeed total quality management is becoming part and parcel of our lives. More and more successful organisations are customer driven, and there is a great change in the strategies being adopted from telling and selling, to communication and sharing knowledge [(9)]. What our customers want determines the success of the library's services. Doing it in such a way that they like what took place in the library and that they want to come back again, is also vital. The availability of technology and our users attitude towards it, together with their level of aptitude in using it, is always significant in medical school libraries. Modern technology is transforming the very way we work. We are providing more and more technology in our medical school libraries. Our roles as librarians are changing as a result; many of us have become teachers of these new technologies, consultants and advisors in the selection of information technology systems, not only for our libraries, but also for our institutions. I came across an interesting reference to librarians of the future with the advent of the Internet, librarians of the future will be cybrarians - navigators of cyberspace [(9)]. Cybrarians will perform three main functions (i) infomapping, acting as an institution's memory, and knowing where knowledge and expertise lie in the organisation (ii) acting as gateways to external sources and (iii) networking, networking, networking.

Besides being aware of and advocates for the use of technology, we must also be aware of what is happening in our medical schools. We must be aware of curriculum changes, or other educational changes in the direction of the medical school. For example, are there any plans to move towards a problem based learning curriculum? And, if so, how will that influence the library and the services on offer. As librarians we should not simply react to service demands by our readers, but we should be attempting to stimulate awareness of our services among as broad a user base as possible. If the library is doing a good marketing job, user satisfaction should be increased, and the Library's case for extra funding should be strengthened, and indeed, the job satisfaction of Library staff should also be increased.

What are they doing at the Royal College of Surgeons in Ireland, you may very well ask, in the way of marketing the medical school library. A new library, The Mercer Library opened three years ago behind the facade of one of Dublin's oldest hospitals. It covers an area of 27,000 square feet, contains 250 reader places, a medical informatics laboratory where students are taught computer literacy, an integrated library computer system called URICA a network of CD ROMs and cavity floors. In other words, we are a high tech library. We were preparing for the 21st century with our cavity floors when every reader place may be a computer workstation. As Librarian of the Royal College of Surgeons in Ireland, I sit on all the major committees within the College, like the Academic council, the Medical Faculty etc. where I represent the Library. I try never to miss an opportunity to promote the Library and its service at these meetings. I have recently been appointed Chairman of the College IT Committee and I am very pleased that my academic colleagues have seen fit to recognise the librarian as someone with some expertise in information technology.

Marketing the New Technologies

I am particularly interested in the applications of computer technology to library and information work. Today a modern library is far more than a collection of books and journals. The emphasis is on access to information, and increasingly that access is provided by electronic means. Information technology is truly at home in the library, and we must market it. The future of libraries depends heavily on our ability to apply technology effectively to fill the information needs of our users. It is important for libraries to be seen to provide a useful service in an electronic information age. With the increasing availability of networks and access to the Internet, more and more demand for electronic resources and their delivery to the desktop, what is our future in this type of environment? We have to become more innovative, and reposition ourselves on the growth curve of the electronic information revolution [10]. Multi media products have opened up new service areas for libraries and these too require marketing. Librarians must act as teachers and guides helping students through the new technology and the vast number of databases and teaching programs becoming available over the Internet.

Library tours and user education programmes: Library tours are another form of marketing we use in the RCSI Library to introduce new students to the Library. Tours of the Library are given to our new lst year students every October when term starts. I also address the students during a series of introductory talks during Freshers week. Orientation tours are quite effective marketing methods; they help to spread the word about what is available. In addition we provide library instruction for specific groups of users. For example, the lst Med students have to do a project each year. In conjunction with the academic staff of the Department of Physiology, a topic is chosen and seminars on literature searching methods are given by library staff, and students are introduced to electronic information resources.

Library publications as marketing devices: The content and style of library publications is of considerable importance in marketing the Library. Publications should be tailored to the audience and to promoting the Library's goals. The choice of the design of publications is of equal importance. We had a graphic designer in to produce a brochure for the Mercer Library. The graphic artist also produced a house style which we use on all our stationery. Most of our internal leaflets are designed in-house and they are simple and cheap to produce and, we think, quite effective! More recently, we have started packaging a range of the services we offer under the heading Medical Information Services and we use an attractive folder to send out the results of online searches or other information we are providing to our customers.

Annual Report as a marketing tool: The Library's Annual Report can be one of any institution's most effective promotional mediums. They are a means of not only informing our public of our activities but also of proposing what we mean to do. Telling the world what you are doing can be as important in creating and maintaining an image, as anything you do. Annual Reports are particularly effective when enhanced by statistical analysis summaries and by well prepared charts and graphs. At the RCSI, the Library's Annual Report is normally part of the College's annual report.

However, I also produce it as a separate document with its own cover and I send it out to the academic staff and to colleagues working in other medical libraries. We present our statistics in the form of graphs showing the key indicators of library activity. What I am trying to do with this is to emphasise the Library's value to the College, which extends far beyond the funds spent on it.

Exhibitions: Exhibitions are another important marketing tool for medical school libraries and, in conjunction with the Department of the History of Medicine, we have organised quite a number of exhibitions of material held in the Library. Part of the fun of exhibitions is the opening reception and this can be important in terms of marketing the Library. Often as a direct result of these pleasant gatherings, people offer collections to the Library or new sponsors come forward. Goodwill is generated towards the Library as a result of these exhibitions.

Friends of the Library groups: Support groups such as a Friends of the Library Group are good promoters of any Library. We had a very active Friends of the Library Group for almost three years. We held a number of special events which were quite glittering occasions and we managed to raise just under £30,000. This has been written up in Health Libraries Review [11].

Articles and notices in medical and professional journals: I try to market of our Library and its services in the local medical press even though you have no guarantee that they will publish exactly what you have given them. I also contributed articles to both medical and library journals regarding services offered by our library. My publications in professional library journals help keep the name of the College before my peers. This is all marketing our library, and drawing people's attention to our activities.

Major bibliographies: Another important step in marketing the Library is to ensure that your holdings get recorded in the major bibliographies. It is important to do this since it draws attention to the availability of important collections to potential researchers. We have managed to get our early printed books into the *18th century Short Title Catalogue of Printed Books*, an international machine readable catalogue containing bibliographical descriptions of hundreds of thousands of items. Another good idea is to publish the holdings of your special collections or rare books as a separate publication, like that of the library at the Karolinska Institute. I plan to do this for the RCSI Special Collections.

Library newsletters and library surveys: Future plans include the production of a library newsletter and a survey of our readers' needs in relation to the services we offer. Publicising the Library's, and indeed the Library staff's, accomplishments and needs through a Library newsletter is a useful marketing tool. Carrying out Library surveys of our readers to determine their needs - is also good public relations - just to let our readers know we care. We are also working on a strategic plan for the library and this, again, will be a marketing device for us when it is completed.

Conclusion

To conclude, marketing medical school libraries is an integral part of our work as librarians and is not, in my view, a separate activity. At Surgeons, we have concentrated on the marketing of the new technologies, in library tours for new students and in user education programmes. We have used our in house library publications as marketing devices, and we are paying particular attention to the packaging of information. I also believe the annual report is a very important marketing tool. We are committed, too, to the holding of exhibitions as a good public relations exercise for the Library. I hope to continue to write for professional journals about the library's activities. Our aim in the RCSI Library all the time is to improve our services to our readers, in an atmosphere and surroundings conducive to study and research.

References

1. Teuton, L.B. Marketing the College library. *College and Research Library News*, Dec 1990, 1073-1074.
2. Smith, G. and J. Saker. Developing marketing strategy in the Not-for-Profit sector. *Library Management* 1992, **13**(4), 6-21
3. Weingand, D.E. Marketing/Planning Library and Information Services, Littleton, Colorado: Libraries Unlimited, 1987

4. McCarthy, E.J. Basic Marketing: a managerial approach. 6th ed. R.D. Irwin, Homewood, Ill, 1978
5. Leeburger, B. Promoting and marketing the library, rev. ed. Boston, Mass.: G.K. Hall, 1989.
6. McCarthy, G. Promoting the in-house library. *ASLIB Proceedings*, 1992, **44 (7/8)**, 289-293
7. Leerburger, B. Marketing academic and special libraries. In: Issues in Library Management. London: Knowledge Industry Publications, 1989
8. Jones, T. Online to customer care. *Aslib Information* , 1991,**19 (2)**, 50-51
9. McKenna, Regis. Marketing is everywhere. *Harvard Business Review*, 1991, **69 (1)**, 65-79
10 Brauwens, M. Corporate library networks: an idea whose time has come. *The Internet Business Journal* **1 (1)**), p.25
11 Doran, B. Fund raising for libraries: a case study. *Health Libraries Review* 1990; **7**, 1-7.

FORMATION ET ACCOMPAGNEMENT DU CHANGEMENT: le cas de la bibliothèque de l'Institut Pasteur de Paris

Corinne Verry-Jolivet, Institut Pasteur, 25 rue du Docteur Roux, 75724 Paris CEDEX 15, France

1 - Processus de modernisation

La bibliothèque de l'Institut Pasteur est située à Paris sur un campus de 2500 personnes, comprenant 10 départements de recherches (180 unités de recherche), un hôpital, un centre d'enseignement, un service d'archives, une bibliothèque centrale... Cette bibliothèque est ancienne, et hébergée encore dans les bâtiments historiques de l'Institut, près des appartements de Louis Pasteur transformés en musée. Cette situation, depuis quelques années, empêche toute évolution réelle de la bibliothèque : locaux mal adaptés et saturés, équipement obsolète, accès difficile, dispersion des collections. De plus, elle a accumulé des retards importants, dont la Direction a pris conscience ; aussi a-t'il été décidé de déménager complètement la bibliothèque dans un nouveau bâtiment, dont la construction s'achève. Ce déménagement commence mi-août. Il amènera de nombreux changements et améliorations - rendus nécessaires - dans l'accès aux collections, les services documentaires, la qualité des prestations, l'extension des horaires d'ouverture, etc.

Les dysfonctionnements constatés ont été mis à plat lors de la phase de projet de cette nouvelle bibliothèque. Ils sont de plusieurs ordres, et nous nous attelons depuis 3 ans à les réduire :

- inadéquation entre l'aménagement des locaux et les besoins des utilisateurs. (Ceux-ci sont aux trois quarts les chercheurs de l'Institut Pasteur, les stagiaires, les techniciens, les médecins de l'hôpital ; et le quart restant les chercheurs extérieurs, documentalistes d'organismes de recherche ou de sociétés pharmaceutiques, des étudiants en thèse, etc.)
- insuffisance dans l'offre de "produits" et dans les moyens d'accès à l'information
- absence d'un espace réservé à l'ACCUEIL, qui ne permettait pas au personnel au contact des utilisateurs de séparer leur rôle opérationnel (travail interne, traitement des documents, rangements, etc.) de leur rôle relationnel, ni de rendre les services attendus par les utilisateurs.
- une hétérogénéité du personnel, tant au niveau de l'ancienneté que de la qualification (une équipe longtemps resteinte, peu qualifiée, et essentiellement formée sur le tas).
- un état d'esprit, bien que fortement attaché à l'institution et à la dimension culturelle et scientifique de la bibliothèque, peu orientée vers les notions de service.

2 - Etat actuel de la bibliothèque

Le développement engagé depuis 3 ans s'est traduit par des modifications de structure qui *Préparent* le changement:

- informatisation
- remise à niveau des collections (très lacunaires dans les monographies et références)
- recrutements de personnel qualifié
- extension des horaires d'ouverture
- réorganisation des collections (accès, plan de classement, etc.)
- création de nouveaux services (prêt, interrogation de bases de données sur CD-ROM, formation des utilisateurs, accès au catalogue en ligne, utilisation du réseau INTERNET, etc.)

3 - Formation et accompagnement du changement

Compte tenu de ce contexte favorable, il a paru intéressant d'intervenir sur plusieurs fronts en matière De *Formation Du Personnel*:

- recensement des besoins individuels
- mise à jour des connaissances techniques, adapté à chaque niveau de compétence
- plan de formation sur 3 ans

Nous avons dû partir du constat que le personnel n'avait jusque-là bénéficié de quasiment aucune formation, faute d'objectifs plus que de moyens ; faute d'un projet réel pour la bibliothèque ; et par crainte d'investir en formation pour un personnel partant d'assez bas.

A) Mise en place d'une formation "sur-mesure" : accueil-communication-service aux usagers. Il a paru surtout intéressant de mettre l'accent sur une formation collective de toute l'équipe orientée vers le *Service Aux Usagers* et principalement sur la *Notion D'accueil*, notion jusque-là plutôt étrangère à la "culture" de la bibliothèque. Le principal changement dans le nouveau bâtiment sera le mode D'*acces* à l'information, et l'accueil, les renseignements, la qualité du service au lecteur, en seront forcément le *Pivot*. Il fallait donc dès le départ agir sur ce front-là et créer de toutes pièces une *Fonction-Accueil* qui n'existait pas. Un des objectisf sous-jacents était d'obtenir une meilleure *Cohesion De L'equipe* et, en matière d'accueil, des *Methodes De Travail Communes Et Partagees*. A défaut, le risque était celui d'une monopolisation de la fonction-accueil par certaines personnes. Il fallait donc opérer une rotation du personnel sur les postes d'accueil, en faire une fonction commune à tous les personnels (au même titre que les fonctions bibliothéconomiques de traitement du document, fonctions transversales partagées par l'ensemble des bibliothécaires, même si chacun garde une responsabilité particulière sur une fonction donnée).Il s'agissait de faire de tous les personnels des *Facilitateurs* d'accès à l'information.

Pour gagner cette opération, il fallait monter un formation sur mesure, e, consultyant des sociétés spécialisées, en collaboration étroite avec le service formation de la Direction des Ressources Humaines, consciente des enjeux liés à la fonction documentaire à l'Institut pasteur. Les éléments principaux du cahier des charges ont été :

- les notions de base à intégrer (communication, service, clientèles, etc.)
- la spécificité de l'accueil en bibliothèque
- le contexte de développement futur de la bibliothèque
- la fonction accueil
- la cohésion de l'équipe autour de "valeurs partagées"

B) Programme de la formation. Il se déroule en 4 modules :

- Eléments de marketing des services
- Communication
- Fonction accueil
- Synthèse et bilan

Les participants ont bien intégré les concepts de marketing du service et ont été sensibilisés au fait que la qualité du service dépend d'eux, et doit être le fruit d'un effort permanent résolument tourné vers l'utilisateur. En matière de communication, ils ont reconnu avoir obtenu des gains, et la formation a été un terrain privilégié de prise de parole et d'échanges, tout en faisant ressortir les clivages existants au sein de l'équipe. Un travail de fond a été mené parallèlement à une analyse en situation réelle avec l'animatrice, qui enchaîne avec la partie "fonction-accueil", centrale et plus concrète, et qui s'appuie sur les acquis des 2 premiers modules. Le programme complet comporte au total 10 journées de formation, alternativement en groupe complet ou en 1/2 groupe, à raison d'une session tous les 2 mois, entrecoupées de journées de suivi.

4 - Conclusion

L'accueil est une fonction partagée par tous les membres de l'équipe. Nous l'organisons de façon à équilibrer les niveaux de compétence représentées pendant les permanences à l'accueil. (Par exemple, il est nécessaire d'avoir toujours quelqu'un capable d'assurer le service de recherche bibliographique sur MEDLINE ou d'autres bases, d'orienter les utilisateurs vers d'autres sources documentaires, de répondre à une demande pointue, etc.) Il est alors évident que la formation est une aide pour acquérir une pratique commune, mais aussi relever les niveaux de compétence et les rendre complémentaires. Néanmoins ce problème de la formation n'est pas simple : il touche à des questions de valorisation de carrière pour les personnes formées. Ce point est d'autant plus sensible dans une structure scientifique comme la nôtre où les niveaux de compétences sont élevés, et où la fonction documentaire demande une pratique et des connaissances approfondies des domaines traités.

La formation vise principalement à aider le personnel à participer à l'évolution des services rendus aux utilisateurs de la bibliothèque ; elle vise aussi à accompagner les changements successifs et aider le personnel à s'adapter à des méthodes de travail nouvelles. Mais il est bien évident que cette formation n'est pas une fin en soi. Elle ne se suffit pas à elle-même et ne résoudra pas tous les problèmes. Elle me semble en revanche être un excellent soutien à toutes les autres formations. Elle ne peut en effet que soutenir un plan de formation global visant à améliorer la qualification professionnelle et technique dans ce contexte de changement, surtout dans des domaines aussi évolutifs que la biologie et la médecine à un haut niveau de recherche.

PERCEPTIONS OF QUALITY AND THE USE OF QUALITY INDICATORS
a survey of health libraries in the Trent Regional Health Authority, England

John R Clark, Tutor Librarian, Retford, Nottinghamshire, England

Abstract
The factors that service users use to evaluate service quality are considered. The findings of a survey into the collection and use of data on quality in health libraries in the Trent Regional Health Authority's geographical area are reported.

Introduction
This paper will examine definitions of quality used in the management literature and assess their application to services. It will examine the work of Parasuraman et al and their five categories that constitute their "*service quality determinants*". The way in which consumer's expectations of services are formed and how they are used to evaluate those services will be examined. It will then report the findings of a survey in libraries in the Trent Regional Health Authority (RHA) into the collection and use of data on quality and their relationship to the five categories. Methodological issues will not be addressed due to lack of space.

Quality, Some Definitions
Definitions of quality have tended to be linked to manufactured goods. These range from: "*Fitness for purpose*" *(Juran)* "Zero *defects*", "*Conformance to requirements*" *(Crosby)* and "*No failures*" *(Garvin)* "*Meeting customer specifications or needs*" *(De Souza).* Even with manufactured goods the precision of these definitions can be misleading. What is precisely meant by "*Fitness for purpose*"? The use of standards is put forward as one possible way of defining that fitness. It is not foolproof. Ishikawa reported that the newsprint produced by the paper mill that he managed passed all published standards. Unfortunately it kept snapping, when in use. This caused considerable problems to the production of his customers' newspapers. Such problems of definition are minor compared with defining quality in service operations. Most services are consumed as soon as they are produced. (De Souza) This makes measurement and quality control difficult. Definitions of service quality have tended to be even less concrete than those for products. They have tended to be considered from two directions:

> Responding to customer's expectations; " *Meeting customer requirements and expectations*" *(Allyne et al) matching* "*customer expectations with actual performance*" *(Parasuraman et al)* "*Meeting customer's expectations*" *(Price)*

> Management's attempts to ensure consistency of service; "*Controlling the variability of the service produced*" *(Allyne)*, "*Service will be dispensed with no customer being favoured or disfavoured over others*" *(Mills).*

De Souza voiced much of management's frustration over the control of service quality by suggesting that "*What is not measured will not be managed.*"

Service Quality Determinants
Parasuraman et al conducted a series of interviews with customers of services about what they perceived to be the key attributes of quality in those services. They found that the attributes could all be included in the following areas:

Tangibles;	Physical facilities and equipment,
Reliability;	Ability to perform the promised service dependably and accurately,
Responsiveness;	Willingness to help customers and provide prompt service,
Assurance;	Knowledge and courtesy of employees and their ability to inspire trust and confidence,
Empathy;	Caring individualised attention the organisation provides to the customers.

These categories provide a way of breaking down the different aspects of a service to assess where performance is good and where more attention is required.

Customer's Expectations of Services

These are formed by publicity, advertising, their own or their friends' previous experiences of the service or similar services and the service's image. Much of a service is hidden from the customer. eg. How can a reader know what you have done to obtain an inter-library loan? This does not prevent the customer inferring "facts" about the hidden parts of the service from the visible parts. eg. a Swissair executive claimed that "*the customer judges how well our engines are maintained by the coffee stains on the flip down tray*" *(De Souza)*. The customer then makes value judgements on how well the (perceived) service received matches expectations (no matter how unrealistic those are.)

The Collection of Data on Library Service Quality

All health libraries in the Trent RHA were surveyed to discover what data was collected on quality issues and performance indicators (PI's). Van Loo has covered the issue of PI's, so they will not be considered here. The 25 (75%) libraries' responses were categorised using Parasuraman et al's categories. Only 30% of the responding libraries collected data on quality standards, compared with 44% collecting PI's. 38% of the data related to tangibles, 36% to reliability, 17% to assurance, 9% to empathy and none to responsiveness. Only 4 libraries used user surveys to assess the quality of their service. Comments from a number of libraries suggested that the data was not used as the basis for any report to management.

Discussion

Data that is easy to collect seems to form the bulk of the quality measures. This usually relates to tangibles and reliability. Responsiveness, which might be expected to be a major feature of an information service, is simply not measured. It is hard to believe that it is not an important issue in providing a quality library service. Failure to collect and report this data means that there is a missed opportunity to demonstrate that meaningful quality measures are being used to assess and audit library services. In a time of cutbacks and change towards a manager led health service, such a lack of information and evidence that a service is delivering a quality service could have serious implications for its future funding and survival.

Recommendations

Data on PI's and quality standards should be routinely collected. Raw data should be interpreted and used as the basis of reports to the body responsible for managing the library.

The use of quality standards and the information gathered should be used as the basis for agreed change and improvements in the service.

The reporting timetable should fit in with the timetable for budget setting so that planned changes can at least have a chance of attracting funding, where necessary.

Where possible the librarian should produce a widely circulated annual report, including information on quality issues and measures.

Bibliography

ALLEYNE, A et al (1985) Controlling Service Quality, Business Quarterly, Vol 50 (Winter) P. 62-7

CROSBY, P. B. (1979) Quality is Free :the Art of Making Quality Certain, New York, New American Library

DE SOUZA, G. (1989) Now Service Businesses Must Manage Quality, Jnl of Business Strategy, Vol 10 (May/June) P. 21-5

GARVIN, D. A. (1983) Quality on the Line, Harvard Business Review Vol 61 (Sept-Oct) P. 588-601

ISHIKAWA, K. (1985) What is Total Quality Control? The Japanese Way, Englewood Cliffs, Prentice

JURAN, J.M. (1988) Juran on Planning for Quality, London, Collier

MILLS, P.K. (1990) On the Quality of Services in Encounters Jnl of Business Research, Vol 20 P. 31-41

PARASURAMAN, A et al (1985) A Conceptual Model of service Quality and its Implications for Future Research, Jnl of Marketing, Vol 49 (Fall) P. 41-50

PRICE, D.(Ed) (1989) Gower Handbook of Quality Management, Aldershot, Gower

VAN LOO, J. (1990) Performance Indicators for the Health Care Library : the Macro Dimension in TAYLOR, M.H. & WILSON, T. Q.A. Quality Assurance in Libraries ,London, Library Association

TENDERING FOR PERIODICALS SUPPLY: Experiences from the United Medical and Dental School

John van Loo, Librarian, UMDS, Medical Library, St Thomas's Hospital, London SE1 7EH, UK

Abstract
The United Medical and Dental School is a single faculty school of the University of London. In student terms it is the largest medical school in the United Kingdom with 1500 undergraduate and 300 postgraduate students. The Library Services have a periodicals budget, in 1994, of £230,000. The library takes c.900 subscriptions and runs two medical libraries and two specialist dental and dermatology libraries. This paper will deal primarily with the financial aspects of the tendering process, looking at why the library went to tender, the contents of the tender specification, the outcomes of the tender and some general conclusions.

Why Tender?
There were three specific reasons for tendering. Firstly, the Library Service underwent an 'Internal Audit Review' early in 1993, which concluded, with or without a proper understanding of the journals market, that the library must place their journal subscriptions out to tender. Secondly, the Medical School Finance Department wished to explore the option of phased payments to improve its cash flow. The Librarian was advised that any early payment discount could be matched by a better return on investment by the School of the remaining balances. Thirdly, it was considered good management practice to 'test the market' and obtain information on a range of subscription agents' services and financial deals.

Tender Specification
There had been some activity in periodicals tendering in the UK and the library obtained specifications from two library consortia[1]. Its own specification was based on these and consisted of five sections.

1. Background information about the library; size of collection, number of sites, automated system, period of contact (3 years), complete list of all titles.
2. Financial requirements; a quotation was requested for percentage discount (or handling charge) based on publishers' list prices, and an itemised list of all titles indicating publishers' price and for non-UK titles foreign currency price, exchange rate and sterling price. The policy on invoicing for 'not-yet-known' prices was requested. Finally quotations for invoicing on an early payment and phased payment process were requested.
3. Service requirements: minimum service standards for handling of orders, claims, cancellations and other communications were stated (48 hour urgent action, 5 day action others, acknowledgement within 10 days), agents were also asked to identify what support services they offered with regard to new title alerts, notification of price, frequency and title changes, provision of stationery and support with taking on a new contract.
4. Management reports; agents were asked to confirm that analysis by site, subject codes, price ranking and three year historical price survey could be provided.
5. Value Added Services: finally agents were asked to provide information on electronic table of contents page services, automated serials management systems, online access to agent's databases, missing issue collections and any publications produced.

This specification was then circulated to six subscriptions agents with a request to tender for the supply of journals to UMDS. The process was handled by our Finance Department, and was therefore a formal process seen as a 'final offer', ie: there would be no post tender negotiation. The quotation was in the form of a written document rather than oral presentation.

Outcome of the Tender Process

As previously stated, the major concern of this paper is the financial aspect of tendering, but some analysis of the service differences is appropriate. The primary conclusion is that there is very little difference between what agents offer except in the quality of service, which can really only be assessed in action, and not in a tender response. Until comparative evaluations are made of agents' services within a research context, selection will be based on discount levels, personal relationships between librarian and agent, and of course, historical inertia. Some minor differences were noted in how supplementary charges were dealt with, methods of notifying new titles and title changes, the scale of missing issue collections and supply of back runs, and whether the agent offered a named contact in a Medical Division. As CASIAS services develop, this may add another factor in the selection criteria. With regard to phased payments, only three agents were able to negotiate on this.

Discounts (and handling charges) are commercially confidential, so will not be revealed. It can be stated, though, that significant discounts are available if the right commercial conditions prevail. Four of the six agents were able to offer discounts. The subscription market place does appear to be becoming more competitive, the number of agents has reduced and we now have the 'gang of four' chasing a reducing market. It may well be in the interests of networks to develop co-operative purchasing arrangements in order to secure improved deals through volume business.

Fig I Single Line Prices

AGENT	COST	TITLES
A	£152,444	698
B	£176,131	692
C	£185,877*	863
D	£204,612	795
E	£241,602	867
F	£251,208**	854

My major comments about tendering are concerned with the use of the 'Single Line Price' and the disparity in publishers prices quoted by agents. A single line price for each tender was provided by the six agents, as follows (Fig I). The large difference between the most expensive' and the 'cheapest' is immediately apparent. It took a considerable time to unravel this. The first reason was that each Agent quoted for a different number of titles. Two agents did not quote for the second of our c.150 duplicate titles, and each agent had a number of titles which were not on their database. Only three of the Agents listed the titles they had not quoted for! Two agents included their discount/handling charge in the bottom line price, the others did not and finally there were a variety of exchange rates used for foreign currency titles. A sample of 24 US titles was taken from five of the Agents to assess the impact of foreign exchange rates (Fig II), which indicated that there was a 25% range in prices, which exactly matched the range in the exchange rates used. There were also minor difference in US $ publisher prices.

Fig II SAMPLE OF 24 US JOURNALS

AGENT	£PRICE	$EXCHANGE	$PRICE
A	4212	1.92	8088
B	5545	1.47	8151
C	4444	1.82	8089
D	4284	1.90	8139
E	5594	1.44	8041
Range	25%	25%	1.3%

A sample of 55 UK titles (from five of the Agents quotations) was taken to identify any anomalies in listing of UK publishers' prices. Of the 55 titles, 9 (16%) had at least one Agent quoting a different price. Of the 275 individual prices, 20 (7%) were different from the norm. This may be caused by quoting the previous year's price, excluding postage charges where applicable, or clerical error. In any case, libraries should be aware that there is a potential problem here.

Conclusions

Firstly, it must be stated that a Tender does not necessarily produce an answer. The highest discount may not mean the best service. Qualitative assessments of service, the potential cost of transferring records and personal recommendations must all be sought. The major conclusions from undertaking the tender process were:

a) Variable response to tender: not all of the specifications could be fulfilled, only three agents offered phased payments, only two agents presented data on foreign titles as requested, only one agent stated policy on "not yet known" prices.

b) Confusing financial data: the single line price is an unhelpful measure for comparison. The only, and best, measure for financial comparison is a single discount/handling charge to be levied on publishers' list prices for a 'package' of journals.

c) Competitive market place: the bargaining power of the librarian, especially if volume business is created by co-operative purchase, may be marginally increasing and therefore improved financial deals are possible. It needs to be understood though that there are implications in moving away from the professional relationship between librarian and agent (working as partners in the information communication chain) to a Customer-supplier relationship where a contract is the defining factor[2] .

d) Role of the Agent: Agents are looking to redefine their role (in order to survive in a decreasing market!) as an article supply rather than journal supply business. All the major suppliers are moving into electronic contents page and document delivery service. In addition there is an opportunity for Agents to act as 'one stop shops' and supply <u>all</u> materials to libraries (CD's, official publications, books, newspapers) as a consolidation service, thereby receiving, processing, labelling, delivery and even shelving (on a daily basis). Selection for journals supply could therefore be an aspect of a much larger and more complex portfolio of services provided by the Agent.

e) Further research: there is very little published evaluation of agents' services, it is recommended that research is required into supply problems, claims responses, speed of acknowledgement of communications, benefits of named contacts and finally criteria based comparisons of CASIAS services.

References

1. Queen's University of Belfast and University of Ulster (jointly) and the Agricultural and Food Research Council.
2. Managing Acquisitions and Vendor Relations Miller, HS Neal-Schuman Publishers, 1992.

HEALTH POLICY, STRATEGIC DEVELOPMENT & INFORMATION: towards a new partnership

S M Nayee,South Thames RHA, 40 Eastbourne Terrace, London W2 3QR, UK

The World Health Oranisation in 1985 formulated a strategy which clearly defined targets for the promotion of "Health for all by the year 2000". Its aims were to increase life expectancy and reduce premature death around the world. Following this lead, the U.K. Government in 1992 launched the new "Health of the Nation" strategy nation-wide. The lead role in this new initiative was given to the National Health Service. Five initial key areas for action were selected in which it was thought that substantial (and measurable) improvements in health could be achieved. These are coronary heart disease and stroke, cancers, mental illness, HIV/AIDS and sexual health, and accidents. Each of these areas represent major causes of premature death or avoidable ill-health in the U.K. They are also costly.

The importance of active partnerships between the many organisations and individuals who can come together to help improve health ("healthy alliances") was highlighted. These include Government departments, local authorities, voluntary organisations, employers, the media and particularly health professionals of all kinds. The development of health policies and strategies must be based on sound scientific research. The NHS Research and Development strategy, launched in 1991, reflected the priorities of the health strategy. Information about health outcomes, service and treatment effectiveness was acknowledged to be partial or incomplete. Work is now underway nationally to address this through such initiatives as the Cochrane Collaboration and NHS Centre for Reviews and Dissemination.

The reforms of the National Health Service set in motion in 1991 by the Government white paper "Working for Patients" had already set the scene for major changes in the way that health services in Britain are managed and delivered. Health authorities ("purchasers") assess the health needs of their residents and develop health strategies to meet those needs. They must ensure through contracts with local "providers" that the most relevant and cost-effective services are purchased for their populations. The need for robust information about the health status of local populations and for monitoring the effective delivery of healthcare has drawn attention to the hitherto partial and incomplete nature of information which is routinely available. Government attention has focussed recently on better use of the NHS "knowledge base" as one of the key "stepping stones" for purchasing.

Focus Groups

Regional Health Authorities were given the lead in ensuring that national objectives and targets were achieved locally. A Forum for the development of health strategy regionally was already in existance in the South West Thames Regional Health Authority under the leadership of the Director of Public Health. Work had already begun on producing regional health strategies in the key areas of mental heatlh, sexual health, and heart health. New "Focus Groups" were established in the other two key areas (cancers and accidents), and two additional areas (child health and disability). The groups were set up as working groups, establishing and maintaining links between district health authorities and region, identifying and sharing information and good practice and acting as a resource for local groups in target setting for health gain. The membership of the groups reflected a commitment to region-wide and multi-disciplinary working, with high-level managerial and health professional input, as well as invited local representatives from other sectors (voluntary groups, local authority, social services). Those with known special expertise were invited to attend.

Library Links

A new library was established within the SWT Regional Health Authority Library in 1992. It has developed into a unique resource for health management, serving primarily the needs of the RHQ. However, the Librarian also has a region-wide role within the Regional Library Service for the development of library services to purchasing authorities (primarily DHAs). The principle of district-wide NHS library services in Great Britain is well established, though development has been inconsistent. In practice, libraries have largely developed within hospital, or provider settings, and are primarily perceived as educational and practical resources for clinicians. Health Service managers have little history of library use, or knowledge and understanding of the skills and resources involved. The establishment of a new library within the Regional Health Authority itself provided an opportunity for changing attitudes. The Department of Health DHA Project had focussed attention in 1991 on the many different types of information which can help purchasers in their new role in assessing the needs of their population and evaluating options for change. Although attention was drawn to the potential of library skills and resources in this respect, progress was slow.

The Director of Library Services for the region had already established a good working relationship with the Regional Director of Public Health, and was a member of the Needs Forum. As the regional Focus Groups were forming, reporting to the Needs Forum, the suggestion was put forward and accepted that each Focus Group should have a librarian as a member. The RHA Librarian, as a member of the Needs Forum, would coordinate their work. Volunteer professional librarians from within the Regional Library Service were found, overcoming initial hesitation about their lack of experience regarding health strategy work. In fact, the policy behind the setting up of the Focus Groups was at a very early stage of development, and a good deal of confusion was in evidence about their role. It was an illuminating experience for librarians to find that not only did they not know quite why they were there, but no-one else did either!

Progress within each of the Focus Groups was different, reflecting the remit which each group perceived itself to have, and the collective experience of its members. According to their own personality and skills, librarians were able to make direct contributions to the information gathering and analysis which each group undertook in its special subject area. This included databases of key documents, contacts or good practice, alerting services and literature searching.

The experience of this initative for librarians has had positive and sometimes unexpected results:-

1. The contribution of librarians in supporting Health of the Nation development work was recognised and apprectiated by the Regional Director of Public Health and other senior managers
2. Librarians experienced working as part of strategic development teams in health management
3. There was an opportunity for librarians to learn directly about policy development in key areas
4. Librarians were able to contribute possible solutions to a variety of information problems
5. Libraries and professional skills were promoted on a wider scale and in a different light
6. Experience was gained in managing change

Unique opportunities were created, through close working relationships with managers, which may not arise in a library setting. Librarians brought information skills into the picture and offered support in ways which managers would not necessarily have thought of and would therefore not have sought Two initiatives, arising directly from the close involvement of librarians with policy-makers **as the policy was developing,** illustrate this in particular.

Healthguide

The dissemination of policy and other information within the NHS has traditionally consisted of the "cascading down" of paper-based documents via letters normally addressed to the chief executives of health authorities or other organisations within it. Real understanding of how effective dissemination may be achieved, particularly through the use of modern technology, still eludes the service. The SWT Healthguide Compendium, the "brainchild" of the Regional Director of Public Health, was intended to be a "readily available accessible" source of information for district health authorities and their colleagues who were working on various aspects of health strategy for their local populations. It would bring together health strategy papers issued by South West Thames, but it would also list "resource documents" such as health policy papers issued by other health authorities, epidemiologically based needs assessments, service reviews and reports. It would contain references to relevant research published in the literature. The RHA Librarian's participation in the project ensured that each document within the Compendium was individually and permanently accessible via the Regional Library Service database. An overview of new national resources such as the Outcomes Database in Leeds was included in the Compendium.

Health of the Nation Database

Following the involvement of the RHA Librarian with a heart health data working group, a pilot project was funded by a new Health Promotion Unit, the Jocelyn Chamberlain Unit. A database was set up to facilitate information sharing about local project work aimed at promoting health. It is now available in all SWT healthcare libraries, and within the Jocelyn Chamberlain Unit itself. The database is intended as a small contribution towards the national NHS initiative on Research and Development. We have recently produced a newsletter which we hope will inform a wider audience about our project, and help to encourage others to contribute information. A trainee project is at present underway to begin to examine the potential for an "integrated resources database" which would bring together the documents, project and other information which the Regional Library Service collectively holds.

Recent major changes in the structure of the NHS at regional level have had an impact on the developments described in this paper. The work of Focus Groups has ceased, and the Health Guide Compendium process has been discontinued. However, the experience gained by librarians in working with managers on health strategy development region-wide still informs our work. Accountability for the regional "knowledge base" is at the moment assured via the Library Service database. The importance of the region-wide library network has never been greater. A tension now exists however with the forthcoming demise of NHS regions in 1996. The Regional Library Service database, with its unique collection of regional grey literature has a significant contribution to make to "knowledge-based" working. Our ultimate goal must be to ensure that an integrated network of library information resources is at the heart of the IM & T and research infrastructure of the NHS into the next century.

DESIGNING A LIBRARY: the Dream of Every Librarian

Rita ZANGANI, Scientific Library, Glaxo S.p.A. - Via Fleming 2 - 37100 VERONA, Italy.

1. Introduction

Every librarian, at least once in his or her professional life, has to design a new library. This is certainly a great challenge, in meeting which the librarian can make full use of all his or her professional skill and creativity. There are many commercially available manuals, offering useful indications about arrangement of spaces, suitable distances between shelves and model libraries to be taken as examples. However, it is quite difficult to find books or papers providing detailed illustration of the entire design process and of the analytical techniques which can prove useful in the overall planning of a library The building of the new Research Centre at Glaxo S.p.A. gave me the opportunity to design the present facility, a specialised biomedical library which constitutes a dynamic structure within Glaxo, fulfilling demand for documentation both within the Company and among the medical community.

2. Materials and Methods

The fundamental requirement was therefore to guarantee that the efficiency of the future library would be based on its capacity to become an open system, offering a range of services, tailoring its efforts to clients' needs and adapting to the probable changes and increases in their requirements. The stages in the implementation of the model of library envisaged are as follows:

i) Redefinition of functions and functional policies
ii) Analysis of users' requirements
iii) Visits to Italian and European libraries
iv) Analysis of collections and their use, to rationalise space allocation
v) Study of the areas of the Library
vi) Choice of furniture and fittings.

3. Description of the Stages in the Design Process

Redefinition of functions and functional policies When planning a new library, this first point is of considerable strategic importance, since definition of functional policies will provide the basis for the type of stucture to be implemented. It is therefore essential to incorporate these requirements in a document, to be approved by the managers whose departments will be most directly involved in using the library's services. In terms of the Library at Glaxo, the following functions and functional policies were approved:

Functions:
- acquire, conserve and manage all scientific and technical material (books and audiovisual materials) needed as documentary support throughout the Company;
- acquire, handle and distribute all scientific and technical periodicals useful for keeping in-house users abreast of the latest developments;
- produce - or obtain from other libraries, in Italy or abroad - photocopies of scientific publications, for both in-house researchers and the medical community.

Functional policies:
- creative implementation of the above functions, planning activities to integrate the scientific - and Company - objectives pursued by the various Directorates;
- keen awareness of the needs of the main client, the researcher, who provides a fundamental contribution to the development of research;
- active rôle as a qualified partner of the user in the search for relevant information;
- commitment to encouraging and facilitating the use of the Library's documents and services;
- optimisation of the cost/benefit ratio throughout the acquisition of documentary material;
- willingness to receive requests from the local and national scientific community.

Analysis of users' requirements The library must be geared towards the client's needs - the client has documentation problems, and the library must solve them. Services must therefore be based on a perfect understanding of users' requirements and tailored to meet these needs. To ensure this, a survey was carried out. This consisted of interviews with users from the Directorates most involved. Interviewees were asked two types of question:

those requiring an answer to be chosen from a number of alternatives, to confirm the librarian's basic idea of the type of library required;
- those to be answered as the user wanted, from his/her specific perspective.

All responses were analysed and subdivided by Directorate, so that needs could be highlighted and appropriate solutions identified.

Visits to libraries Planning of the new Library included visits to European biomedical libraries. The purpose of these visits was to examine: (i) organisation, (ii) archiving criteria, and (iii) new technology, with a view to possible application in our Library The following libraries were visited: WHO Library, Geneva, Library of the Faculty of Medicine, University of Geneva, Smith, Kline and French Library at Welwyn, GGR Library, Greenford. Following these visits, a report was drafted. For each library, the three parameters listed were considered in relation to fulfilment of our needs. This report, as well as confirming that our choices were consistent with those implemented by the most up-to-date facilities, provided stimulating new ideas.

Analysis of collections and their use, to rationalise space allocation Immediate access to information is essential for a library which sets out to guarantee its clients an optimal service. It is therefore important to keep in the Reading Room not only the current year's issues of periodicals received on subscription, but also back numbers for the previous few years. The archive, generally not adjacent to the library (basement, etc.), will be used to store other yearly collections which are less in demand. A sample of 1000 requests for photocopies received from users was analysed, with a view to highlighting the years of major interest. The breakdown was as follows:

- 83% for issues covering the last decade
- 13% covering the decade 1972-82
- 3% spanning the decade 1961-71
- 1% for the 3 previous decades.

On the basis of these data, it was decided to keep scientific periodicals for the last 10 years in the Reading Room - meaning that related space requirements had to be met. The analysis of trends was also useful as a basis on which to evaluate space requirements for the general periodicals archive. In this respect, the major innovation was to identify a number of criteria for the setting up of an archive designed to provide documentation of greatest interest to Company users. For material whose storage could not be justified in cost/benefit terms, it was decided to forward any requests to outside suppliers (B.L.). The criteria for inclusion in the in-house archive were:

- 50 years for high-interest periodicals
- 20 years for medium-interst periodicals
- 5 years for periodicals of limited interest
- local archiving (on user's premises) for extremely specialised periodicals.

Study of the areas of the Library The organisational model for implementation of functional policies relevant to the Library is as follows:

i) reception and information area
ii) area for outside users and for rapid consultation by in-house users
iii) specialised area for Chemistry Directorate
iv) area containing display of periodicals for reading and consultation
v) mediathèque.

Reception and information area: situated immediately inside the main entrance, this is the area which provides the user's first contact with the Library. Queries can be answered, and information provided, on the Library's services and how to use them. It is also here that access by in-house and outside users is controlled.

Area for outside users and for rapid consultation by in-house users: this is a specialised area, meeting documentation requirements of outside users and providing a means of rapid consultation by in-house users. This room houses catalogues and periodicals, books for general consultation and Medline on CD.

Specialised area for Chemistry Directorate: given the importance of chemistry in a pharmaceutical Research Centre for the discovery of new molecules, a specific area has been set aside for chemists. Users can access STN International for searches on the Chemical Abstracts Data Bank. The area also houses a microfilm collection of C.A. and a printed collection of Beilstein, efficiently fulfilling the Chemistry Directorate's requirements in terms of documentation and bibliographical searches.

Area containing display of periodicals for reading and consultation: this is the classic periodical reading room, with collections of scientific periodicals going back over the last 10 years. It is a readily accessible, open area. Periodicals and information bulletins are displayed for ease and convenience of consultation, encouraging and satisfying the scientific "curiosity" of users. This area is divided into two sections: one for display of the most recent issue and archiving of back-numbers for the current year, the other for consultation and archiving of issues for the previous 9 years.

Mediathèque: this innovative area provides facilities for storage and consultation of audiovisual materials produced in house, concerning scientific topics. Video cassettes can be viewed on the spot.

Choice of furniture and fittings Names of suppliers specialising in library furniture and fittings can be found in periodicals specific to librarianship issues. A short list of at least three suppliers should be drawn up, and their catalogues inspected. It is then important to have each supplier included in this short list send sample shelving, so that products can be examined and the final choice made "in situ". This also allows managers of other directorates taking a close interest in the library project to see the shelving. The librarian should obviously "guide" the final choice, reporting and explaining the different suppliers' offers to the management level responsible for the ultimate decision on the library.

4. Conclusions

Since an efficient, intelligently rationalised library is a major resource for any organisation, I have attempted in this short presentation to share with colleagues a professional experience which I found most rewarding and enriching.

MEDICAL SCHOOL LIBRARIES AND EXAMINATION RESULTS

Hugh Brazier, The Mercer Library, Royal College of Surgeons in Ireland, Mercer Street Lower, Dublin 2, Ireland

Abstract
A study of the number of books borrowed from the library by undergraduate medical students showed significant differences between students in different years of the medical course, students from different regions of the world, and male and female students. In the first year of the medical course, students who borrowed most also performed best in their end-of-year examinations, and this association was only partly explained by regional differences. No such association was found among final-year students.

Much has been written in recent years on the changing role of the academic medical library. It is argued that changes in the undergraduate medical curriculum, including the development of problem-based learning and other student-centred methods, give the library an enlarged role in the educational process. We hear a great deal about the need for students to acquire information handling skills, and to learn how to use the range of information systems available in libraries. Such skills are seen as essential to the practice of medicine in the late twentieth century. But what contribution does the medical school library in fact make to medical education? Do students who make good use of the library become better doctors? Do they perform better in their college examinations? In a rapidly changing educational environment it is important to be able to answer such questions. It is also important because of the high cost of maintaining library services. Are medical colleges getting value for money from their libraries?

Surprisingly little has been published on this subject. The considerable literature on factors affecting student performance in examinations contains almost no reference to level of library use as a factor. The library journals, in spite of extensive coverage of fashionable topics such as performance indicators, focus almost entirely on measuring internal library performance, and omit any reference to the performance of the students who use the library. In this study I examine the extent to which undergraduate medical students use the borrowing facilities of their college library, and ask whether there is a relationship between book borrowing and examination performance.

Materials and Methods
The study was undertaken in the Medical School of the Royal College of Surgeons in Ireland. The RCSI Medical School attracts students from all parts of the world, and has 46 nationalities represented among its total of approximately 950 students. The undergraduate medical course is a six-year one. It starts with a pre-medical year in which the students study biology, chemistry and physics, followed by two pre-clinical years and three clinical years. For the first three years (from the pre-medical year to second medical year) the students are based in the College; for the three clinical years (third to fifth medical year) they are based largely in one or more of the College's associated teaching hospitals. Except in fourth medical year (when the students spend much of their time in a number of widely scattered hospitals), all students have ready access to the College's library facilities throughout their course.

To measure levels of library use, I used data generated by the library's URICA integrated library system. I recorded the number of books and other items borrowed by each student. These data count only the first issue of an item to a student, and exclude renewals of items already on loan. Examination scores were obtained from the RCSI Examinations Office. I analysed results from the first and last years' examinations: the end-of-year biology, chemistry and physics results from pre-medical year, and the final medicine and surgery results from the end of fifth medical year (the students' final examination). Data on students' countries of origin were also obtained from the Examinations Office, and each student was assigned to one of four regions (A - D).

Overall borrowing levels were obtained from the two academic years 1992/93 and 1993/94 (n = 1,899). The pre-medical student data used in the analysis were from 1991/92 and 1992/93 (n = 316). The fifth medical year student data were from 1992/93 and 1993/94 (n = 286). The analyses were carried out using the Data Desk statistical package. The factors which predicted number of books borrowed, the effect of number of books borrowed on examination results, and the effect of confounding variables on this relationship were calculated using a general linear models approach. Because number of books borrowed showed a skewed distribution, and its relationship with examination results are curvilinear, a book borrowing score was derived which was the square root of the number of items borrowed. This was normally distributed and associated linearly with examination marks.

Results

The number of items borrowed by a student in an academic year varied widely, from zero to 103. The median number of items borrowed was 6, and one fifth of students (20.4%) borrowed nothing. Figure 1 shows the median number of items borrowed in an academic year by students in each of the six years of the medical course. There was no difference in borrowing level between the pre-clinical and clinical years. Borrowing rose in fourth medical year and fell again in fifth medical year.

FIGURE 1. The median number of items borrowed in an academic year by students in each of the six years of the undergraduate medical course at RCSI. Data from 1992/93 and 1993/94 ($n = 1899$).

A general linear model was used to test for the effects of sex, region and year on borrowing score. There was a significant difference in borrowing level by year of course ($F = 7.5$, $df = 5, 1899$, $p < 0.001$) but Scheffé post-hoc tests showed that this was due to a higher level of borrowing by fourth medical year students; all differences between 4th medical year and other individual years were statistically significant at p _ 0.001, while no other years differed significantly from each other.

Women borrowed more books than men. The median number of books borrowed by female students was eight, while the median for male students was four. The difference in borrowing was statistically significant even when adjusted for the effects of different years and regions ($F = 11.6$, $df = 1, 1899$, $p < 0.001$). Likewise, students from the four regions had different borrowing habits ($F = 56.8$, $df = 3, 1899$, $p < 0.001$).

I examined the relationship between borrowing levels and achievement in two years, pre-medical and fifth medical years. In the pre-medical year, total end-of-year examination marks ranged from 79 to 484, with a median score of 348 marks. Marks were significantly positively related with the number of books borrowed from the library during the year. A regression analysis showed that marks rose 7.9 for each 1-unit increase of book borrowing score (Figure 2); that is, you would expect a difference of about 8 marks between a student borrowing 4 books and one borrowing 9 books, or between students borrowing 16 and 25 books.

FIGURE 2. The relationship between total end-of-year examination mark and library borrowing score (square root of items borrowed) among RCSI pre-medical year students. Data from 1991/92 and 1992/93 ($n = 316$). Total mark increases by 7.9 for each one-unit increase in the borrowing score ($p < 0.001$).

In pre-medical year, borrowing level was significantly related to region, with students from region A borrowing least and students from region D borrowing most ($F = 11.3$, $df = 3, 307$, $p < 0.001$). There was no difference in level of borrowing between men and women when adjusted for differences between regions ($F = 1.8$, $df = 1, 307$, $p = 0.428$) nor was there any evidence of the male-female difference being different in different regions. Because marks differed between students from various regions, the linear model was extended to adjust the effect for regional and sex differences in marks. Adjusting for these reduced the gain in marks for a 1-unit increase in borrowing score to 4.8 marks, but this was still statistically significant ($F = 6.2$, $df = 1, 307$, $p = 0.013$).

In fifth medical year, the pattern was different (Figure 3). There was a slight relationship between borrowing score and marks, but there was no evidence of a significant association between level of student borrowing and examination marks ($F = 1.1$, $df = 1, 272$, $p = 0.303$).

FIGURE 3. The relationship between total end-of-year examination mark and library borrowing score (square root of items borrowed) among RCSI fifth medical year students. Data from 1992/93 and 1993/94 (n = 286). The association is not significant (p = 0.303).

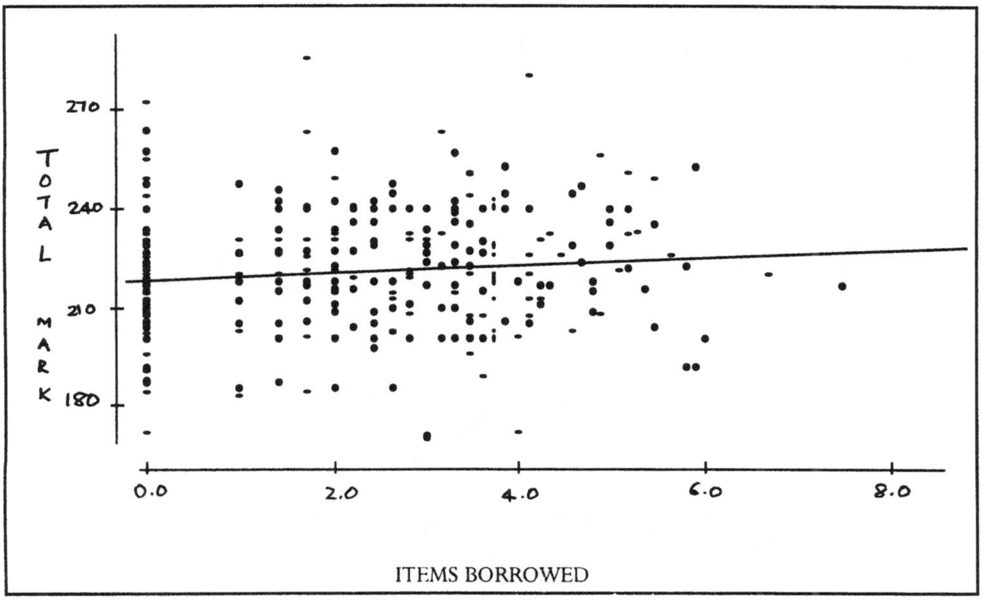

Discussion

The use of number of books borrowed as a proxy for library use is clearly only a first approximation. The present analysis does not take into account appropriateness of books borrowed, nor use of books within the library, nor buying of books by students. Nor does it measure the extent to which students make use of the whole range of other library services. Nevertheless it shows a number of interesting associations. The higher book borrowing score in fourth medical year occurs in spite of the fact that fourth-year students are physically most remote from library facilities, and presumably shows that these students find it worth making an effort to get to the library and borrow books. The number of subjects in which the students are examined is greatest in the fourth medical year (9 subjects, compared with 3-4 in each of the other years), and the higher borrowing score reflects this.

The relationship between examination results and borrowing found in pre-medical year is not surprising, since students from a wide variety of educational backgrounds enter medical school with very different experiences of library use as part of coursework. What is more surprising is that the relationship between borrowing levels and marks is only partly explained by the differences between regions. Within any region, marks go up with increasing levels of book borrowing. This is not necessarily a causal relationship, of course. It could well be that more motivated students borrow more books, rather than that the students who borrow more books learn more.

The relationship between book borrowing and results is not present in fifth medical year. This may be because of the more practical nature of the skills required in final year. It may also be that borrowing levels are simply too crude an index of study to be a useful predictor of performance. This study represents a first step in an investigation of the use made of library facilities by medical students, and of the relationship between level of library use and examination performance. There are many factors affecting students' use of the library, and their examination performance. The analysis carried out so far has only scratched the surface of a subject which deserves considerable further study.

Section 4

The Library in the Learning Environment

DEVELOPING A PASSPORT TO LEARNING RESOURCES FOR NURSES

Margaret Ashcroft, Library and Information Consultant, Capital Planning Information Ltd,52 High St, St Martin's, Stamford, Lincs PE9 2LG, UK

Abstract

This presentation discusses the vision, the process and the reality of developing a "passport", to improve access to library and information services and other essential learning resources for nurses.

The Vision - the needs to be addressed

The needs of nursing students for access to learning resources were researched in a national survey carried out in 1992 [4]. The survey confirmed the inadequacies of many nursing college libraries but also helped to identify the needs (and some examples of ways to solve the problems): the need for strategic planning of learning resource provision, the need for a whole series of management improvements, including increased budget allocations, the integration of learning resource provision with curriculum delivery and organisation structures, and the need for management guidelines to enable all the `key players':- funders, college managers, teachers and those responsible for validating educational delivery and professional standards - to ensure effective learning resource provision.

The English National Board for Nursing, Midwifery and Health Visiting (the ENB) took up that challenge and commissioned a project to draw up Management Guidelines for Library and Information Service provision to nursing professionals [1]. The project involved extensive consultation between all the groups of key players. A series of regional focus groups aimed to achieve a national consensus, to encourage a sense of ownership as opposed to prescriptiveness, and to find co-operative, constructive solutions as to how to manage provision for nursing professionals. Discussion focused on how to remove barriers to access for users, how to promote access and how to manage access cost effectively and efficiently.

The keys to any form of solution were the need to clarify historical `muddles', by reviewing provision in terms of current users' needs and efficient management methods, and the need to replace inaccurate assumptions with clear statements. The key needs which led to the idea of a user's passport were identification and awareness: for learning resource services to identify clearly to their users what is offered and to whom it is available and promote awareness among existing and potential users; and for users to be able to identify themselves and their reason or right of access and to be aware of what services are available to them.

A complete "passport" package would ideally include:

- identification of the holder of the passport at any point of access in a networked group
- a guide to the availability of sources and services of learning resource, library and information providers
- a user's `charter' (a means of informing users of their rights to access)
- a means of channelling users to the appropriate initial point of access
- a means to educate and develop users as independent learners
- a system to monitor the take-up of learning resource services
- a system of recording the individual's use of learning resources services and charge or account to the appropriate budget holder

The result aimed for, with the right balance of components, and with the right supporting systems in place, is empowerment, of not only users but also of service providers.

The Process

The various stages of strategic and operational planning and implementation necessary to the development of a passport were identified and discussed in a report for the British Library Research and Development Department [3]. At all stages there is an implicit requirement for co-operation and negotiation between participants. The development of a users' passport is not a process to be undertaken by one library service in isolation, nor in an organisational environment in which crucial decisions about higher education linkages have not yet been finalised.

Each of the following areas for consideration need to be inter-related and to some extent concurrent.

- Informing and empowering users includes processes necessary to produce at the very minimum a guide or directory of access points. Identifying and comparing what is available can progress to the setting of common standards or at least to agreement of differences. Service objectives and performance measurement can be developed into statements of users' rights, and quality assurance programmes provide opportunities for user participation in policy-making.
- Supporting curriculum delivery implies the processes necessary for consultation between library managers, teachers and students, in developing user education programmes, in ensuring that appropriate management information is used to inform service provision to satisfy curriculum requirements are met - in terms of stock, and services, as well as appropriate user access policies.
- Technology and library automation issues include the processes necessary to ensure compatibility of library systems to enable, at the very least, interchange of users' registration information. Bar code systems, magnetic swipe and smart card technology need to be investigated further to test charging systems, use-monitoring for managers and the facility to provide users with an individual record of library use. Processes will be needed to ensure user feedback on the technology and to ensure that the passport does increase user empowerment rather than become a resource management system.
- Organisational and management issues include the process of strategic planning necessary to decide upon a passport mechanism. Representation and joint commitment of all potential participants is crucial. The development of service level agreements between participants will offer managers opportunities to lead the field in specifying and monitoring, and making more transparent the systems by which libraries operate. Possibilities for recording `personalised' management statistics lead to more detailed costing of services and more realistic budgets?

The Reality

The reality is only a small part of the vision, as yet. The Institute of Health and Community Services at Bournemouth University has produced a passport to learning resources provision for students. Many other institutions undoubtedly have similar guides to services but this example has been chosen to illustrate the practical reality of developing a passport because of its history and its future potential [2]. The "Student Passport to Library Services" comprises a single guide with sections (using a common structure) on the University Library, and on each of the four hospital library services to which students may have access while on clinical placement. The information given is what one would expect of any library guide: hours of opening, study facilities, loans and sanctions policy, request service, reader assistance, special reference collections, library stock, photocopying, opportunities for student feedback and further information about library services.

The passport was launched in early 1994 but is actually the result of common policy-making and agreements dating back to 1980, and liaison and trust which was built up between the separate library services. It was the formalising of that liaison which contributed to the current co-operative and collaborative policies over provision of learning resources that the passport represents. In this case liaison was actually stimulated by many of the changes in the organisational and funding environment which have hindered progress for other colleges of nursing. The amalgamation of nursing colleges, their integration with higher education, the formation of National Health Service Trusts and the development of purchaser/provider relationships have contributed in a positive way to the current co-operative policies on learning resources provision. The change of funding arrangements which developed from the allocation of Project 2000 funding and Working Paper 10 regional training budgets necessitated the development of discussion between the Institute and the hospital library services.

There are many areas still to be tackled in depth. Access policies for health personnel who are not registered students with Bournemouth University need urgent attention, as do policies for students studying away from the `network' libraries. Standards and monitoring across all the services, student charter issues and opportunities for feedback are hardly developed beyond the embryonic stage. Not yet addressed are the relationships between service levels and funding; or all the issues around accounting and cross-charging for service provision: until service providers can account for all costs, funding levels, the real crux of the problem of improving access, cannot improve.

Evaluation of this apparently straightforward and relatively unsophisticated passport must recognise that it has only been possible because of a long history of liaison, that it represents a substantial amount of professional collaborative effort, and that it is only the starting point for formalising other aspects of library service management. What the passport achieves, even as it stands, is a set of very clear statements to students about the services to which they have a right to access.

Conclusion

The concept of co-operation between library services has a long history, and none of the processes or operations discussed here is new; neither has the project developed yet to its full potential. However, the idea of combining processes and operating systems, to develop a "passport" mechanism or package, has been received with great enthusiasm by many service managers and potential users, people who are looking for solutions to access problems.

References

[1] Ashcroft, M: *Management Guidelines for the provision of Library and Information services for Nursing Professionals*; English National Board for Nursing, Midwifery and Health. 1993. £10.00. isbn: 0 946810 51 6

[2] Beard, Jill *Developing Access: towards a passport for learning resources* Unpublished paper presented at an English National Board workshop 24th May 1994

[3] Capital Planning Information: *Developing a passport to learning resources for nurses; [draft] report to the British Library Research and Development Department*. March 1994 [unpublished]

[4] Capital Planning Information: *Library and Information Services to support Project 2000, British Library R&D Report 6088*. CPI. 1992. £19.90. isbn: 0906011 85 X

A FLEXIBLE MODEL FOR INFORMATION SKILLS EDUCATION FOR NURSING STUDENTS

Jacqueline M. Barker, University of Wales College of Medicine, Heath Park, Cardiff, CF4 4XN, Wales

This paper examines the underlying reasons why any information skills course for nursing students needs to be flexible, basing the objectives of such a course on the needs of the participants. The content of such a course offered at the University of Wales College of Medicine is presented in detail along with methods of delivery, timing and ideas for supporting documentation stressing how all of these are designed to be flexible. Finally, methods of evaluation and feedback are discussed.

The Main Library University of Wales College of Medicine (UWCM) is an academic, multidisciplinary library located in a general hospital and offering services to all staff and students of UWCM as well as staff of the local Health Authority. UWCM has a very active Nursing Studies Department offering a wide range of courses and undertaking nursing research programmes. The nursing profession is undergoing major change in its drive for professionalisation. Nursing education is responding to this by increasing specialisation, research and reliance on scientific literature(Tyler and Switzer, 1991).

Any information skills course supporting nursing education must accommodate the full range of nursing specialities, e.g. community health, midwifery, geriatric, psychiatric nursing and so on, as well as the specific level of education being offered. At UWCM the information retrieval course aims to meet the needs of undergraduate, postgraduate (doctoral and non-doctoral), diploma and professional upgrading students. The number of part-time and distance learning courses is increasing dramatically. Many students are more mature, returnees to study with jobs and families as well as courses to complete. Information skills course must meet the needs of these students as well as the traditional full-time undergraduate entering nursing from straight from school. Modern information retrieval is firmly technology based. Each student has an individual combination of experience, expertise and indeed, preference, with regard to libraries and computer technology which must be recognised and accounted for within user education programmes.

Underpinning all of these is the very nature of nursing itself - multidisciplinary and interdisciplinary. Nursing students need a wide range of subject knowledge - biology, psychology, social science, health policy, medicine as well as nursing practice and nursing research. General educational trends have been welcomed and taken up by nursing tutors. The move toward student centred learning with its reliance of research and self-direction satisfies the drive for educational and professional acceptance (O'Brien, Proctor and Walton, 1990). Finally, but certainly not least the amount of information available and the number of potential sources of information has grown considerably in recent years. Effective access to this information is vital to the individual nurse and to the nursing profession as a whole.

Any information skills course must fulfil all of the above criteria. The skills learnt should be source and system independent, transferable and user specific. It should allow each individual student to begin with different needs, background and experience, take an appropriate route through but achieve the same result- lifelong information literacy, confidence and effectiveness. Opinion on how to teach information skills tends to be divided into two schools of thought(King,1987). The first is the conceptual school which emphasises the theory of information retrieval and its educational significance. The other viewpoint is the skills-based school emphasising practical searching, maintaining that modern computer software should dispense with the need to understand the principles(Reichel and Ramey, 1987).The course devised at UWCM aims to draw on the advantages of each of these viewpoints. The conceptual school (giving system independence, transferability, and encouraging critical thinking) is carefully blended with skills based learning (giving practical hands-on expertise, using real searches to increase personal relevance) in order to meet the course objectives listed below:

1. To give students an understanding of the practical importance of text-based (and other) information in the health sciences and in the acquisition and transfer of knowledge.

2. To provide students with the knowledge and skills they need to gain relevant, timely and appropriate information to meet their present and future needs i.e. to be able to select appropriate sources; to understand the principles on which these sources are based in order to make the best possible use of them; to develop the practical skills necessary to extract the information they need from a variety of sources and media; to record and store the information they have found

3. To ensure that students are aware of the systems and services available through UWCM library and are able to use them to their full potential to improve the quality of their academic performance in the short term and their professional competence in the long term.

4. To ensure that students feel confident and comfortable about using these systems.

The course at UWCM is split into four one hour sessions as follows:

Session One. Library Induction.

Library Registration. Form filling

Library Induction. A short talk on basic library services emphasising what can be done rather than what should not be done.

Library tour. A guided tour pointing out main features to enable students to start using the facilities immediately including practical hands-on use of the OPAC.

Session Two. An Introduction to the Literature

Scientific information literature knowledge

Types of literature

Book classification scheme- UWCM OPAC revisited.

Journal based information- its scope and usefulness particularly in relation to nursing

Tools for finding journal information-indexing and abstracting journals. What do they cover? How are they used?

Citations What? How? Styles.

Keeping records

Actual examples of UWCM printed indexing journals.

Session Three Principles of Information Retrieval

Print vs computerised

Which database?

Which medium?

UWCM sources

Searching principles- index terms, tree structures and thesauri

Boolean operators, broadening and narrowing a search

Devising real search strategies using examples

Session Four Practical Workshop

Practical hands-on workshops- small group

Some groups of student receive all four sessions as outlined above(e.g. first year degree students). Others may have sessions one and two amalgamated. This is decided in close liaison with nursing teachers.Subject wise the course is molded to fit the needs of each specific group. All the examples used to demonstrate principles are course specific and in fact frequently the participants own examples are used. While this does increase the burden on the course instructor it does give students a much greater sense of ownership and relevance. Close liaison with nursing studies staff helps to be better prepared. Databases for practical searching are chosen in relation to specific needs although Cumulated Index to Nursing and Allied Health Literature (CINAHL) is usually the first example. Degree level midwifery students may begin with MEDLINE. All the students are actively encouraged to return for more database training on a voluntary basis. Databases currently on offer through UWCM include CINAHL, MEDLINE, ASSIA(Applied Social Science Index and

Abstracts), CLINPSYC, Cochrane Pregnancy and Childbirth Database, Science Citation Index, Social Science Citation Index and EMBASE.Nursing students may not use all of these but it is the experience at UWCM that they use at least two or three. This supports the conceptual core of the course which ensures that information skills are transferable across databases and media.

A variety of teaching methods are employed with large group formal sessions kept to a minimum. Methods include traditional talks, tours, interactive discussion, use of audiovisual aids and video. Great emphasis is placed on a hands-on approach in small groups. One-to-one training is given when necessary and the importance of informal opportunities to reinforce skills is recognised and encouraged. In house documentation prepared to support the course ranges from formal lecture notes through quick reference guides to interactive search strategy sheets. Appropriate timing of information skills courses is probably one of the most important aspects but also one of the most difficult to achieve. Nursing students arrive at UWCM at the same time as hundreds of other students who also require user education courses. Very close liaison with teaching staff is required to match course requirement with information retrieval skills. Library staffing commitment at this time is immense in order to provide student with the necessary skills at the time and point of need. Evaluation of the course takes two forms. Firstly user satisfaction is measured in the short term by the completion of a very simple questionnaire. Users are asked what they think course organisers should STOP, START and CONTINUE including in the course. In the longer term a Student Library User Group provides feedback. More formal evaluation methods are under investigation.

Secondly, user proficiency needs to be measured. User workbooks proved too time consuming to prepare and tend to be rigid in format and content. Certain student groups will this year undertake a course integrated evaluation exercise. They will be require to submit an information log or commentary outlining the steps they take to find information for a particular piece of work, the databases used and search strategies employed. This will be assessed by the User Education Librarian and will represent a proportion of the overall grade for that piece of work. UWCM is currently investigating the possibility of a study to measure the quality of information retrieval as a result of user education (Barker,1992).

References

Barker, J.M. (1993) *End-user education and computerised information retrieval systems in a health care library.* M.Sc. Dissertation. University of Wales, Aberystwyth.

King, D.N. (1987) Creating educational programs in libraries. Introduction and Part 1: Training and education. *Medical Reference Services Quarterly,* **6,** 3, 83-90.

O'Brien, D., Proctor, S. and Walton,G. (1990) Towards a strategy for teaching information skills to student nurses. *Nurse Education Today,* **10,** 125-129.

Reichel, M. and Ramey, M.A.(eds) (1987) *Conceptual frameworks for bibliographic education: Theory into practice.* Littleton, Colorado:Libraries Unlimited,Inc.

Tyler, J.K. and Switzer, J.A.H. (1991) Meeting the needs of nursing students: a library instruction model for a nursing research class. *Medical Reference Services Quarterly,* **10,** 3, 39-44.

The author wishes to acknowledge that the presentation of this paper was aided by generous financial assistance from the University of Wales College of Medicine William Morgan Thomas Fund.

THE LIBRARY'S ROLE IN THE PROBLEM-BASED EDUCATION AT THE ZAGREB SCHOOL OF MEDICINE

Jelka Petrak, Zagreb University School of Medicine, Central Medical Library, 41000 Zagreb, Salata 3, Croatia

Abstract
Zagreb School of Medicine has adopted PBL in 1990 for the electives in the preclinical years. Its central library has joined the program directly and indirectly. The first year experiences and the results obtained by the analysis of students' questionnaires are described.

Introduction
Zagreb University School of Medicine has adopted problem- based learning (PBL) in 1990 for the electives in the preclinical years. The elective courses started in the second semester. They were organized in three blocks, 4 weeks a block. Students could choose three out of 13 courses (1). The program was carried out in the groups of 20-25, in the form of tutorial sessions. The students of each elective used, as a sort of guidance, their respective manuals written by all faculty members participating in the course. The final testing was in the written form. The students' evaluation of the faculty and the course was performed in the form of an anonymous questionnaire. The Central Medical Library, Zagreb School of Medicine, has joined the program:(1) directly - by integrating library instructional module as a separate teaching unit into the elective "How to Study Medicine"; (2) indirectly - by satisfying the growing information needs of PBL students, usually not identified as a separate user group.

1. Direct Experience
The main goals of the elective "How to Study Medicine" are:

- teaching students to recognize the principal aims and methods of medical education, and to become aware of the way they have to go from medical student to full medical professional;

- helping students to formulate their own learning goals and to adopt the process of acquiring knowledge by contextualising and elaborating their learning;
- understand the specific features of their future profession;
- acquire essential skills needed to locate and evaluate appropriate information independently (2).

The case analyzing was the very foundation of each session, and, as an illustration, one of the three teaching cases used during the period, is described. The scenario was the simulation of a plenary session during a conference "The Physician for the 21st Century". The students were divided into the groups of 4-5, each group being assigned the role of a specific group of the conference participants:

1. Dean and vice-deans for teaching and research, representing the School of Medicine,
2. University Chancellor and vice-chancellors for teaching and research, representing University,
3. Government vice-president for social affairs, ministers of health and education, and their assistants for financial matters,
4. Presidents of the Croatian Medical Association and Physicians Chamber, and representatives of other medical professional associations and trade unions,
5. WHO representative and a representative of the European Community Committee for Health Education,
6. journalists.

Each group was assigned the task to find and describe shortly at least one article dealing with the future aims of medical education, but representing strictly the positions of their specific groups. "Aims of the undergraduate medical education at the Zagreb School of Medicine" was used as a basic material for discussion of the changes needed in the near future. The library part of the program was discussed and defined during the joint meetings of all faculty participants in the course. Two librarians, involved directly in the program, participated in the process of formulating test questions and manual writing.

The library part of the program (5 hours) was defined on the levels of:

A. *Knowledge* - formal and informal information flow; the role of the library in the information transfer, especially in the peripheral scientific communities, dependent mainly on the import of information (3); different information resources and their accessibility; scientific paper and its structure, etc.

B. *Attitude* - the affirmative attitude toward the use of a larger number and wider variety of information sources to support learning; stimulation of critical opinion, etc.

C. *Skills* - organization and use of the library and its resources, retrieving and finding of relevant information, etc.

The first session in the library (1 hour) was a sort of lecture dealing with the level A. problems: growing volume of knowledge required to practice medicine, the importance of biomedical information, etc. It was followed by three hours of "library work". Using different tools (card catalogue, printed Index Medicus, MEDLINE in CD-ROM version, local database in CDS- ISIS format), the students tried to find a paper (or a monograph) relevant for the solving of their problem, i.e. for supporting their position in the conference discussion. Students were guided through the process of formulating a search question, translating it into key words and searching. The second lecture (1 hour) shortly analyzed the key components of a scientific paper (IMRAD), with special emphasis on citation style and cited literature.

Two questions regarding "library matters" were included in the final written test: the structure of the scientific paper, and the classification of information sources into the primary, secondary and tertiary groups. Each student was also required to analyze in written form the paper found in the library formulating his/her impressions and attitudes (if any!), and explaining shortly the aims, methods and main results of the paper. In the final discussion with the course tutor (oral evaluation) some students mentioned "benefits of the library" and disappearance of their "library fear". These elements belong to the level B, rather than A and C. But, being the first year students we consider their attitudes to be very important as an essential prerequisite for their future learning habits.

2. Indirect Experience

Since most PBL programs are designed to encourage students to locate appropriate literature independently, it has been shown in some recent studies (4,5) that PBL students use the library more frequently, especially some services, like journal collection and photocopying. Our experiences show that primarily we had to make some changes in staffing: small groups of PBL students were coming to the library with their tutors and they needed some organized reference assistance.

Changes in Library Organization

Trying to get some elements for our future decisions on further changes in library organization, staffing and services, we analyzed the students' final anonymous questionnaires in the 1990/1991, the first year of the new program. These questionnaires, completed by each student, are supposed to be the means for students to express their opinions and remarks on the whole of elective program, and, on the other hand, of providing some insight for comparison of the "traditional" and new parts of the curriculum. We analyzed 284 questionnaires. Three questions were of our special interest, evaluating in a way the work of the library.

1. The access to the suggested reading was measured by the 1-5 scale, 5 being "easily accessible" and 1 "difficult to access".

Year	5	4	3	2	1	No answer	Total
1990/91	112	58	58	26	16	14	284

Absolute frequencies

Over half of the students (59%) answered that the literature was easily accessible (marks 5 and 4), and only 5% (mark 1) that it was difficult. This shows that the suggested sources are well covered, and that the students are satisfied with the service.

2. The analysis of the question on the use of literature in foreign languages showed that only 25.4% (72) of the students have been using it, and that even 75.6% (212) of the students did not use any of the information sources in a foreign language. Though expected in the freshmen population, the analysis indicates that faculty, first of all, but also the librarians, have to emphasize from the very beginning the internationality of the biomedical communication process and the importance of international biomedical journals as the key element in the communication of the new information.

3. Answering the question on the main source of knowledge needed in the elective course they took, 36% of the students found the strongest support in their tutor, 27% in the manual, and less than 25% in other literature.

Source of knowledge	5	4	3	2	1	No answer
group	37	63	81	59	25	24
tutor	102	95	48	11	7	21
manual	36	80	65	50	30	23
other publications	68	61	40	29	40	46

Absolute frequencies

The students evaluated the sources by the 1-5 scale, 5 being the most reliable source. One or more sources could have been marked. Summing up the last two figures, the library, though not directly mentioned, proved to be a very important point of support, being the place where in most cases these published sources could be found.The analysis of the free form comments has really been encouraging for us. Answering the question: what did you like in the program, 47.8% of the students mentioned the work in the library. Among the answers as to what was unsatisfactory or not to the expectations, no one mentioned the library. These questions did not deal with the issues that could give us a reliable answer on the students' use of library services and their satisfaction or dissatisfaction with the quality of these services. Nevertheless, the results of the analysis do give us some hints of students' use of suggested sources of information. The degree of their reliance on tutors and respective manuals (question 3) indicates that it is necessary to help students to find the way toward numerous other sources of information. The high percentage of students who pointed at the library part of the program as exceptionally useful, shows that such help is really needed.

Conclusions

The experiences of the librarians as well as of the teaching staff, the analysis of tests and course evaluations by the students, show that the students are interested in acquiring training and instruction in information-seeking skills. Therefore, Zagreb School of Medicine has recently decided for library instructional module to be a separate teaching unit in the 4th semester for all undergraduate medical students, starting with the new academic year 1994/95.

References

1. Pokrajac N. Nastava elektivnih predmeta prve godine (The first year electives). Glasnik 1991:17:1-4.
2. Jaksic Z. "Rjesavanje problema" kao nastavna metoda i kao nacin ucenja ("Problem solving" as a teaching and learning method). Zagreb: Medicinski fakultet, 1990.
3. Royaltey HH. The information needs of health care professionals and consumers in developing countries. Bull Med Libr Assoc 1988;76(1):35-43.
4. Marshall JG, Fitzgerald D, Busby L, Heaton G. A study of library use in problem-based and traditional medical curricula. Bull Med Libr Assoc 1993;81(3):299-305.
5. Rankin JA. Preparing medical libraries for use by students in PBL curricula. Acad Med 1993;68(3):205-6.

DELIVERING OPEN LEARNING: the Flexible Library

Jean Yeoh. St George's Hospital Medical School Library, London SW17, UK

Abstract

Open learning is now widespread in nurse education and making new demands on library services. A model of open learning provision is proposed with suggestions for the library's contribution to this form of educational delivery. The model is then compared to the reality of provision in a recently established Open Learning Centre.

Open learning is a philosophy of learning which is based around improving access to education and training for people who may have difficulty in attending traditionally organised courses. The term is often used interchangeably with distance learning but open learning also involves a philosophy of learning which places the student at the centre of the learning process. Open learning is perhaps more accurately described as individualised learning in the context of this presentation. The teacher becomes a facilitator of learning and the student develops independence and self direction in learning. These processes can be difficult for students and painful for teachers. Distance learning has been available in the guise of correspondence courses for many years but the last ten years have seen a rapid growth. Public libraries are becoming involved in open learning and many commercial companies offer in-house open learning systems for staff training.

Perhaps the distinguishing characteristic of open learning is that course materials tend to be specially designed for the purpose. The Open University has long been an ideal role model for the production of good quality learning materials but there are now a number of producers of excellent interactive learning packages in the health sciences field. Initially, many individual teachers enthusiastically created their own in-house materials although the results were often amateur in appearance and lacked the facility for interaction between text and student needed for distance learning. Many teachers also underestimated the huge amount of time required to produce and test good quality materials. There was also some evidence of ignorance concerning copyright law with reproduction of printed materials without permission being sought from copyright owners.

Nursing education has increasingly adopted open learning as a method of delivering courses. There are a number of reasons for this but primarily it has been used with nurses who already have a nursing qualification and are undertaking further professional development. Many encounter difficulties in obtaining time off for course attendance and distance learning packages provide an obvious solution. In some cases teachers have adopted an 'outreach' approach and go to the students for tutorials, rather than students coming to an educational centre. For instance, outreach courses may be run for Health Visitors in health centres, cervical screening updates for practice nurses can be set up in family doctor practices and cancer or terminal care courses run on a series of hospital sites. Some courses use the educational institution as the main base for tutorials while others are entirely distance learning based with communication being through the marking of coursework and contact with individual personal tutors at the end of a phone. The high quality of open learning materials now available has also encouraged teachers to integrate learning packages into traditionally taught courses. Courses may use a single pack or a combination of different packages.

Open learning has changed the way in which students learn and has radically altered the role of teachers who are no longer the sole source of knowledge. This now comes from the learning materials and teachers are there to provide a framework for the organisation of learning and offer tutorial support. Librarians also need to adapt to this new philosophy of learning which offers a tremendous opportunity for extending the librarian's role. Librarians often have a wealth of expertise about open learning that is unrecognised This could include evaluation of packages, development of new packages, advice on sources, course planning and running courses. Some libraries have already developed user education packages in various formats that are based on individualised and independent approaches to learning, and librarians could also become involved in running distance learning study skills programmes where a number of commercial packages already exist. However open learning should also mean a close examination of library systems that may not meet the needs of this new breed of student.

I propose to develop an ideal model of library provision for open learning. St George's Library established an Open Learning Centre just over a year ago and I will assess how far this provision has actually matched my proposed model.

The key to successful open learning provision is a strong partnership between the library and the teaching departments. Both will need development in the provision of open learning and student support and it is important that librarians have access to development programmes offered to teachers. I have made the assumption that the library is the logical base for an open learning centre. This view is not necessarily widespread. For example, some open learning centres in the further education system are based around resource centres, staffed by lecturers, which have no links with the library or even other teaching departments. Nevertheless there are many advantages in basing open learning provision in the library. These include:

1. Longer opening hours and therefore better access for students.
2. Security systems so that expensive packages do not disappear.
3. Efficient systems for the issue and return of materials already exist.
4. Considerable expertise in handling multi media materials.
5. Librarians have experience in a counselling role.
6. Libraries are service based organisations.
7. Availability of the whole library collection to support open learning packages.
8. Access to computers for assignment writing.
9. Up to date knowledge of availability of new learning materials.
10. Sharing of resources across departments with accompanying cost benefits.

Traditional education courses have often survived without a great deal of administrative support. In open learning educational support is important but solid administrative support is also vital. Provision of the packages alone is not enough and organisations that have tried to run open learning without support have encountered a high drop out rate and delays in course completion. The human element is still important and counselling and support play a key role however good the learning materials. Open learning centres need to be centrally located in the institution and provided with sufficient equipment and resources. While students no longer need classrooms they may need quiet study places. There needs to be a system for managing financial information, dealing with enquiries, providing course information and organising the storage, distribution and maintenance of stock. Libraries easily meet these criteria.

Library routines may need to be adapted to meet the needs of open learners and large academic libraries with more bureaucratic structures could have difficulty in this area. Students will find it helpful to have a 'drop in' centre or focal point to meet colleagues and tutors and this centre can double as a tutorial base. While the administrative base should be in the library, outreach facilities may be needed. Postal loans systems are one option, but another may be for the librarian to go to the students, rather than waiting for students to come to the library. Distance learning students work in isolation and the library staff may be among the few contacts they make during a course. It helps if the library has a designated person who is able to empathise with the particular problems of adult learners so that students know who to ask for, whether the contact is face to face or by other means. Students need to be confident that they are dealing with people who understand the difficulties they are facing. Librarians have had to develop skills of guidance as a necessary part of their ordinary role but counselling and advisory skills will be even more important when dealing with open learners. Rowntree (1), quoting Dixon (2) recognises the contribution of librarians:

> "...librarians provide first-level tutorial support - in the form of counselling, encouragement, motivation and study skills - leaving second-level support in the form of advice on subject content and assessment to tutorial staff."

This shifting role is recognised in a recent report on academic libraries(3) which notes the support that will be required from librarians will include some of the tutorial skills normally provided by the teaching staff. Of course, this also has implications for the level of library staffing. In the nursing sector open learners are often studying in their own time and paying for courses themselves. In juggling the needs of their course, their work and their family commitments they will need to make efficient use of library resources so that user education and other information skills must have a high priority. Many will find the library a convenient meeting place for group work and discussion and libraries having computer facilities for word-processing and multimedia use will be at an advantage. Although most experts would suggest that it is not cost effective to produce in-house materials there are curriculum areas not covered by commercial packages. Writing open learning materials demands a particular skill which is not always dependent on subject knowledge and librarians should be considered as part of the writing team. Decisions relating to the format of course materials will benefit from a librarian's experience in handling different types of media and their advantages and disadvantages in daily use, storage and exploitation. If an institution decides to publish a package commercially librarians have considerable knowledge of possible publishers and potential copyright issues.

The Open Learning Centre at St George's is based in a multidisciplinary health sciences library and it was established as a result of a close relationship between nursing lecturers and the library. When the idea of open learning provision was first raised the library had not been considered as the location for learning support. Close links between the library and the nursing college, established by involvement in course development committees, made it easy to suggest the direction in which open learning support might go. Once the advantages of this proposal were recognised it was taken up enthusiastically by teaching staff and a working party including librarians and lecturers was established to develop the idea. A suitable room within the library was converted into a 'drop in' Open Learning Centre and a part-time administrator, who happened to be an ex-teacher, was appointed from within the current library staff. It was decided at the outset that the Centre would concentrate on teacher supported courses which would be properly validated although the Centre was available for people who wanted to work through materials by themselves. A reference collection of open learning materials is provided in the Centre. These are available for teachers wishing to use open learning materials to examine what is available and select materials for new courses. They are also available for potential students who want to know what courses are available, and they can then either opt for a course run by the nursing college or contact open learning institutions direct and make their own arrangements. A leaflet explaining how the Centre operates is available and there is questionnaire for potential students to complete to indicate interest in areas of study. The Administrator can proffer advice on courses available but she will also refer nurses on to designated lecturers if further counselling is required. Following these contacts, and using completed questionnaires, the College then will attempt to set up appropriate courses if there are sufficient students or will advise them how their needs could be met.

Once materials have been chosen and purchased for a course they are stored in a closed access system. Students usually pay for course materials, but if they return packages in good condition 90% of their payment is refunded. The remaining 10% is retained and used to purchase materials for the Centre and returned packs are re-used. Alternatively students can opt to purchase materials outright. Individualised learning courses are now also part of mainstream classroom based nurse education and some have a flexible element allowing students to work at their own pace and choose finishing dates, although there are strict deadlines for coursework submission. Their use has rapidly spread to traditional courses once lecturers have seen the quality of open learning materials on offer. For example a traditionally taught nursing course contains modules and assignments on research. Many found this part of the course intimidating and the use of open learning materials on research to supplement traditional lectures has helped students enormously. Materials are also used where students may need to be brought up to standard before beginning a course. Clearly the library has to be closely involved in course development and planning so that sample materials for evaluation are obtained and then ordered in time for courses to begin. It is hoped that eventually the Open Learning Centre will be funded and used by disciplines other than nursing.

How far does the Open Learning Centre at St George's match the ideal of library based open learning provision I described earlier? The library's computerised issue system has not coped with the multiplicity of issue periods required for open learning packages as easily as had been anticipated. Some imaginative adaptations by the administrator have produced a workable system, although it is rather time consuming and not the slick operation that was expected. For example open learning students and teachers have separate open learning library tickets to record loans in addition to their ordinary library tickets. Some general library routines do not meet the needs of qualified nurses. For example an overnight loans system, designed to be a convenience, works well for medical students and staff working office hours. However it is actually highly inconvenient for most nurses and the library is probably insufficiently sensitive to nursing shift systems and changes in work patterns. So far the Centre has relied on students collecting course materials from the library and this has been co-ordinated with library user education sessions. It is certain that we will need to examine this practice and look at postal delivery or outreach visits to other centres. It was intended that the Centre would be available for nurses to work on packages. However other library user groups have realised that it offers a quiet study area and to some extent their presence prevents use by some of the more diffident nursing users. This has exposed a general lack of provision for group work and discussion.

The Centre has been operational for about fifteen months and there are some unresolved issues. One of these is the re-use of packages. The concept of sale or return was devised so as not disadvantage students on low incomes and to avoid packs being chosen on the basis of cost rather than educational suitability. We may have to offer a sliding scale as we begin to re-use materials which have become a little worn at the edges. Other issues arise from the fact that the Centre was established at a time of significant reorganisation in the nursing college. The Centre was a 'grass roots' development rather than a directive from the top. While official recognition has been forthcoming in terms of increased funding the college has not appointed an academic leader for open learning. This has created difficulties for the library when there has not been an obvious focus for communication. Although the Centre has an Administrator it is clear that the library needs good backup systems to cover absences.

However on the positive side, teaching staff involved in open learning courses have developed a very friendly relationship with the library with resulting mutual benefits. Similarly, the Centre Administrator has developed excellent relationships with students, many of whom are not traditional library users, and this has improved their confidence in their general use of the library. Because the Centre is based in the library, learning packages have been shared across different teaching departments resulting in considerable cost savings. Previously materials had been kept in locked cupboards or had simply not been collected from students once courses were completed. Although there are some reservations about the adaptability of the computerised system there is no doubt that as open learning expands even an imperfect system is needed to cope with the complexities and size of open learning cataloguing, loan and recall requirements. As well as generally maintaining the Centre the administrator performs most of the clerical work although teachers could still pass on more of these tasks. We have not persuaded all teaching staff of the value of centralised holdings and resource sharing. However the overall benefits of basing open learning provision in the library outweigh any disadvantages and this view is generally supported by the teachers who have been involved in course delivery.

References

1. Rowntree K Exploring open and distance learning. London: Kogan Page, 1992.
2. Dixon K Implementing open learning in local authority institutions. London: Further Education Unit, 1987.
3. Fielden J Supporting expansion: a report on human resource management in academic libraries for the Joint Funding Councils' Review Group. Bristol: John Fielden Consultancy, 1993

EXERCISES IN CRITICAL THINKING:
Library User Education for Biomedical Students

Chris Atton, Napier University, 10 Colinton Rd, Edinburgh EH10 5DT, Scotland

Abstract
The author describes how he encouraged critical thinking skills in library user education. Exercises were designed to introduce students to finding and assessing information, and communicating the results appropriately. In the first year of the course the research was undertaken in small groups, where discussion played a significant part. In the second year, where the work was completed individually, the emphasis on dialogue was retained as the primary learning method. By learning to ask questions, by thinking critically and taking responsibility for their own learning, the students became effective and enthusiastic users of information.

The Value of Critical Thinking
As the interests of commerce and industry increasingly influence the content of syllabuses in higher education, so we see an increase in the formal teaching of transferable skills, particularly in colleges and the "new universities". But the promotion of such skills by the business interest should not blind us to the fact that they are of inestimable social import. They might also be used to further students' understanding of the society in which they live, to evaluate what they are being told, to decide for themselves what they need to know. Yet students find it hard to value such skills when they are taught separately from the core curriculum: however transferable they might appear to the educator, the students will mostly consider them as more hoops to jump through. Transferable skills work most successfully where they an integral part of the core curriculum. Unfortunately library user education is mostly still taught as a separate subject; even when team-taught with a subject specialist, the students are rarely encouraged to work out for themselves the relevance of what is being studied.

As a result, I find that my work is increasingly to do with teaching people to think for themselves, to think critically, to examine and reflect on what they do. I am moving away from the "how to find a book" mentality of much library instruction towards a properly educative model of teaching. In some instances I'm not developing "student-centred" learning anymore, but "student-led" learning. This is hard since many students are not encouraged to think for themselves (whether this comes from school, other parts of their life or other parts of their current education). They don't look kindly on being given control over a course.

The work I want to discuss here developed from applying critical thinking to bibliographic instruction in an attempt to make the skills learned and the research undertaken more relevant both to the students' core subjects and to their lives. Critical thinking may be defined as:

1. A readiness to question all assumptions
2. An ability to recognise when it is necessary to question
3. An ability to evaluate and analyse

(After Bodi, 1988)

Critical Thinking in Groups
Much library user education still focusses on the mechanics of information retrieval, concentrating on using catalogues, navigating classification schemes and exploiting abstracts and indexes. This approach tends to produce a student with the technical knowledge of the information retrieval systems of a single library. In my experience the mechanics of librarianship mean little to students, even when they are applied to tasks the students regard as essential, such as completing a seminar paper or an essay. I firmly believe that the skills learnt in bibliographic instruction are secondary to the cognitive, intellectual processes of examination, reflection and criticism. If students can be stimulated to consider these primary processes, then the processes by which they might find information on which to practice these cognitive and intellectual skills should follow.

In fact, this is precisely what I found when I designed a series of critical thinking exercises to replace the standard first term, first year undergraduate bibliographic instruction for the part-time BSc Life Sciences at Napier University. In order to encourage mutual support and discussion of what for many (mostly mature) students would be their first introduction to academic work, the exercises were all undertaken in small groups. Each group was presented with a paragraph about an aspect of scientific study (topics included Nobel Prize winners, Buckminsterfullerene, global warming). Each paragraph replicated a number of aspects from published writing: bias, inaccuracies, incomplete information, assumed prior knowledge. The task of each group was to research the content of its paragraph. They would have to identify all the aspects outlined above, explain contexts, justify arguments. To do this they would need to devise their own plan of research and undertake this research in the university library (and beyond, if necessary). The aim of the exercise was to encourage each member of the group to think critically about information. If the exercise could give the students experience of the research process *at whatever level*, then the contours of research would be recognisable and applicable at any educational level.

The critical thinking exercise succeeded in developing a questioning approach amongst the students and encouraged them to analyse and evaluate the information they found and the methods for its retrieval and presentation. It was clear throughout the exercise that the students were stimulated and enthusiastic; they were able to develop sophisticated and effective research strategies with minimal guidance from me; they were able to critically assess their own and others' approaches in the light of such work. There was no reason to suppose (on the contrary, it would be counter-productive to attempt it otherwise) that similar methods might not be used when introducing more advanced research techniques in the use of specialist journals, abstracts and indexes.

Critical Thinking and Critical Teaching

The next stage then was to transfer the skills learned here to the individual research and writing of a scientific report, based on the exploitation of journal literature, which was a significant part of the students' work in their second year. During the completion of the previous year's critical thinking exercises I had found myself asking questions such as: "What right do I have to assess others' experiences?" and "Should I not be assessing effort rather than results?" It is fitting that the development of critical thinking skills in students should be accompanied by a critique of one's own skills, to produce a relationship with students (as Ronald Sultana put it) "with sharing and critical reflection on knowledge as being the normal practice" (Sultana, 1990).

The most fulfilling parts of the exercise had come when the groups presented their results and discussed with each other the various methods employed and the information found. Since the report writing exercise was an individual piece of work, I felt it was important to sustain the obvious advantages of class discussion. During my planning for the second year I had been reading Ira Shor's book "Critical Teaching And Everyday Life", in which he stresses the crucial role of dialogue in the classroom. In building on the work of Paolo Freire, Shor identifies "a political economy of schooling", comprising three processes:

1. Learning through dialogue
2. Critical literacy as the foundation for studying any discipline

Teaching Modes That Challenge the Social Limits of Thought and Action

I had already engaged in 1. and 2. to limited degrees. The third element I had hardly considered. This is ironic, since much of my time is spent writing and speaking on the role of the library and the librarian as agents for social change, and on wider social issues such as the mass media and world development. In what now appeared an increasingly unnatural separation, I endeavoured to look at my role as a professional information worker and my life outside that role more holistically. Certainly this is what students do: "being a student" cannot be separated from "being a parent"or "being a worker", certainly not for mature students.

According to Shor, the value of the dialogue form for learning lies in its egalitarian, non-hierarchical nature, where students and teachers are equals in the classroom. By doing away with such symbols of control as the lectern, the teacher's desk, the teacher's monopoly over the instruments of communication (the lone voice, the blackboard) students can be encouraged to take part more in their own learning, to be self-educating in a non-authoritarian environment.

Learning Through Dialogue

The first meeting of the class in the second year began wth me reading out from the syllabus the details of the report writing assignment which the students would have to complete. As with many course documents, this was more in the language of academics than that of students. The first thing the class wanted to do was to have these terms of reference explained to them. Instead I suggested they identify what was unclear. One student homed in on the phrase: "The report must be of a scientific nature" and there followed this exchange:

> Student: What do you mean by "scientific nature"? Do you mean science pure and simple?
> Teacher: What is "science pure and simple"?
> Student: How gravity works?
> Teacher: O.K. Where would you research that?
> Student: A physics book.
> Teacher: What kind of physics book?
> Student: Any one: the one we used at school would do.
> Teacher: And what would you do with the stuff in the book?
> Student: Just write it out: it'd be easy!
> Teacher: Would you learn anything about research, then?
> Student: No. You'd just learn how to copy things out.
> Teacher: Which you already know. So take gravity as the scientific principle and ...
> Student: Find out how it affects aircraft...
> Teacher: Or...
> Student: Dancing...
> Teacher: What happens when you dance?
> Student: You get excited... You get dizzy...? I don't know!
> Teacher: That's O.K. But if you were interested enough, you could do your research on what happens to you when you dance. You'd be investigating a subject scientifically, the report would be of "a scientific nature". Now, what science would you need?

Through this discussion the students were able to examine the purposes of the report, potential topics and approaches to research. No questions were considered out of bounds; neither were "absolute" answers supplied. Methods and problems of applying the skills gained in the previous year's work were also discussed. The results of this discussion were used to frame and inform the more formal tuition that followed, which concentrated on methods of finding and assessing journal literature. Crucially they came to understand that there were no absolutes in the acquisition of knowledge. The students were encouraged to think critically about planning their work, why they were doing it and what they hoped to achieve. In addition, the students began to understand that knowing *what* questions to ask *when* was more important than mere questioning. For us as librarians, this is similar to the way in which we are taught how to conduct a reference interview. I reveal those methods to the students and encourage them to take responsibility to critically examine their own questions and, by implication, their own assumptions about the information they expect to find.

Critical Literacy

The students decided that they would spend the next week thinking about a topic and, if necessary, doing some reading to give them basic ideas. Everyone would be prepared to give a brief talk (a minute) about their topic: its subject, what approach they were going to take, why they had chosen it. The students then asked for help on finding information in journals, since journal use was one of the prerequisites of the report. Once again, this work was done using dialogue. In fact, the topic was addressed inadvertently, growing from a discussion about report writing (a good example of flexibility and spontaneity at work; a fixed agenda would have prevented this from happening.)

I was asked how anyone could "sort out all the stuff on AIDS". How can you be sure that all aspects of a topic have been explored by the publications you have access to? How do you know what the conclusions are when the research is still going on? In response to these questions, I referred to the current controversy over Peter Duesberg's hypothesis that HIV is not a necessary cause of AIDS. None of the students knew Duesberg by name, though one or two remembered seeing "something in the paper". By discussing articles in *Nature*, *Sunday Times*, *New Statesman and Society* and the less sensationalist coverage by the alternative press in such titles as *Open Eye* and *Steamshovel Press,* I was able to discuss with the students the wide range of perspectives available on what for many academics is a clear cut case. We then examined the reading habits of the group, which were largely popular press. We talked about bias in the mass media, and the divide between the popular and the scholarly press; strategies for keeping up to date with subjects being studied at university, and their social and political context.

In short, the students identified that they needed to: recognise bias and emphasis in journals; balance the need to read widely with the need to select appropriate information; choose and evaluate information. By learning to ask questions, by learning from each other, by thinking critically and taking responsibility for their own learning, the students became effective and confident users of information.

But if critical thinking is to mean anything it must be preceded by critical teaching. This means constantly refining, experimenting and taking risks. If you're expecting students to do it you must be prepared to do it yourself. Such processes should inform everyone's search for information and what we do with it. Such processes should inform our practice of librarianship. Our decisions on what to buy, how to arrange it and how to educate people to use it should not simply be unthinking, clerical activities. They too need to be conscious, critical decisions.

References

Bodi, Sonia (1988) Critical thinking and bibliographic instruction: the relationship, *Journal of Academic Librarianship* 14(3), 150-153.

Shor, Ira (1980) Critical teaching and everyday life. Boston, Mass.: South End Press.

Sultana, R. (1990) Towards a critical teaching practice: notes for the teacher educator, *Journal of Further and Higher Education* 14(1), Spring 1990, 14-30.

MEDICAL INFORMATION SERVICES AT TARTU UNIVERSITY

Aili Norberg, Tartu University Library, Struve 1, EE 2400, Tartu, Estonia

The present paper aims at giving a survey of the status of medical information services in Estonia and at Tartu University in particular. Some background information about the Republic of Estonia will be given as well as data about the Medical Faculty of Tartu University (TU). The paper will focus on the role of TU Library in establishing and development of an information base for medical training and scientific research and the problems of creating and maintaining an efficient system of communication.

Estonia is a small North-European country which after a period of silence of 50 years began to be mentioned in the world press in connection with the national liberation movement. In 1991 the independent Republic of Estonia was restored. The population of Estonia is about 1.5 million whereas 800,000 (55%) of it are Estonians. There are 7 higher educational establishments in Estonia. The oldest of them is Tartu University, founded in 1632 by the Swedish king Gustaf Adolf II. In 1919 (in connection with the establishment of independence), it became a national university and a symbol of national culture. The recent social development has also brought about significant changes in the life of this ancient university. These changes have been most considerable in teaching and research of the humanities and social sciences, but have also been important in science and applied sciences.

The Medical Faculty is the second largest faculty in TU after the Faculty of Philosophy. It comprises 9 institutes, 18 clinics (together called the Clinicum) and a professional training centre for doctors and pharmacists. There are 1500 students taught by 230 teachers in this faculty. The Medical Faculty has been and still is the only institution educating future doctors in Estonia. 130 young doctors are released annually. The Medical Faculty is also the republic's only centre for advanced professional training in the field of medicine. All doctors are tested every 5 years in Estonia and prior to that they take professional training courses. Totally, there are about 6000 doctors in Estonia, which is about 1 doctor per 250 persons. In 1993, for example, 2800 doctors participated in the above-mentioned courses. In general, doctors in Estonia spend 3% of their total number of working hours on additional professional training. The Medical Faculty and the Clinicum are the centre of scientific research in the field of medicine. The teaching staff of the faculty includes 56 PhDs and 112 MSs. An average number of 20 dissertations are defended by Estonian doctors in this faculty annually. The Medical Faculty publishes 3 series of transactions which are appreciated by 120 exchange partners all over the world.

It is the Department of Scientific Information of TU Library which renders the Medical Faculty the necessary bibliographic services, offers professional publications as well as access to a number of computerised databases. Doctors are practical and determined people also as library users. They are intensive consumers of information in case the library is able to offer:

a) bibliographic information systematised in the best possible way;
b) necessary professional journals;
c) monographs;
d) good handbooks (especially full-text databases);
e) copying facilities.

Nowadays a significant part of this task is fulfilled by the Information Centre of the Clinicum which was established in 1994. The history of medical information services at TU Library can be divided into 2 periods according to the methods of information retrieval:

1) the use of printed sources of information;
2) the use of computerised databases.

Up to 1991 TU Library was a part of the huge Soviet information system which meant that all bibliographic information, with the exception of publications obtained through exchange, came via the Central Institute of Medical Information in Moscow. This was due to a peculiar centralised communication system in the former Soviet Union. To get a copy of an article in a western professional journal was a complicated and time-consuming task. A description of all the hinders of the scientists' search for information would deserve a separate treatment. However, with a certain time lag, it was possible to follow the development in the field of study. The active use of that kind of information services by the Medical Faculty reveals its great importance at the time. The amount of information, more or less satisfactory for research up to masters degree was provided. The development of the more advanced branches of medicine was based upon numerous personal contacts of the researchers (information exchange of the so-called invisible councils), etc.

Certainly, every possible step was taken to provide the top scientists with information as well (exchange of literature with Western libraries, purchases, inter-library exchange, copying, etc.). These activities were managed by the information specialists of TU Library. The major fields of research of Tartu University were and still are each supervised by one worker of this department (10 persons altogether), whereas 2 of them deal with medical sciences.

As a consumer of information each person is unique. The best way to deal with the situation is to know the customers and their needs as thoroughly as possible. The customers must get the right information at the right time. The information workers of TU Library have usually been bibliographers-humanitarians, i.e. they have no medical background. Therefore it is of vital importance to develop a reliable feedback system to offer the consumer of information the relevant data and enable the librarian to keep in touch with the new trends in the specific field of study and thus develop an equal partnership. The beginning of the movement towards an open information community (1990-1991) was particularly difficult as the former sources of information ceased to function whereas the new ones were not yet open mostly due to economic recession, but partly also because of inability to use them. Aided by colleagues from many countries who have given TU Library both economic support and advice, it has been possible to implement Western information technology. Public organisations, colleagues from libraries and private persons from many countries have offered their help in subscription to professional journals, study aids and valuable handbooks in various fields of science, incl. the field of medicine. At present the information services of TU Library can offer access to 30 computerised databases, incl. the whole set of CCOD, the series of which "Life Sciences" and "Clinical Medicine" are very popular with doctors in Tartu, as well as "Medline", "Medline Professional", "Consult" and other databases.

The new system of government financing of libraries is also taking shape. In the current year various institutions of Estonia subscribe to 445 medical journals, incl. 315 ones by TU Library. Also the problems are levelling out in educating library staff as well as the users of the library to be able to work with the new information carriers. Computerised databases have become regular sources of information and it may be said that a break-through to a new technology of information has been accomplished. But the role of an academic library as a centre of communication is not only to collect, sort out and make the existing information accessible, but also to deal with the questions of newly generated information, internal problems of the academic community, its creative activity and output, connections between various scientific communities, etc. It is also an important question for the medical information services of TU. The productivity of the workers of an academic institution also reflects their access to information, i.e. the quality of information services. The opportunity to use CCOD which presents materials carried by world's high-impact journals has enabled the librarians to follow the activities of the Estonian doctors in the world circulation of information. In 1993 40 articles by Estonian physicians were published in the journals of CC.

Is it enough or not? To get an approximate answer we must compare our data with that of some other country. It would be reasonable to compare the three Baltic states. In 1993 the number of publications in the field of medicine seems to be nearly the same. Traditions in science are very viable. For example, Riga was the city where the grandfathers of the present generation of all the Baltic nations went to get their education in technology and engineering and it has remained the centre of these sciences up to now. For example, in 1993 87% of the Baltic publications on technical engineering were published by Latvian authors. On the other hand, Tartu was and still is the centre of humanities (68.4% of publications) and educated land-cultivators (66.6% of publications) of the Baltics. The priorities of Baltic science inherited from the previous century are still actual. A common topic today in Estonia are the problems brought about by the future integration into European context of culture and science. Its success depends first and foremost on the quality of the country's own contribution to the partnership. The national and international co-operation in this context is very important. This can be carried out in many ways, but in the field of information through developing library networks with integrated databases and mutual facilities for document delivery.

Lastly, the library development policy should be considered as a distinctive part of the over-all national information policy. A library network cannot be planned separately from the development of all other information resources of the country. As it is said, only a healthy and well-informed nation will cope with its problems. This is essential for a small nation.

THE IMPACT OF PROFESSIONAL DEVELOPMENT REQUIREMENTS ON THE USE OF INFORMATION SOURCES BY NURSES: a survey

Christine Urquhart and **Sophie Crane**, University of Wales, Aberystwyth SY23 3AS, UK

Abstract

A survey of 5% of the qualified nursing staff was undertaken in late 1992/early 1993 in Plymouth to ascertain how the College library should support the proposed national continuing education requirements for nurses, midwives and health visitors. A structured interview, plus vignette study indicated the need for networking and/or integration of local health libraries, improved journal collection and current awareness services. One third of the sample appeared lacking in information-seeking skills. A self-access library and study skills package was proposed.

Survey Aims

Aim 1: to examine how PREP might affect nursing staff in Plymouth.

The proposed changes in continuing education (PREP) for nursing staff in the UK (UKCC 1990 and 1993, ENB 1990) are likely to affect the organisation and delivery of library and information services. The demands of PREP on library services were seen by many College principals and learning resource managers in the NURLIS study to be greater than those of Project 2000 (Capital Planning Information 1992). As the College (TSWCH) library services were already fully stretched by the demands of Project 2000 (diploma level nursing education) planning information was required on the type of resources and support services that would be required by the trained nursing staff in the future.

Aim 2: to examine preferred methods of learning, use made of journals and need for current awareness.

The requirements for advanced professional practice are likely to require access to research resources and improved information-seeking skills (LA/NIS subgroup 1991). Continuing education will be varied in format, and provided both by the conventional providers (colleges, universities offering formal courses) and also by organisations, including journal publishers, offering open learning schemes. Nurses may wish to use their local libraries for courses organised elsewhere.

Aim 3: to examine perceptions of local health libraries.

Trained nursing staff have had to rely on libraries devoted to the needs of medical staff or nursing students (Holdsworth,J 1991). There are several libraries in Plymouth which trained staff could use, but which would they choose to use?

Aim 4: to determine information-seeking skills and strategies, use made of formal and informal sources

In a study (Wakeham, M et al 1992) which reviewed the information-seeking behaviour of nurses, difficulties in obtaining information appear to affect use of resources. These difficulties may include poor information retrieval skills.

Method

The survey involved a structured interview plus vignette ("case study") information problem. Choice of method was partly governed by time restraints. The staff were selected by asking team leaders in the community, and a random selection of ward sisters/charge nurses to suggest members of staff prepared to participate in the survey. College tutors were asked to suggest names: in this way a number of clinical specialists and practice nurses who might have been overlooked were included. A check of the participants showed that the selection was not quite as random as had been hoped, but the response rate from arranged interviews was satisfactorily high (86.9%, return rate from original letters, 56.8%).

The structured interview used a combination of open and closed questions to obtain information on professional development plans and preferences, use and views of journals, times when access to the library would have been possible, and some personal background information. After the interview the participants were presented with a vignette, and asked to write how they would tackle the particular "information problem". Several vignettes were designed, based on "problems" derived from the recent nursing literature or from genuine queries in the College library. The vignette content was related to the area of practice.

Results

Over the sample as a whole, 86.3% (63/73) of nursing staff had attended two or more courses in the past two years, with many attending four or more. In Plymouth, the indications are that many nurses are exceeding the PREP minimum, particularly as some nurses are doing a University(Plymouth) degree (part-time). Chapman and Hall (1992) found figures for study day attendance nearer the PREP minimum. The main problems associated with course attendance were the problem of study leave, or lack of places available on the course. Most seemed to receive adequate information about courses. The most popular method of learning was attendance at a study day, indicating a preference for some direction in learning, and (possibly) easier accreditation of learning. Next in popularity were reading, and discussing. The most popular combination of learning styles, study day followed by reading, seems to contradict the stated lack of popularity of library methods for continuing education. Presumably reading is only popular when some direction is given.

Only 6.9% (5/73) read a journal cover-to-cover, most (84.9%, 62/73) reading specific items only, and nearly half (43.8%, 32/73) omitting non-relevant clinical articles. Journal reading is therefore quite selective. However, journals are used for more than clinical updating, 64.4% (47/73) using them for professional news. Only two formal journal clubs were revealed in the survey, most staff relying on "word of mouth". Community and practice nurses did particularly well in this respect, general practitioners often pointing out material in the medical journals. Although 41.1% (16/39) wards/units surveyed were considering new journal subscriptions, only four of those units were considering subscriptions to new (or revamped) journals. Typically, the units would be subscribing to 1) an established specialised journal or 2) a general journal with Open Learning units, e.g. *Nursing Times,* to support staff on the ward doing that Open Learning course. Units appear to assume that the College library would subscribe to new journals.

Nursing Times, was overall, the most widely read journal with 67.1% of participants seeing it. However, it is closely followed in the number of personal subscriptions by *Professional Nurse* (23 and 21 respectively). There were 24 workplace subscriptions for *Nursing Times,* and 17 for *Nursing Standard.* The best general journal appeared to be *Professional Nurse,* with 50% of its readers liking it and 41% "quite liking" it. Out of the community nursing journals, the *Journal of Community Nursing* was most popular, with 61% of its readers liking it and 39% "quite liking" it. Nursing staff valued relevant and reputable clinical journals. The idea of receiving a specialised current awareness service was very popular, although most of the subjects mentioned were very general. Many of the desired topics were multi-disciplinary, which would make service provision difficult from any single library. The vignettes were analysed first by a coding process. Four mutually exclusive categories of information-seeking strategy emerged. These were:

1. Use of more than two sources, with information-seeking strategy evident (30%)
2. Use of more than two sources, no information-seeking strategy evident (22%)
3. Use of two or fewer sources, with information-seeking strategy evident (13%)
4. Use of two or fewer sources, no information-seeking strategy evident (36%)

Although nearly one third appeared competent at finding information, over one third appeared to lack information-seeking skills. The remainder either knew about sources (but lacked strategy) or had a strategy (but lacked knowledge of sources). The relationship between number of sources used and use of a strategy was found to be significant (Chi-squared=5.38). For analysis the sample was divided into: *Group A (Use of more than two sources)* and *Group B (Use of two or fewer sources).* The types of sources mentioned were listed and divided into informal(personal) and formal (published) sources. Study of the use of informal sources showed that very few (6%, 4/64) of the participants would not use informal sources. Examination of the pattern of use of colleagues/managers and specialists(nursing and allied health) showed, however, that there was no difference between Group A and Group B. Most nurses were aware of the resources offered by patient support groups.

Study of the use of formal sources, including specific mention of particular libraries, showed that (unsurprisingly) the College library was mentioned most. Of more interest, perhaps, the University library, public library, HEA library and the Staff (largely medical) library all had similar rankings. Analysis showed that Group A were significantly more likely to mention use of a library than Group B. Of those people in Group A who had an information-seeking strategy, only one did not use a library. However, when studying mention of journals and literature searching, the findings suggest that most staff are aware of journal resources, even though many lack skills in using these resources. Around 30% did not mention use of a library, or library resources, in their solution of the vignette information problem.

Conclusions

The main recommendations were:

1. The College needs to take a leading role in the provision of specialist clinical journals and supporting secondary services (e.g. CD-ROM). Access to the journal literature should be promoted by cost-effective current awareness services.
2. An self-access information skills package should be designed for distribution at study days, and the variety of information skills instruction greatly improved and extended.
3. Networking and/or integration of library resources needs urgent review.

References

Capital Planning Information (1992) *Library and Information Services to support Project 2000, NURLIS Phase 1,* Boston Spa, British Library, R&D Report 6088, ISBN 090601185X

Chapman,R and Hall, B (1992) Post-registration education in three fields of clinical practice, *Nursing Times,* 88 (43) 53-56

Crane,S and Urquhart,C (1994) Preparing for PREP: the impact of changes in continuing education for nurses on library provision of journals and current awareness services: a case study, *Health Libraries Review,* 11, 29-38

ENB (1990) *Framework for Continuing Professional Education and Training for Mangers (series of reports),* London, ENB, ISBNs 0946810265, 0946810287

Holdsworth,J (1991) *The Provision of Health Care Information in the UK: a summary report.* Boston Spa, British Library, Research Paper 98, ISBN 0712332626

Library Association and NIS subgroup (1991) Implications of PREPP for library and information services, *NIS Newsletter,* 11(3) 10-13

UKCC (1990 and 1993) *Report of the PREPP Project & The Council's Proposed Standards for Post-registration Education,* London, UKCC

Urquhart,C and Crane,S (1994) Nurses' information seeking skills and perceptions of information sources: assessment using vignettes, *Journal of Information Science* 20(4) (in press)

Wakeham,M, Houghton,J and Beard,S (1992) *The Information Needs and Information-seeking Behaviour of Nurses,* Boston Spa, British Library R&D Report 6078

HUNGARIAN COLLEGE LIBRARIES IN NURSING EDUCATION

Eva Bakos, Haynal University of Health Sciences, Library of the Faculty of Health Sciences, Budapest, Hungary

Abstract
Study on the role of Hungarian college libraries in nursing education by comparing demands of training on library with the level of library services.

Where are we coming from?
What are we?
Where are we going to?

It was Gauguin's famous painting that gave me the quotation to my presentation. The structure of my lecture is based on these three questions. Though the title of my presentation is "Hungarian College Libraries in Nursing Education" - I must tell you that in Hungary at the faculties of health sciences not only nurses, but other paramedics, for example physiotherapists, dietitians, optometrists, and other health professionals are also trained.

In Hungary education of registered nurses begun not so long ago in 1990. We have four Faculties of Health Sciences belonging to our four medical universities but branches of these faculties can be found in several Hungarian cities. It is necessary to explain the structure of the Hungarian health professionals' education because the college libraries' work depends on it. Each Faculty of Health Sciences has their own department for training registered nurses, but departments for other professions are not so common, new departments have been started by local needs. The first Faculty of Health Sciences was founded in 1975 in Budapest. Formerly there was no higher education for physiotherapists, dietitians, home care nurses, health visitors.

Health professionals were trained in four secondary level institutions. In 1975 our Faculty was established by uniting of these institutions. The library of the faculty has been based on the collection of the formerly independent schools' libraries. Nowadays the collection has 40000 books and 180 titles of periodicals on the field of nursing, allied health, physiotherapy etc. The other three Faculties of Health Sciences in Hungary were established in 1990 or later. As a matter of fact they were established under much better conditions than the Faculty in Budapest.

Our Faculty of Health Sciences has had trouble with educational buildings from the very beginning. I mean there are not enough rooms even for lectures, and the library lies also under the pressure of room-shortage. Our Faculty has four educational buildings in Budapest lying rather far from each other. In the first decade each department had its own library under the supervision of the central library. The library wasn't able to satisfy the demands of high level services owing to dispersion and underfinancing of collection development. The recently started faculties don't have to struggle with these handicaps. These institutions are situated in appropriate buildings and have obtained initial financial fundings. The number of students is not much at the new faculties, its average not more than 500, and branches to choose are also fewer. The Faculty of Health Sciences in Budapest attracts the most students in Hungary, not only regular but correspondent students as well, altogether 1700 students in 1993/94. Starting registered nurses' education brought new demands on the services of the library. The methods and curriculum were worked out with the help of international experiences.

The library wants to be a partner in the cooperation with lecturers and students: it provides access to literature and new information. At the same time the new administration of the faculty demanded higher levels of library services. The challenge of the new demands could be satisfied with the following methods :

Collection analysis according to subject-matter and the data of circulation. It was very hard work for each colleague of the library, because we had to evaluate the role of each piece of the collection two times at least. Parallel to this work we discussed the importance of books with the lecturers, because we didn't want to withdraw compulsory readings from circulation.

Creating a well applicable collection demands to eliminate inert materials from the stock. It was very important for our library, because since the foundation of the faculty library this work had always been postponed. While collection analysis was realized department libraries were eliminated in agreement with the heads of departments. Access to the collection of these department libraries was unsure owing to the lack of library hours. The collections of department libraries were integrated with the collection of our central library, and we provided steady access to them.

In the future our endeavour is still to concentrate the fundings of acquisition for books and periodicals. The level of library services can be raised only with the help of this method. About periodicals: We did the collection analysis and elimination of duplicates, the same was done to the text-books and lecture notes. The state of the library catalogues were miserable, cards of new books were rarely filed into their places. The collection of the library had been arranged by accession numbers, so the catalogues can't be neglected. We had to find a solution to complete catalogues quickly: automation stepped into the library work at that point. In 1991 there was some technological development introduced in the library: a PC with CD-ROM. To complete our catalogues Hungarian Book Database on computer has been chosen. It contains the bibliographic data of all the books edited between 1964 and 1989 in Hungary. A full catalogue card can be made with the attachment of accession number, so it is very quick to complete the card-catalogue and to create a new computerized library database.

We had planned to finish catalogue completing within a year, but the problems of human resources didn't let us to manage our work according to the plan. The work with computer cataloguing seems to be very simple under certain conditions : A librarian with computer-using and cataloguing skills is essential. This problem of our work is going to be solved slowly, as my colleagues are learning how to work with PC-s and cataloguing programs. New tasks involve more new tasks: bibliographical information or literary research have been supported by a CD-ROM and Database on Nursing and Allied Health from Silver/Platter. This database and its use was introduced to lecturers and students. But I have to tell you, the popularity of it could be increased, specially with the increasing number of students with good command of English language. The most attention to the database is shown by students of nursing and physiotherapy. In the meanwhile our library had an opportunity to buy a copy machine by support of Soros Foundation. Formerly there was a great demand for this service, and could be hardly fulfilled.

One more step forward in information services: our library has joined the Hungarian Information Infrastructure Project. It means that our library has become a part of the national and international information network. Students as end-users can become adept at information skills, even at the ones that are not only library-specific. World is open for us with the help of international information network, but I mean not only databases but colleagues abroad. Norway became very close to us as we frequently change messages with my colleague, Maria F. Lund from Sykepleierhogskolen i Lorenskog. I'd like to thank her for the help she has given to me and our library. The librarians are proud of the technical advancements but the new information tools have to meet the new demands of the lecturers and students as well. The number of library users has increased with 80 percentages in the last four years. But we librarians know that this percentage could be improved under better conditions, e.g. adequate library rooms and open access system.

There is another problem for college libraries of higher health education: the method of education is not based on students' library work. Direct connection between library and training is still missing. In the English-speaking world the method of teaching is based on students' library work, so the libraries have became noisy. Librarians from those countries always make complaints against noise. I wish their trouble were mine. For all that there is a rapidly increasing demand for library services. One of our goals is the elimination of blank areas in the collection, such as a collection of works by Florence Nightingale and books on her life and work. The recently started libraries have also trouble with collection organizing. Their small collections can't fulfil the demands of the lecturers and students. That's why cooperation among libraries is very important, services can be improved without extra costs.Faculty library in Budapest helped the new libraries in the country with small collections of handbooks and periodicals. Professional meetings of librarians are useful in connections and cooperation, library users make benefit of good cooperations among librarians as well.

To fulfil our tasks we , librarians have to find new sponsors for the library and new sources for the acquisition of books and periodicals. We have achieved certain success: there are foundation, both national and international (e.g.Soros and Sabre Foundations) supporting the library and training with lots of books. Whenever applications or other foundations are invited, our library applies for them as well. Our goals are common with the ones of other librarians: to give library users adequate information as qiuckly as possible.

WHAT DO MEDICAL STUDENTS KNOW ABOUT LIBRARY CONCEPTS? A pre- and post-test study of students participating in the problem-based curriculum at Lund University.

Rabow A I & Akerblom H,UB2 - Lund University , Box 3, S-22100 Lund, Sweden

"*Education is an admirable thing, but it is well to remember from time to time that nothing that is worth knowing can be taught*" *(Oscar Wilde).*

Abstract
A test of medical students' definitions of library concepts has shown scant basal knowledge - on an average 30% correct answers. The practical implications are discussed.

Introduction
In connection with the recent development of a problem-based medical curriculum at Lund University a continuing library instruction (LI) course was planned in cooperation with the medical faculty. This course has three levels gradually exposing the students to more complicated information retrieval and has become an integrated part of the curriculum during the first five terms for a total of ten hours. In accordance with the ideology of problem-based learning we have aimed at making the library instruction more process-orientated instead of traditionally resource-orientated, ie, we try to focus on the conceptual process of using information rather than on sources and locations but of course we teach both skills and concepts. Our goal is Information Literacy not Library Rules.

Purpose
A pretest with a dual purpose was developed. A review of the literature has shown that there is a scarcity of applicable test instruments. We decided to test the students' knowledge of a number of frequently used library concepts. Our primary objectives were to adjust the LI course to the level of pre-understanding of the students, to identify possible misperceptions and to find the right terminology level of written and oral instructions. "Communication has to be simple and build upon the knowledge of the recipients to be able to get through".[1] Part of these objectives was also to diminish "library anxiety" or rather "information anxiety", which has been found a problem for students faced with PBL and its demands on self-directed information searching from a variety of sources. C. A. Mellon[2] found 1986 that 75 to 80% of students described their initial and continuing response to library research in terms of fear and anxiety and this has a potentially negative effect on library instruction. Our secondary objective was to check whether the pretest had an educational value of its own, ie, if it would focus the students' attention on library concepts and make them aware of their lack of knowledge, which might increase their interest in LI. A pretest might also serve as an advanced organizer of context.[3]

Methods
29 concepts were selected from authoritative lists of library terms. Their relevance was thoroughly discussed with experienced librarians, as were their definitions. The total number of medical students tested was 267. Before the first library instruction session the main students group (A; n=199) was asked to write a short definition of the concepts on pre-printed forms. The students were explicitly informed that all the definitions should refer to the use of these concepts in a library and information retrieval context. We deliberately chose this method over the multiple choice method so as not to give the students any hints at all about the meaning of the terms and also to explore how they spontaneously conceived these concepts, ie, we were interested in the cognitive processes of the students. The tests were individual and anonymous, and each student worked alone. The reliability of the test was measured and found satisfactory.

Another group (B; n=68) was tested after one previous library institution session including a written compendium. The test was later repeated (with the same concepts rearranged) as a post-test on a part of the first group (C; n=53) **after LI** in order to see if the awareness from the pretest of lack of knowledge had made them more susceptible to instruction. The post-test was given half a year after library instruction. It is to be noted that no right answers were distributed after the first test although many of the concepts appeared during the first LI session,

The results were corrected according to a given list of definitions and each answer was graded either correct or wrong, ie, we accepted no in-betweens.

Results

All participating students completed the pretest forms. There was a statistically significant difference between those students who had received LI before the test (B) and those who had not (A). Group A had 28.6% correct answers and Group B, 32.4%. Mean for A was 8.3 and B, 9.4 (Table A). Group C had 26.6% (mean 7.7) correct answers before LI and 33.8% (mean 9.8) after LI, which is significant at the 1% level (Table A)

TABLE A

STUDENT GROUPS	CORRECT ANSWERS	(%)
Group A n=199 no previous LI	8.3 ± 3.7	(28.6)
Group B n=68 one previous LI session	9.4 ± 1.8	(32.4)
Group C: CI (before LI) n=73 CII (after 1 LI session) n=53	7.7 ± 0.5 9.8 ± 3.8	(26.6) (33.8)
The differences between Groups A & B between CI and CII are both significant ($p < 0.05$ and $p < 0.01$ resp.) The difference between Groups A & CI and between Groups B & CII is not significant		

However, even if both groups B and C who had received LI before the test were significally better than group A who had not, the difference between groups C and B did not reach statistical significance, indicating that the pretest had not significantly influenced the results after LI.

Discussion

The results show that medical students seem to have scant knowledge of basal library concepts - on an average 30% correct answers. Only one out of 267 medical students could define the meaning of Thesaurus - not even after one LI lecture. Nobody knew the meaning of Descriptors. Many definitions were surprisingly in a group of this kind, eg, the very common misconceptions of the terms BIBLIOGRAPHY (confused with BIOGRAPHY)and MONOGRAPHY. (Table B).

The concept DATABASE clearly has more associations of technology or hardware than of content which unnecessarily complicates our common explanations of bibliographic database as being electronic versions of their printed counterparts and also sheds new light upon the common belief of the end user that database-searching is a technological rather than a conceptual process, the success of which is due to the searchers skills and knowledge of the database contents and structure. (Table B)

TABLE B. Examples of student definitions given before LI:

BIBLIOGRAPHY	**Novel about the author himself A story about my life A story about a person's life Library knowledge The knowledge of books Overview of contents in a library A story about somebody's life written by another person**
MONOGRAPHY	**Collected works A word to use for computer searching a specific subject Written by ONE person about ONE person Written by myself without help A picture Written by a person about herself The history of your own life Book about eg the life of the tree frog but no other frogs**
DATABASE	**Computers for use in the library A computer (monitor, hard disk) Terminal for storing data Main computer with extensive information Memory bank in a computer system All programs in a computer The computer memory where you can search for references An information bank in software form Memory accessible from many stations A harddisk with a basic material to be searched A collection of computers with information A search station Central unit with a large memory connected to many other units Datacentre with main memory The programming Information centre for computers**

ONLINE CATALOGUE	**Catalogue of available computer programs** **Contents of a computer** **Catalogue of recent articles** **Catalogue of computer information** **Everything fed into the computer** **Quick reference index** **Catalogue published regularly**
PERIODICALS	**A journal during a specific time period** **An encyclopedia - *many students gave this answer*** **Journals published more seldom** **Journals in chronological order** **List of articles in annual order** **List of published articles on certain subject over a given time period** **The most current articles**
REFERENCE DEPARTMENT	**Where you can find references - many *students gave this answer*** **Where you find published articles** **Where you find journals** **Department with books with only references**

When analysing the fairly bad results even after LI you have to bear in mind that (a) although the concepts were touched upon in LI most of them were only defined in passing during their first session and the (b) the students did not know that they would have to reproduce this knowledge in a test, and seem to have acted according to Senecas epigram " non vitae sed scholae discimus". Obviously it is not enough with only one lecture on library use and information retrieval. Students need more sessions with problem-solving approached to internalise their knowledge of these concepts. Even so, some of the concepts will probably remain obscure until they have to realise their significance in relation to their own needs.[4] Our results can be compared to Naismith and Stein who 1989[5] published a test of library's user's comprehension of the terminology used in hand-outs and in librarian's speech. They found that their users only understood half of the commonly used terms. Librarians often tend to use a vertical relationship in their interactions with their patrons-clients instead of a horizontal one.[6]

These results also have implications for the production of user-friendly computer manuals, online held screens and library instructions. One example is the introduction page to Silver Platter MEDLINE Express. It is hardly meaningful to point the user's attention to the thesaurus when almost nobody has the faintest idea of what it represents. Our results show the necessity of adapting point-of-use instructions to a language that can be understood and to explicitly incorporate them into bibliographic instruction sessions. A Library instruction curriculum planned with our results taken into consideration will hopefully improve the situation for new generations of medical students but it may be assumed that many active physicians today lack this kind of knowledge.

References

1. Nöklebye Heiberg,A Personal communication.
2. Mellon, C A. Library anxiety: a grounded theory & its development, Coll& Red Lib 1986 Mar; 47(2): 160-5
3. Tievel, V. Evaluating library user education program. Coll & Res Lib 1989 Mar; 50(2):249-59.
4. Snow, B. What jargon is really necessary when teaching (& learning) online skills? Online 1985July;10(4):100-7.
5. Naismith, R, Stein, J.Library jargon. Coll & Res Lib 1989 Sept; 50(5); 543-52.
6. Smith, NM, Fitt, SD. Vertical-horizontal relationship. Spec Lib 1975 November; 66; 11; 528-31.

SECTION 5

DEVELOPING NEW SERVICES & RÔLES

INTEGRATION AND THE INTELLIGENCE FUNCTION

Dorothy Husband, Librarian/Intelligence Coordinator, North West Anglia Health Commission, St John's, Thorpe Road, Peterborough, Cambridgeshire PE3 6JG, UK

The early 1990s have been a time of enormous change for health services and health service staff in the United Kingdom. Throughout the state-funded National Health Service (NHS) policy decisions have been implemented which rearrange management structures. The basis of this activity has been the "purchaser-provider split". This separation of the management of local health service providers has produced local policy makers who commission care - the purchasers, and hospitals and community health services which enter into contracts with the purchasers to provide care. The tendency has been for local health authorities, the purchasers, to combine with each other to allow more strategic use of their purchasing power. Increasingly the district health authorities in England and Wales are also combining their expertise and priorities with those of the Family Health Service Authorities, the bodies which commission and support the local services of family doctors and dentists, community pharmacists and optometrists.

In April 1992, a merged health authority, North West Anglia Health Authority, was formed of parts of two counties - the north of Cambridgeshire and the west of Norfolk. The population of this area is about 404000, and it is about 3070 square kilometres. This is important to information people because the basic statistics from which we work - such as population projections, census data and unemployment rates are based on the counties of England. There is also a strong feeling among people of each county that the others are somehow "different" - so the bringing together of staff and knowledge from each of the previous health authorities was not a painless process!

In April 1994, the responsibility for family doctors, primary health care, community pharmacists and optometrists was given to a new body which carried forward the work of the two year old health authority but also took in some of the staff from each of the Family Health Services Authorities for the counties of Cambridgeshire and Norfolk. This was the second major change, involving different ways of working and areas of expertise, and forms part of my motivation to ensure my work feeds into processes of integration. I think it is important that library and information staff should be recognised as part of the "team" - and I recommend being in there at the creation of a new organisation to promote this! I was appointed about two months before the first merger, which meant that I experienced some of the changes as an existing member of staff. I hope that I therefore understood a little of the uncertainty felt by the staff, and could start to identify with them.

My job title is Librarian/Intelligence Coordinator, and this probably needs a little explanation. At the time when the NHS reforms were being planned, a report was produced by the NHS Management Executive, which is the supervisory link between Department of Health policy and local implementation. This was called "Purchasing intelligence"[4] and proposed a need for staff and skills development in the new health service purchasers which would bring together the areas of textual and numerical information to provide the knowledge base for planning health care. This paper recognised that, in the past, the libraries and the data management of health care in the NHS have been entirely separate, and that this was unhelpful in developing new ways of working. Since I was appointed, my aim has been to become the source of information, or at least referral, for people who need "intelligence", whether this is "traditional" library information or something new. I was also, in a sense, able to start with a clean sheet of paper, since there were few existing cooperative arrangements to blend in with. I investigated how we fitted into a local network of library provision, both within health service organisations and in the local community. My immediate priority was to rationalise expenditure on books and journal subscriptions, so that these were coordinated and there was no unintentional duplication. I also set up ordering arrangements with specialist booksellers and a periodicals agent. However, there were limits to what I could do, and setting further priorities was difficult. When I remembered part of a long-gone management course I had undertaken, I tried to diagram my way out of this situation. It was clear that there were two priorities which had to be fulfilled before I could really get my teeth into the "traditional" library work - which I still saw a need for. One was that I had to have a way of managing records of information resources held within the authority,

---

[4]NHS Management Executive Purchasing intelligence London: Department of Health, 1991

and I didn't yet have a computer or a text management package. It took time to sort this out, but eventually I had a new Dell PC and we implemented Inmagic Plus. I also needed the physical storage space - shelves - for books, journal stock and reports. The Authority was due to move to newly refurbished offices early in 1993, so that side of my work was constricted by a lack of space for many months.

It was thus a combination of two factors which led to my development, in personal and organisational terms, into an active participant in change management. I didn't have a physical Library, and my managers had other needs. In August 1992 the reactions of staff to the merger process seemed unenthusiastic in some quarters, and senior managers wanted to know why. I was available, though investigating priorities and planning for my information work, to attempt to help with organisational issues. I was therefore approached and asked if I would work with one of the Executive Directors to identify staff perceptions of their workplace and report on areas which needed improvement. I was pleased to do this, as it was a new sort of work for me, but one which I was well placed to try. My position working across the new authority, and, I hope, my personality, meant that I was well-placed to talk to every member of staff. So in the space of three weeks I spoke to about seventy people, in a semi-structured interview format. Examples of the questions are shown on the slide:

What do you think are the main strengths of North West Anglia Health Authority? How can we build on them.

What advice would you offer to the organisation that might help it to run more effectively?

I recommend this process as a way of getting to know your Library users - not just what their job title is, but also what they think is important in and important about their work. I also talked to all the staff members except four, which meant I was able to try to demonstrate to them that I as the Librarian was an approachable and professional person (confidentiality was VERY important in this process). One of the questions was "What would help you to do your job better?" - and in quite a few cases the response was about information resources, which I was able to feed into my priorities for the Library and Intelligence Service. I was also enabled to look at corporate reality - for the most senior managers, the strategic level of managing the new Authority took priority, but my interviews kept me very much in touch with how the full range of staff were thinking, and the sort of information they needed about both internal and external developments.

From this point onwards, my role in the organisation has had two sides - though they are intimately linked! For instance, the interviews with staff showed a need for a regular newsletter with internal information such as new employees, retirements, social events and charity fund-raising. I took on the editorship of this newsletter, since it allowed me to investigate what was happening in the organisation - which was very good for learning about new projects, and beginning to support them in information terms - and I was also able to have a list of new additions to the library stock published in a news sheet where people were likely to read it.

Our authority is also concerned to develop into a "learning organisation" - which can be defined as on organisation which constantly obtains information and feedback from its environment, and has the capability to transform itself to meet new challenges and opportunities which are identified. In this context, the role of current awareness services and, particularly, the supply of national and health service news to policy-making staff, are an integral part of developing appropriate relationships with other bodies. The learning organisation also has implications for personal and managerial development of the staff, and my professional services are important in supporting people in both formal and informal education and training We also took from the results of my interview the basis for an Organisation and Management Development action plan. This was carried forward by a "diagonal slice" group of eight Authority staff - people from each department and a range of seniority. This group met at least monthly for over a year, and carried through some of the ideas proposed by staff. For instance, it changed the planning of lunchtime talks for the entire staff on topics of current importance and development so that they were available to a wider range of those who worked part-time, and helped to develop the list of priority areas which needed to be covered. This group also did a lot of the preparation for the production of a handbook for staff coming to work in the Authority - which may seem like a small thing, but was very important in an organisation lacking a personnel or human resources coordinating function.

In the preparation for our second merger, and in the integration process since our groups of staff have been working together, action learning groups have been set up. These are sets of about ten people, and all staff members are members of one of these groups. Each group includes staff from a range of jobs, and offers an opportunity to learn about both what we as an organisation do, and how we do it. We meet to talk every month about recent developments. I facilitate one of these groups, and while there have been practical problems in organising our meetings, they have formed a very useful channel of communication. We are currently working on a new way to manage organisational development in our current management structure, and held a half-day seminar for all staff (about 100 people) two weeks ago, which looked at our current priorities, such as project management methods.

I also think that it is important to see my work as an integral part of the local provision of health care. The people who form my core users are those who make policy decisions based on public health medicine, government priorities and local political situations, and much of this relies on the printed word for effective communication. My role is to organise those textual materials so that they can be used by internal users - in this way I am working very much as a special or business library. While I have not yet done much about internal documents except start a collection of those items we publish for external use, the policy guidance and reports (known as "the circulars") we get from the Department of Health need a lot of bibliographic management, and we are constantly developing better ways of ensuring that these publications are both widely available and also targeted at those who must take action on the organisation's behalf. I now allocate a suggested "lead officer" for actions which must be taken to satisfy our national management, and record this on the bibliographic database which holds records of each circular. The Head of Performance Review then uses the database to follow up those circulars which need action and ensure that we fulfil our responsibilities.

I am also keen that, as a service provider, I mirror good practice in health care. The East Anglian Region of the NHS adopted some qualities as necessary for good quality health services. These were, in turn, developed from Maxwell's six dimensions of health service quality which were published in the British Medical Journal in 1984[5]. I think that these are also ideals for information services:

Health services should be:

Effective	Accessible
Efficient	Appropriate
Equitable	Responsive [6]

Effective - people should get the best possible service from resources available

Efficient - services should achieve the intended quality for the most economic use of resources

Equitable - aiming to improve everyone's access to information, focusing attention and benefits on those with the greatest needs

Accessible - everyone should be able to obtain services when and where they are needed

Appropriate - services will balance best professional practice with sensitivity to individual and group preferences

Responsive - services should address what people want and expect

---

[5] Maxwell, R J Quality assessment in health British Medical Journal 288, 1470-1472

[6] East Anglian Regional health Authority Health in perspective 1992/93: annual report Cambridge: EARHA, 1993

To work towards these objectives is obviously ambitious, but it would be entirely impossible without constant feedback from users. Involvement in organisational development has given lots of opportunities to get feedback , and has enabled me to respond to many needs expressed by the staff.

These are, then, very interesting times. The work which I do has broadened considerably from that which I thought I was appointed to do. I think this is because a willingness to try new roles and to motivate others to develop the organisation are valuable to that organisation, and senior management would like to benefit from that energy wherever it is in the staff. Librarians do not just have technical knowledge and experience, but also have many other skills and valuable experience which often seem to be overlooked. In the case of our new organisation, which has been self-consciously considering its internal development, the roles were made explicit, and the experience was there to be taken. While time constraints mean that my Library services are inevitably less developed than they would be if I had spent all my time working on those, I hope that my organisation development role, and my involvement in the many changes which are continuously taking place, have tied my professional work more closely to the objectives, the staff and the policy-makers of my part of the National Health Service.

IMPORTANCE OF HOSPITAL LIBRARY FACILITIES TO CLINICAL DECISION-MAKING BY MEDICAL STAFF

M Casado Uriguen, M A Garcia Martin, P M La Torre, M I Montes del Olmo, T Mas Vilardell, M F Ribes Cot, [For correspondence] Biblioteca Hospital Universitario "Marques de Valdecilla, ave de Valdecilla s/n 39008, Santander, Espana

Annual budgets for hospital library services in Spain are beginning to show a series of restrictions which present a threat to the relative well-being over the last few years of library services and collections, which have not in any case reached minimum internationally accepted standards. It must be borne in mind that as regards structure and planning. Spanish hospital libraries present a lack of organization which, as mentioned, fails to reach minimum standards. Nevertheless, these libraries provide a professionally interested and concerned human network, involved in a series of activities aimed at providing the use with a fast, efficient, and relevant service at reasonable cost. Those of us involved are concerned about the future of our library services and aim to demonstrate the importance of these services within the global context of hospital and, in particular, in the day-to-day work of the physician.

Methodology

In order to evaluate the importance of hospital libraries to clinical decision-making by medical staff, a survey was sent to all doctors at five Spanish University Hospitals: Cruces Hospital (Bilbao), Basurto Hospital (Bilbao), Virgen del Rocio Hospital (Sevilla), Santa Creu i San Pau Hospital (Barcelona) and Marques de Valdecilla Hospital (Santander). These five Hospitals all have over one thousand beds and provide training programmes for Medical Residents. Table 1 shows the characteristics of participating Libraries.

Table 1 Selected characteristics of participating hospital libraries

HOSPITALS	BOOKS	JOURNALS	ON-LINE	CD-ROM	LIBRARIANS	SUPPORT STAFF
Cruces	3000	800	Yes	Yes	1	3
Basurto	1387	395	No	Yes	3	0
Valdecilla	6900	593	Yes	Yes	1	3
San Pau	9208	350	Yes	Yes	2	1
V Rocio	8000	332	No	Yes	1	6

The design of the questionnaire was based on the Rochester report. We also used the survey designed by Wolff and Benson, as this included concepts which coincided with our interest in whether physicians consider that new technologies in library services improve access to information necessary for clinical decision-making. In the first place, the aim was to assess the degree to which information obtained by physicians from the library influences clinical decision-making, but we also took the opportunity to investigate through the survey which sources are used most and valued most by the user.

Results

A total of 3877 questionnaires were sent, of which 799 (20%) were returned. The percentage of replies received according to professional status was: Senior medical staff 27.6%, Physicians 51% and Residents 20.3%. Table II shows the results of the survey.

TABLE II Items selected as a percentage of the total for each question. In questions 1, 7, 8 and 12, only one item can be selected; the other questions allow several items to be selected.

1. FREQUENCY OF USE OF THE LIBRARY	
- Daily	4.1
- Weekly	38.9
- Fortnightly	19.6
- Monthly	19.3
- Others	18.1

2. WHAT TYPE OF INFORMATION ARE YOU USUALLY LOOKING FOR?	
- Interpretation of signs and symptoms	27.4
- Differential diagnosis	58.1
- Treatment	60.5
- Drug information	25.5

3. AVOIDANCE OF ADVERSE EVENTS REPORTED BY PHYSICIANS	
- Hospital admission criteria	17.1
- Hospital acquired infection	25
- Additional tests	28.2
- Surgery	33.7
- Follow-up outpatients visits	40.1

4. IMPORTANCE OF THE DIFFERENT INFORMATION SOURCES	
- Library	78
- Diagnostic imaging	83
- Lab tests	78.7
- Discussion with colleagues	87

5. ASSESSMENTS OF CLINICAL VALUE OF INFORMATION BY PHYSICIANS	
- Accurate and relevant	81
- Better medical decisions	79.7
- Memory refresher	72
- Contributed to higher quality care	69.2
- Saved physicians time	49.3
- Substantiated prior knowledge	40.9

6. USE OF SELECTED INFORMATION SOURCES BY PHYSICIANS	Never	Always
- Textbooks	19.1	58.2
- Journals	2.9	90.7
- Indexes	27.9	39.3
- CD-Rom	14.3	65
- Online	42	12.3
- Others	33.4	6.2

7. IS THE INFORMATION PROVIDED BY THE LIBRARY USEFUL FOR YOUR CLINICAL DECISION-MAKING?	
- Yes	87.4
- No	12.6

8. FREQUENCY OF USE OF CD-ROM	
- Bimonthly	38.5
- Monthly	27.9
- Weekly	10.7
- Daily	0.4
- Others	22.5

9. AIM OF CD-ROM SEARCHES	
- Bibliographic search	66
- Read abstracts	49.4
- Author search	35.2

10. CD-ROM SEARCHES ADVANTAGES	
- Speed of searching	72.2
- Large collection of journals	43.7
- Updated information	51.1
- Convenience	26.9
- Availability	27.4

11. CD-ROM DISADVANTAGES	
- Time required to learn use	23.8
- Incorrect information	5.3
- Inability to read the text	5.4

12. DO YOU THINK THAT CD-ROM IS USEFUL FOR CLINICAL DECISION MAKING	
- Yes	86.2
- No	13.8

Discussion

The principal aim of our study was to develop a method for analysing the service offered by the Hospital Library to its users, with a view to establishing the fundamental role of library-obtained information to clinical decision making and day-to-day patient care, and demonstrating the importance of the library to the Hospital Authorities responsible for funding. Several authors have emphasised that at present the most important line of investigation for Hospital Libraries is undoubtedly the analysis of the impact of the library on clinical decision-making and the measurement of its direct contribution to health-care. The results of our survey show that for doctors at the five hospitals studied, and in particular for hospital physicians, the hospital library provides information which is useful in improving patient care, in agreement with the results of the Chicago and Rochester reports. Moreover, the library provides an information service which is an integral part of the day-to-day work of the doctor, on a par with discussion with colleagues and laboratory tests. The areas for which information was most frequently sought, treatment and diagnostic interpretation, coincide with Woolf and Benson and also confirm our hypothesis as to the decisive role of the library in patient care and clinical decision-making.

It is important to note that medical journals are the most frequently consulted sources of information, followed by bibliographic indexes and above all CD-ROM, which provides the doctor with a frequently-used and positively-value service, despite the negative opinion about the time required to learn how to use the system. This suggest that we should continue training users in computer-search, and computer system designers should develop more user friendly products.

In order to safeguard the future of hospital libraries and to protect existing facilities, we need to demonstrate that the library is an integral and essential part of the daily work of the professionals involved in health care. How can we establish the necessary symbiosis between the user and the library, and provide the facilities of this interaction? By creating individualised reference services, streamlining interlibrary loans, continually improving and updating by collection and, if necessary, restructuring the library to meet the needs of the hospital staff. It is important to remember that is in fact the medical staff who are best able to demonstrate to the Hospital Authorities the important role of the library in improving the quality of patient care and clinical decision-making. For this reason the use of the library services should be periodically measured and analysed, and the results made available to the management so that they can evaluate the impact of these services on the quality of patient care. It is our view that the demonstration of the impact of the hospital library service on clinical-decision making is one of the most important responsibilities of the professional librarian.

Acknowledgements

The authors gratefully acknowledge the support of Ms J G Marshall, who provision of the Questionnaire was fundamental to this study.

Bibliography

- Woolf SH, Benson DA. The medical information needs of internists and pediatricians at an academic medical centre. Bull Med Lib Assoc. 1989. 77(4). P372-80.
- Marshall JG. The impact of the hospital library on clinical decision making: the Rochester study. Bull Med Libr Assoc. 1992. 80(2). P169-78.
- Joynt RJ, Marshall JG, McClure LW. Financial threats to hospital libraries (letter). JAMA. 1991. 4. 266(9). P1219-20.
- Veenstra RJ. Clinical medical librarian impact on patient care: a one-year analysis. Bull Med Libr Assoc. 1992. 80(1). P19-22.
- Scura G, Davidoff F. Case-related use of the medical literature. Clinical librarian services for improving patient care. JAMA. 1981. 2. 245(1). P50-2.
- Webster Fuscher W, Reel LB. Total quality management (TQM) in a hospital library: identifying service benghmarks. Bull Med Libr Assoc. 1992. 80(4). P347-352.
- Brandon AN, Hill DR, etal. Selected list of books and journals for the small medical library. Bull Med Libr Asso 1993. 81(2). P141-193.

LES BIBLIOTHEQUES MEDICALES FACE A DES SERVICES NOUVEAUX ET DES ROLES NOUVEAUX : Evaluation à partir d'un exemple celui de la Bibliothèque Interuniversitaire de Médecine de Paris

Madame Pierrette Casseyre, Biblliothèque Interuniversitaire de Médecine, 75270 Paris Cedex 06, France

Résumé

Les nouveaux services mis à disposition dans les bibliothèques médicales, grâce aux nouveaux supports de l'information, tant bibliographiques que catalographiques, ont incité la Bibliothèque Interuniversitaire de Médecine à tenter de faire une évaluation des services rendus et des besoins exprimés. L'introduction de nouvelles technologies, les demandes des médecins, la veille documentaire ont entraîné dans toutes les bibliothèques médicales de nouveaux services et l'émergence de rôles nouveaux. La Bibliothèque Interuniversitaire de Médecine (B. I. U. M.), centre d'acquisitions et de diffusion de l'information scientifique (CADIST) pour la médecine en France, a essayé de faire une évaluation de tous ces nouveaux besoins et de ces nouveaux services. L'inadéquation d'anciens locaux à un libre accès, alors que la richesse de ses collections en cours est incomparable (plus de 4500 titres de périodiques courants), l'ont incité à s'interroger sur le maintien de la qualité et les services nouveaux qu'elle peut promouvoir. Le rôle de Centre Français d'Acquisitions et de Diffusion de l'Information Scientifique et Technique pour le domaine biomédical donne une spécificité très forte à la Bibliothèque Interuniversitaire de Médecine. De ce fait elle s'est vu allouer une subvention particulière, en 1994, de 1.840.000 F., en plus du budget de fonctionnement.

Grâce à cette subvention, de nouveaux abonnements sont pris, et des achats d'ouvrages étrangers effectués. Beaucoup de bibliothèques médicales en province demandent à la B. I. U. M. l'achat d'ouvrages étrangers onéreux. La mission de la B. I. U. M. est ainsi remplie, c'est-à-dire acquérir non seulement en faveur de son propre fonds mais pour aider les autres bibliothèques médicales. Le rôle de veille documentaire est de ce fait très important, surtout en ce qui concerne les acquisitions de nouveaux périodiques (environ une centaine par an). Sont pris en compte divers indicateurs : parution dans les bases de données, (impact factor, développement de certaines spécialités). Le problème se pose quand le périodique vient juste de paraître et qu'on ne connaît pas encore son impact. Faut-il s'abonner ? Si non, sera-t-il possible de récupérer ultérieurement le début de la collection? Le problème des périodiques étant crucial en médecine (90% des communications concernent les périodiques), la B. I. U. M. a porté ses efforts en priorité sur ce secteur.

Les lecteurs ont maintenant à leur disposition dix postes de consultation pour l'interrogation de notre catalogue en ligne de périodiques. Cet OPAC se caractérise par l'introduction des abréviations des titres de périodiques adoptées par les différentes bases de données. En fait, ce sont toujours les informations que possède le lecteur, et non les titres développés des périodiques. Une évaluation de l'OPAC a été faite auprès d'un échantillon de 300 lecteurs ; ceux-ci trouvent à 87%, la consultation très performante ou performante. Les deux critères de performance retenus, c'est-à-dire le gain de temps par rapport au catalogue papier et la facilité d'utilisation ont obtenu 68% et 58%, et ces chiffres atteindraient respectivement 91% et 92% si l'on englobait les réponses "assez de temps", "assez facile". La consultation très aisée de ce catalogue, la rapidité de réponse ont eu une conséquence sur le nombre de communications demandées en un an ; cinq mille demandes supplémentaires ont été effectuées.

La mise sur informatique des statistiques de communications de périodiques tant dans la salle que par le prêt entre bibliothèques nous permet de connaître la circulation des titres de périodiques. Chaque mois le palmarés des titres les plus demandés est constitué. Les deux circuits sont complètement différents, et les titres demandés en prêt inter par d'autres bibliothèques totalement différents de ceux empruntés en salle. L'évaluation des titres de périodiques demandés en salle nous permet donc de voir si les nouveaux abonnements correspondent bien aux demandes des lecteurs. L'importance du prêt entre bibliothèques (63 000 demandes traitées par an) entraîne à une réflexion sur la nécessité ou non d'avoir le système ADONIS au niveau de notre prêt entre bibliothèques. Cela permettrait une usure moindre de nos documents, un déplacement moins important en magasins, une manipulation réduite.

Les demandes de plus en plus fréquentes de télécopies nous ont incité à réfléchir sur le coût pour l'utilisateur. En effet, si la B. I. U. M. est très équipée au point de vue qualité de photocopieur, il n'en est pas de même de toutes les bibliothèques médicales. Les qualités des télécopies sont souvent médiocres, et le surcroît de prix demandé au lecteur pour une télécopie est difficilement admis malgré la rapidité de l'obtention du document. Comme dans toutes les bibliothèques médicales, l'arrivée des réseaux de CD-ROM bibliographiques a révolutionné la manière de travailler tant pour les bibliothécaires que pour les lecteurs. Jusqu'alors, les recherches en ligne se faisaient sur rendez-vous, tout au moins dans toutes les bibliothèques médicales françaises. Il était alors relativement possible de planifier le service des recherches bibliographiques. La mise en place des CD-ROM en libre accès a complètement transformé le service de références bibliographiques. Il est indéniable que, pour l'instant encore, tant que l'antiserveur ne sera pas généralisé, le lecteur ne sait pas utiliser seul les CD-ROM, malgré les menus très assistés, malgré les conseils écrits près des postes de travail. Il ne sait pas pourquoi choisir la recherche sur BIOSIS plutôt que sur MEDLINE, et surtout ne sait pas utiliser les thesaurus. En effet, quoique l'interrogation en langage naturel soit possible, étant donné l'importance des synonymes en médecine, de nombreuses références échappent à cette interrogation.

Tous les conservateurs et bibliothécaires passent désormais plus de temps en service public. Car il y a une assistance constante à l'interrogation des CD-ROM de 10 h à 18 h. Ceci a nécessité une formation très poussée à l'interrogation, de tous les conservateurs et bibliothécaires faisant des permanences dans la salle. Jusqu'alors, seules 4 personnes faisaient l'interrogation des bases de données en ligne. Du fait des réseaux de CD-ROM installés près du bureau de références, en libre-accès, il a fallu modifier tout le service public. Pour l'instant, il y a gratuité totale de l'impression. Certaines bibliothèques médicales ont déjà commencé à facturer ces nouveaux services. Pour l'instant, le problème primordial à résoudre est la liste d'attente aux CD-ROM, le fait même de la gratuité incite à demander à nos lecteurs de ne pas dépasser le temps qui leur est imparti pour la consultation (30 minutes). Cette restriction est, à vrai dire, rarement respectée si le lecteur est livré à lui même ; l'aide du bibliothécaire est alors capitale.

La B. I. U. M. a commencé a réaliser des dossiers de presse sur des sujets très précis, à la pointe de l'actualité médicale. Il est encore trop tôt pour faire une évaluation de ce nouveau service. Jusqu'alors, ce rôle était dévolu aux centres de documentation privés, les bibliothèques, ayant un rôle d'acquisition, de mise à disposition des ouvrages et des périodiques, des bibliographies. Il y a donc eu un nouveau service offert, donc une nouvelle activité créée. La B. I. U. M. travaille actuellement à réaliser un catalogue de congrès répertoriant à la fois ouvrages et dépouillement de périodiques, puisqu'un grand nombre de congrès parait dans les périodiques. La B. I. U. M. catalogue déjà sur un réseau : SIBIL, différent du réseau OCLC. Mais la lourdeur du catalogue ou tout au moins du signalement des congrès dans ces réseaux par rapport aux besoins des lecteurs qui recherchent une entrée matière extrêmement simplifiée, une entrée par ville, par année, mots du titre nous ont amené à repenser complètement le service. Les congrès ouvrages vont rester catalogués dans le réseau. En outre , tous les congrès (y compris les ouvrages) apparaîtront sur un autre support traités grâce à un logiciel documentaire extrêmement simple qui nous permettra d'éditer à l'intention des toutes les bibliothèques médicales françaises un catalogue annuel un peu ressemblant à celui de la B. L. D. S. C. pour la médecine.

En fait, la meilleure évaluation d'une bibliothèque est liée à la satisfaction du public. En ce qui concerne la B. I. U. M. l'inadéquation des locaux à un libre accès aux documents nous pousse à être de plus en plus performant dans l'aide apportée aux lecteurs. Les bibliothèques médicales, sont souvent considérées comme "atypiques" pour les autres bibliothèques, car les besoins très particuliers de leurs lecteurs les poussent à aborder des solutions originales s'écartant souvent des sentiers battus traditionnels en bibliothèques. Il est parfois difficile d'obtenir des crédits sur tel ou tel projet ne rentrant pas dans un cadre bibliothéconomique établi et bien connu. Mais cela n'empêche pas en général les bibliothèques médicales de progresser pour, je crois, la plus grande satisfaction de leur public.

USER NEEDS, SERVICES AND COLLECTION: A strategic triangle for the Library KNAW

R. Brandsma, Library KNAW, P.O. Box 41950, 1009 DD Amsterdam, The Netherlands

Abstract

By means of two user surveys the Library of the Royal Netherlands Academy of Arts and Sciences (KNAW) involved the users in the development of services. The results are described. Libraries can maintain their position by strongly improving their processes for document delivery. Other types of services have to be developed in cooperation with users.

In which way do libraries have to improve their services? What is the opinion of users about the development of services? In this lecture I will treat these questions through our experiences at the Library of the Royal Netherlands Academy of Arts and Sciences (Library KNAW). The Library KNAW is the national focal point library in the Netherlands for the medical and natural sciences. The library has approximately 10,000 current periodicals and serial publications in the fields of medicine, pharmacology, biology and chemistry. The main service of the Library KNAW is document delivery to other libraries, private persons or companies. Document delivery means: delivery of photocopies of articles by mail or lending to customers issues of journals and copies of books. Apart from our Dutch customers we receive requests from 58 foreign countries. In 1993 the Library KNAW received a total number of 190,000 requests. Special services are on-line literature searches and information on current research. 42 % of the requests for documents at our library are received electronically through an automated system created by PICA. The other part (58 %) of the requests for documents are received mostly by post. By means of two different user surveys we involved our customers in the development of our services. The first inquiry was a questionnaire which was send to a random sample of users of the Library KNAW. A second inquiry was started by visiting the most important clients for an interview. The aim was to have more data about our users. To get their opinion about the quality of our services. To examine their needs for new services. The purpose is to supply the optimal package of products and services.

1. Questionnaire

With the questionnaire we collected data concerning external and paying clients. The Library KNAW aimed the questionnaire at all her external users in the Netherlands. Among these are intensive and occasional users, organizations and private persons. This part of the population included 3000 user addresses. By means of a random sample questionnaires were send to 600 addresses. 304 forms were returned. This means a response of 51%. I will start with the results concerning the user categories (Table 1). For the improvement of the services it's useful to gain insight in the categories to which the users belong.

Table 1. Categories of users in %

Companies	22%
Research institutes and universities	23%
Hospitals	19%
Private persons	23%
Remaining government institutions	13%

Which services of the Library KNAW are used by these users? It appears that 90 % of the respondents made use of our document delivery services and only 15% of special services. On the whole companies react most positively to future services. To know which type of document is the first choice, several questions were asked about this subject. The results clearly show that journal articles are by far the most requested type of document. As a consequence the emphasis of the collection building will be put on journals. Specific questions have been asked about the reasons why the users order documents from our library. The 'nature of the collection' (32%), 'only place where the document is available' (32%) and 'speed of delivery' (30%) are the number-one-criteria.

What is the users' opinion about the quality of the document delivery?

Table 2. Quality document delivery in %

	unsatis-factory	satis-factory	good
Shipment document quality	0	38	62
Speed of delivery	5	40	55
Satisfaction rate articles	5	40	55
Copy quality	7	40	53
Satisfaction rate books	8	49	43
Clarity invoice	13	50	37

The users are generally satisfied with the quality of the document delivery (Table 2). The invoicing is valued much lower. As a consequence the invoice has been improved. On the whole 40 % of the respondents valued the aspects of document delivery as 'satisfactory' and 50% as 'good'. However in our opinion the services have to be improved, to enhance the percentage 'good' in the future. The question remained which aspect of document delivery we had to improve. The answer is based on the enormous amount of requested copies of journal articles and the no 1 criteria 'speed of delivery' to choose for our library. Because of these facts our library has to raise the 'satisfaction rate of articles' and the 'speed of delivery'. Another important part of the questionnaire was the feasibility of eleven future services at the Library KNAW. The users could indicate wether they were interested in a particular future service or not. It was clearly stated that all future services should be payed for. They all raised some interest. Four were particulary favourite (Table 3). Three of these four services deal with document delivery. There was moderate or less interest for the rest of the services (Table 4).

Table 3. Use of future services in % (favourite).

	Yes/possible	No
-Document delivery within 24 hours	69	31
-List of documents on specific subject from catalogue Library KNAW	63	37
-Delivery of not available documents through other suppliers	52	48
-Prompt delivery relevant documents from on-line searches	52	48

Table 4. Use of future services in % (moderate/less).

	Yes/possible	No
Tailor made review reports	49	51
Table of contents of journals	48	52
of new books and journals	44	56
Document delivery within 2 hours	40	60
Training courses in information searching	38	62
Advice scientific literature	33	67
Advice indexing systems	28	72

If the results are considered in general, it's memorable that almost all the favoured services deal with document delivery. Other types of services appear to awaken less interest.

2. Interviews

The interviews were held during visits to our most important customers. Among our users a group exists which use our services very frequently. These users, selected on the basis of the number of requests, were interviewed. The group included 38 librarians or information-managers. In the interviews questions were asked about their interest in a number of new and future services as described by us. We also asked for their suggestions about future services. The results of the interviews indicate that electronic networks will become very important. Users should be able to retrieve and order documents in catalogues through networks. Users should also be able to send through networks, files with lists of references for batch-ordering. For batch-ordering, libraries ought to accept all kinds of reference formats from on-line or CD-rom databases. Another interesting subject was the electronic delivery of full text articles with pictures. For the near future users like the idea of electronic document delivery, but fear high prices.

3. Conclusion

So far I have talked about the results separately, but what can we learn from both surveys? We can learn that libraries have to follow two directions for the development of services. One important direction is the improvement of the service 'document delivery'. But to avoid total dependence on document delivery, libraries have to make efforts to develop other types of services. Both surveys prove that there is a slight interest in services, which are not based on document delivery. To increase interest, libraries have to develop these services in close cooperation with individuals or groups of users. An example is the development of a 'Registration System on Current Medical Research' at the Library KNAW in cooperation with a government commission, which gives advice on the amount of money medical research groups should get. Meanwhile the main reason for using a library today is the reliability of a guaranteed delivery of documents. The surveys show what the user in search of biomedical information especially wants. He wants a not too expensive, readable photocopy of an scientific article on his desk within 3 days.

The delivery of photocopies of articles is therefore an important service of libraries, which can not be neglected. Libraries can maintain this market by strongly improving their processes for the delivery of copies of articles Fast and guaranteed delivery are the objectives. Otherwise publishers and subscription agents will take over this market by commercial document delivery services. Libraries can have a head-start on publishers and subscription agents by knowing their users and the services they want. Libraries also form the link between users and information sources. They can reproduce data about the use of specific journal titles. These figures can be used for the building of user orientated collections. This provides them with a position of knowledge which every publisher will envy. Summarized, the strength of libraries is: their knowledge about the relations between 'services','collection' and 'user needs'. These relations form a strategic triangle for libraries. Libraries will be successful by knowing the users needs.

LE ROLE D'UNE BIBLIOTHEQUE SCIENTIFIQUE DANS L'EVALUATION DE LA RECHERCHE DANS LE CADRE D'UN INSTITUT SCIENTIFIQUE POUR L'HOSPITALISATION ET LES SOINS (ISTITUTO DI RICOVERO E CURA A CARATTERE SCIENTIFICO).

M Curti, C Klersy, C Tinelli, S Visentin. Dir. Scientifique IRCCS Hôpital S. Matteo 27100 Pavia, Italia

Résumé
Quantifier et peser les résultats de la Recherche Scientifique apparait être une charge organisative complexe et difficile. Ce travail présente le rôle d'une Bibliothèque Biomédicale dans l'analyse et l'évaluation de la production scientifique en temps qu'indicateur de la Recherche. En particulier seront décrits les aspects méthodologiques utilisés pour évaluer qui a "publié" (analyse par chercheur, par Service ou Institut) ou quels sont les sujets traités (analyse par secteur ou thème de Recherche).

Introduction
Les horizons ouverts par les innovations technologiques font attendre des changements dans le rôle même des Bibliothèques Scientifiques: à côté des nouveaux instruments pour la recherche bibliographique et la documentation scientifique (banques de données en ligne, sur cd-rom, banques de données full-test, etc.), nous trouvons d'intéressantes nouvelles branches d'activité: les services audiovisuels, les multimédia, les services pour la réalisation de présentations scientifiques (Palette, cd kodak, retouches de photos), les téléconférences, etc. Mais parmi ces rôles potentiels et innovatifs, nous tenons à nous arrêter sur celui représenté par l'analyse et l'évaluation de la Recherche. Il s'agit d'un aspect organisatif des plus importants et difficiles. Le manque de moyens plus ou moins chronique d'une part, et les coûts de plus en plus élevés de la Recherche Scientifique d'autre part, font que l'attribution de fonds doive se faire sur la base des résultats obtenus et sur ceux qui sont prévus. Or, si la quantification des ressources affectées est simple à définir (coûts du personnel, de la technologie, du materiel, etc.), la mesure des résultats, leur évaluation quali-quantitative et l'évaluation de l'efficience et de l'efficacité est bien plus complexe. Une méthode indirecte d'évaluation est représentée par l'analyse de la production scientifique: la presse spécialisée, moyen de diffusion fondamental des résultats scientifiques, peut aussi être regardée comme le moyen approprié pour leur qualification et quantification. La revue sur laquelle les travaux scientifiques sont publiés est généralement synonyme de qualité: la reconnaissance internationale, l'inclusion dans des index tels que Index Medicus ou Science Citation Index, la diffusion de la revue et la quantification (Impact Factor) du nombre de fois où les travaux qui y sont publiés, sont à leur fois cités dans d'autres articles publiés sur des revues indexées, représentent des indicateurs bibliométriques parmi les plus utilisés dans le monde scientifique.

Buts
La Direction Scientifique de l'IRCCS-Policlinico S.Matteo de Pavie est chargée, de par sa fonction officielle, de l'organisation de la Recherche dans l'Hôpital. A partir du moment où le Ministère de la Santé Italien affecte à l'hôpital les fonds pour la Recherche, la Direction Scientifique doit activer les nouveaux projets en leur attribuant les ressources parvenues; ceci implique nécessairement de faire des choix. En d'autres termes il s'agit de décider si privilégier telle équipe, tel service, tel chercheur plutôt que tel autre, ou encore, si privilegier un secteur ou un sujet de Recherche par rapport aux autres. Le but de cet article est de présenter et de discuter le rôle de la Bibliothèque Scientifique et les aspects de la méthode qui a été mise au point pour l'évaluation de la production scientifique de l'Institut afin de définir des indicateurs qui serviraient à "choisir" les meilleurs projets et/ou les meilleurs chercheurs.

Matériel et méthode
Le point de départ étant que la qualité d'un article scientifique va de même avec la qualité de la revue sur lequel celui-ci a été publié, nous avons vérifié combien et quelle production scientifique de l'Hôpital San Matteo a paru sur des journaux scientifiques classés dans des index bibliographiques qualifiés et acceptés universellement par le monde scientifique, comme Medline et Science Citation Index (versions sur cd-rom). Les cd-rom consultés ont été: 1) Medline disquette annuelle 1992 et janvier-avril 1993 et 2) Science Citation Index disquette annuelle 1992. Les mots clefs utilisés ont été: 1) dans le champ auteurs: Nom et initiale du prénom des chercheurs du IRCCS et 2) année de

publication = 1992 (Le cd-rom janvier-avril 1993 de Medline a été consulté afin de réduire au maximum les pertes d'information sur les publications de 1992 et mises sur ordinateur début 1993). L'identification certaine des articles publiés par les chercheurs du IRCCS a requis, malgré l'utilisation de mots clefs nominatifs dans la phase de recherche, un contrôle capillaire des nombreuses homonymies. Les informations sur les auteurs, le titre, la revue, et les notes bibliographiques des travaux sélectionnés ont été ensuite insérées dans une base de données créée à ce but et intégrée avec les variables suivantes:

1) Le service d'origine (champ multiple) de chaque auteur à l'intérieur de l'Hôpital; afin de garder une correspondence biunivoque avec celui-ci, le champ des auteurs a été transformé lui-même en champ multiple;
2) l'Impact Factor (IF) - année 1992. Pour chaque revue, l'IF correspondra au nombre de fois, en moyenne, que les articles de cette revue particulière, publiés au cours des deux années précédentes (dans notre cas 1990 et 1991), ont été cités dans d'autres articles publiés au cours de l'année en examen (1992 dans notre cas) par les autres revues du Science Citation Index. Il représente en fait l'importance qu'un certain journal a pour le monde scientifique;
3) un champ multiple qui reporte les disciplines dans lesquelles est classée la revue (le "Subject Category" du Science Citation Index). Le choix du champ multiple est dû à la possibilité qu'a une revue de paraÎtre sous plusieurs disciplines (par exemple le journal: Am. J. of Tropical Medicine and Hygiene est classé dans la discipline "public health" ainsi que dans celle "tropical medicine");
4) un champ multiple lié au précédent, qui attribue au journal de publication et pour chaque discipline où celui-ci est présent, une score dérivé du IF; celui-ci est défini comme impact factor indexé (IFI) et il représente le quotient (multiplié par 100) du IF du journal de publication et de celui du journal le mieux coté dans la même discipline. Le but de l'indexation est de rendre uniforme l'unité de mesure afin de permettre de comparer les scores obtenus dans des disciplines différentes. De cette façon toutes les revues placées au premier rang de chaque discipline auront une valeur de IFI par discipline de 100, indépendemment de la valeur absolue du IF. Les revues classées à un rang inférieur auront des points IFI proportionellement inférieurs à 100. Le différent poids de la même revue dans deux secteurs d'intérêt scientifique différents est mis ainsi en évidence.

Résultats

L'anayse qui s'en est découlée, avait pour but la constitution de classements de la production scientifique à utiliser comme indicateurs de qualité des résultats de la Recherche. Ceux-ci ont été calculés aussi bien par chercheur, que par service, que par discipline scientifique.

Analyse par auteur: Tous les auteurs ont un même poids, indépendant du fait d'être à la première ou à la dernière place, d'être à 10 ou seul auteur. Une première analyse a été faite en comptant le nombre d'articles par auteur; dans ce cas toutes les revues avaient le même poids et la note finale exprime le nombre total de publications faites. Dans une deuxième analyse, chaque auteur a été doté de la valeur de IF du journal dans lequel il a publié. Les deux méthodes sont criticables, car tandis que la première rend uniforme le poids, la seconde fait ressortir des différences énormes due aux variations de IF que l'on observe au passage d'une discipline à l'autre. Pour cette raison, le système de score basé sur le IF uniquement, sera considéré correct seulement si la comparaison entre auteurs se fait à l'intérieur d'une même discipline: la comparaison des 45.12 points obtenus par le dr XY dans la discipline "public health" avec les 30.50 points du dr YZ a un sens, tandis que ces derniers ne peuvent être comparés avec les 20.15 points obtenus par le dr KK dans la discipline "anesthesiology".

Analyse par service d'origine: Un score a été attribuée à chacun des services intéressés par la publication scientifique. Celui-ci sera la même pour tous, indépendemment du nombre de chercheurs du service ayant contribué à l'article. Dans ce cas aussi nous avons effectué deux analyses différentes. La première se base sur le simple décompte des travaux publiés. La seconde fait appel aux points de IF de la revue de publication. Les deux méthodes présentent les limites citées ci-dessus; il ne semble donc pas correct d'utiliser ces scores pour comparer deux services entre eux. L'utilisation du IF se révèle valable uniquement si la comparaison a lieu à l'intérieur d'une même discipline. C'est le cas par example d'un score réalisé par le Service A et d'un score réalisé par le Service B dans le cadre de la discipline "tropical medicine".

Analyse par discipline: L'analyse par discipline est différente des précédentes en ce qu'elle permet d'évaluer le comportement d'un auteur ou d'un service dans le cadre de plusieurs disciplines; les deux autres méthodes ne consentaient par contre que l'analyse et la comparaison de la productivité de plusieurs auteurs ou services à l'intérieur d'une seule discipline; nous avons vu comment un score de IF peut représenter un bon indicateur tant qu'on se limite à une discipline à la fois. Lorsque l'intérêt se porte sur la comparaison de la production scientifique dans plusieurs disciplines il est bon d'utiliser l'IFI. Cet indicateur permet de mettre en évidence si un auteur ou un service a été plus productif dans une ou l'autre discipline.

Discussion et conclusions

La Recherche d'indicateurs capables de décrire avec fidélité et de synthétiser les résultats de l'activité scientifique n'est pas un problème avec une solution évidente. La méthode d'analyse et d'évaluation ici décrite présente elle-même des limitations dont il faut tenir compte: 1) le IF, par exemple, n'est pas calculé pour toutes les revues scientifiques, mais seulement pour celles qui sont citées au Science Citation Index. Ces dernières représentent toutefois les plus importantes et les plus répandues dans le monde scientifique; 2) les revues du SCI analysent surtout la litérature en langue anglaise (considérée cependant comme la langue la plus importante dans le monde scientifique); 3) une bonne partie de la litérature "grise" et d'autres formes de production scientifique (posters, comunications aux congrès, etc.) ne sont pas considérées dans cette analyse; il est vrai aussi, que l'apport qualitatif de ces travaux est d'importance limitée; 4) la valeur du IF est influencée non seulement par l'importance scientifique du journal de publication (importance plus grande, citations plus nombreuses) mais aussi par sa diffusion (diffusion plus grande, citations plus nombreuses) et par le sujet traité (discipline plus vaste, plus de revues, plus de citations). Ces limites, comme nous l'avons vu, sont en parties dépassées par l'indexation (IFI); 5) le score de IF ou IFI attribué à l'auteur ou au service d'origine ne l'a pas été sur la base des citations de ses propres travaux, mais sur la base des citations de tous les articles publiés sur le journal en question; 6) l'intervalle de temps sur lequel construire les indicateurs devrait être supérieur à un an, étant donné que les retombées d'un article scientifique sont à plus long terme.

Il faut enfin signaler que d'autres méthodes d'analyse et d'évaluation, complémentaires de celle que nous présentons ici, peuvent être et doivent être utilisées en bibliométrie, comme l'analyse des citations. Cette technique permet en effet de vérifier à long terme la retombée de l'article publié non plus sur la base des citations du jounal, mais sur la base des citations de l'article même. Naturellement les indicateurs bibliographiques ne sont pas les seuls à devoir être tenus en compte pour la définition des fonds pour la Recherche; il doivent en effet être accompagnés par d'autres indicateurs, tels que le nombre de chercheurs par service, l'existence de projets déjà en cours ou en train de se définir, le potentiel de développement du service, les investissements éventuels déjà effectués et qui doivent être renforcés, etc.

Ceci dit, la description de l'activité scientifique se fondant sur le IF et sur le IFI, peut être considérée comme une méthode robuste, à même d'identifier les aspects les plus importants de la Recherche effectuée, mais surtout de jouer le rôle "d'indicateur" que nous lui avions attribué: mettre en évidence non pas combien un auteur ou un service a produit, mais qui a le mieux travaillé et dans quelle discipline, ou encore quelle discipline ou quel secteur de Recherche a fait le plus de progrès et mérite d'être soutenu. De cette façon la Bibliothèque Scientifique acquiert un rôle précis et influent dans l'évaluation de la Recherche; elle se propose comme un instrument fondamental pour tous ceux qui doivent décider combien, comment et où investir dans la Recherche.

THE COCHRANE COLLABORATION: Electronic Publication of Systematic Reviews of Randomized Controlled Trials (Rcts) in Health Care As A Contribution to Evidence-Based Decision Making

Carol Lefebvre, UK Cochrane Centre, Summertown Pavilion, Middle Way,Oxford OX2 7LG, UK.

The Rationale for Systematic Reviews

Clinicians and policy-makers are increasingly turning to reviews rather than primary research for information to guide decision-making. Reviews are necessary because of the continuing "explosion" in the primary literature, and the difficulty of accessing some primary material. In addition reviews can "create" new evidence. The combination and synthesis of the results of smaller studies can provide answers to questions which have not otherwise been adequately answered by the individual results of small studies. Sound decisions about health care must be based on as high a proportion as possible of the available evidence. For example, a systematic review a decade ago of all the available randomized controlled trials of corticosteroids would have shown that a short course of this inexpensive treatment substantially reduces the risk of neonatal morbidity and death when given to women expected to give birth prematurely. For many years this evidence was not taken into account, and consequently tens of thousands of babies suffered unnecessarily and neonatal care has been more expensive than it need have been.

Are all reviews equally suitable for informing decision-making? Unfortunately, the quality of reviews is often poor, and reviewers do not always strive to be comprehensive in gathering and assessing all relevant data. The poor quality of most reviews has meant that advice on some highly-effective forms of health care has been delayed for many years, and that other forms of care have been recommended long after research has shown them to be either ineffective or harmful. Good quality reviews are being recognized in many different quarters as the way forward for the future. The editor of the BMJ wrote the following comments in the "Editor's choice" section of the BMJ in January 1994, when the journal published a major systematic review on the use of aspirin in cardiovascular disease[1].

> "...many clinical studies are of a low scientific standard. Ironically, our drive to raise our scientific standards has led us to exclude clinical papers that are case reports, uncontrolled series, non-randomised studies, surveys with low response rates, and trawls of case notes ... whether we have done the right thing to devote so many pages to the "aspirin papers" ... overviews that use individual patient data are likely to be the gold standard papers of the future."

Throughout my paper I shall refer to <u>systematic</u> reviews. What are systematic reviews and how do they differ from other reviews? The steps involved in conducting a systematic review are as follows: state the objectives of the review; outline the eligibility criteria; search for eligible studies; assess the quality of each study; apply the eligibility criteria and justify any exclusions; analyse the results of the eligible studies; prepare a structured report of the review, stating the aims, describing the materials and methods, and reporting the results. Systematic reviews are also known as overviews, and meta-analyses are systematic reviews (overviews) incorporating statistical synthesis of data.

The Cochrane Pregnancy and Childbirth Database

The Cochrane Pregnancy and Childbirth Database was first published in May 1993. It contains over 600 systematic reviews of RCTs and is compiled by a team of more than 30 specialists world-wide, including obstetricians, midwives, general practitioners and anaesthetists. Each review consists of the following four elements:

> a cover sheet indicating the title of that particular review; how to cite it; contact details for the reviewer and the editorial group of which they are a part, sources of funding support; and the date the review was last updated a structured report including the objective, criteria for the inclusion and exclusion of trials, comments on the quality of the trials included, the results of the review, implications for practice and implications for research, and the conclusions of the review data from the individual trials displayed both in tables and as graphs showing summary information in the form of meta-analyses where appropriate full bibliographic citations to all the reports of trials included in that particular review.

The database is updated twice-yearly as part of an annual subscription and costs £99 per annum for institutions and £57 for private individuals. The Cochrane Pregnancy and Childbirth Database is well advanced as a result of groundwork done over a period of more than 10 years by Iain Chalmers and his colleagues at the National Perinatal Epidemiology Unit in the UK. Progress within other specialties is encouraging, and systematic reviews in other areas -- notably Stroke, Subfertility and Cancer -- are expected during 1995. The Cochrane Database of Systematic Reviews will eventually provide evidence of the effects of care in all specialties.

Electronic publication offers two major advantages over print publication. First, reviews can be updated easily, not only as data from new trials become available, but also in the light of valid criticism by users of the reviews (thus extending the somewhat limited traditional peer-review process common to hard-copy journal publication). Second, electronic distribution of regular updates to the database is considerably more straightforward than distribution of hard-copy. As the database expands, it will be published on CD-ROM, and the text sections of the Cochrane Reviews will be made available over the INTERNET.

The Cochrane Collaboration

The activities described above are being undertaken within the framework of the Cochrane Collaboration. The Collaboration began with the opening of the UK Cochrane Centre in November 1992 as part of the English National Health Service Research and Development Programme. Financial support and encouragement soon followed from other parts of the United Kingdom and elsewhere throughout the world. Response from individuals has also been extremely encouraging. To reflect this world-wide interest and support together with the contribution of individuals based in other organizations we now refer to our activity as the Cochrane Collaboration. In addition to the enormous growth in individual interest, several other Cochrane Centres have opened elsewhere throughout the world.

Why Randomized Controlled Trials?

Randomized controlled trials (RCTs) have been chosen as the major source of evidence within the Cochrane Database of Systematic Reviews. In order to explain this it may be helpful to consider the following definitions based on Last's *Dictionary of Epidemiology*[2].

Randomization is defined as: ...allocation of individuals to groups, e.g. for experimental and control regimens, by chance. Within the limits of chance variation, randomization should make the control and experimental groups similar at the start of an investigation and ensure that personal judgement and prejudices of the investigator do not influence allocation...

Randomized controlled trials are defined as: ... experiments in which individuals in a population are randomly allocated into groups, usually called "study" and "control" groups, to receive or not to receive an experimental, preventive, or therapeutic procedure, manoeuvre, or intervention. The results are assessed by rigorous comparison rates of disease, death, recovery, or other appropriate outcome in the study and control groups, respectively. Randomized controlled trials are generally regarded as the most scientifically rigorous method of hypothesis testing available...

RCTs are not always necessary to provide reliable assessments of the effects of health care. The good and bad effects of some forms of health care are obvious. Sometimes trials are not feasible. For many, probably most forms of care, however, randomized controlled trials involving sufficient numbers of patients are essential to distinguish reliably between the effects of care and the effects of bias or chance.

Identification of Randomized Controlled Trials

In order to inform decision-making in a reliable way systematic reviews must be based on as high a proportion as possible of relevant RCTs. But how easy is it to identify RCTs, for example in MEDLINE? A recent review summarizes research over the past decade[3]. This has shown that of those reports of RCTs indexed in MEDLINE one can only expect to identify approximately 70%. There are several factors which contribute to this. First, if authors have not adequately described their research, indexers acting for the (US) National Library of Medicine (NLM) will not be able to index the reports satisfactorily. Until recently many authors did not appreciate the significance of describing their research methods adequately, and consequently many RCTs are not identifiable as such from the published reports.

Second, suitable terms must be available within the MeSH vocabulary to enable indexers to reflect a particular aspect of a report. MeSH is constantly updated to reflect developments in health care. Nevertheless, there is an unavoidable delay between the recognition of a new or important concept and the introduction of new terms into MeSH. No suitable descriptor term was available to describe randomization as a methodology until RANDOM-ALLOCATION was introduced in 1978. Thereafter a further descriptor term RANDOMIZED-CONTROLLED-TRIALS was introduced in 1990, together with RANDOMIZED-CONTROLLED-TRIAL as a Publication Type in 1991. Finally, even when suitable descriptor terms have been available, they have not always been consistently applied by NLM indexers. I recently carried out a study of the first six months of MEDLINE for 1993. I identified 432 reports of RCTs with the text-word "random" truncated (i.e. random, randomized, randomly etc.) in the title or abstract, which had not been indexed with any of the controlled vocabulary listed in the above paragraph. The abstracts included such phrases as "in a randomized, multicenter trial", "patients were then randomly assigned", "a randomized placebo-controlled study", and "double-blind placebo-controlled randomized clinical trial". The 432 reports described here were identified by searching for just one term in the title or abstract. How many more reports of RCTs would be identified by a similar search of the Methods section of the original article?

Progress is being made, however, in a number of ways to overcome these problems. First, many authors are now also end-user searchers of MEDLINE and are aware of the difficulties they themselves have faced in retrieving relevant articles. This influences the way in which they write their abstracts, which in turn facilitates the work of the indexers. Also, journal editors and publishers are assisting in the task through the adoption of structured abstracts and improvements in their instructions to authors. Second, with regard to MEDLINE indexing terms, NLM is involved in research which should lead to improvements in retrieval from MEDLINE using controlled vocabulary. Their Unified Medical Language System (UMLS) project to build a so-called Metathesaurus should eventually facilitate searching. More immediately, however, agreement was reached with NLM in December 1993 which will result in a new indexing term (CONTROLLED-CLINICAL-TRIAL as a Publication Type) being added to MeSH from January 1995. This term will be used to index controlled trials where the method of allocation to treatment or control cannot be described with certainty as being randomized. Third, and perhaps most importantly, the NLM is constantly striving to improve the efficiency of its indexing. Efforts have been made within the Indexing Section to make indexers aware of the importance of identifying RCTs. The Library believes that this has resulted in twice as many articles as previously being coded correctly as RCTs. In addition, the research described above (which revealed 432 reports of RCTs that had not been coded correctly despite obvious statements of randomization in the abstracts) also had a positive effect. I presented this evidence at a meeting last December attended by many of the senior staff from the NLM together with their colleagues from other sections of the US National Institutes of Health (NIH)[4]. The findings were well-received and quality control procedures have subsequently been introduced by NLM to prevent this in future. Furthermore, support and encouragement have been received from the Office of Medical Applications of Research of the NIH together with NLM for a project to identify as many RCTs as possible in MEDLINE which have not been coded as such. The NLM has agreed to amend MEDLINE retrospectively back to 1966 by adding the existing Publication Type RANDOMIZED-CONTROLLED-TRIAL and the new Publication Type CONTROLLED-CLINICAL-TRIAL to reports of trials identified by scanning MEDLINE records. I have designed a search strategy for optimal recall of RCTs and so far have run it against MEDLINE for the period 1985-1993. 100,000 records have been downloaded for that period, and the scanning process to identify trials is underway in Oxford, at the UK Cochrane Centre. References which are reports of RCTs will be forwarded electronically to the Baltimore Cochrane Centre in Maryland, USA for further processing and will then be forwarded to the NLM to be re-coded. It is hoped that the re-coding of this section of MEDLINE will be completed by the end of 1994.

The above findings relate specifically to MEDLINE. This is not to suggest, however, that other medical databases do not suffer from similar problems. Indeed, experience with EMBASE is likely to be worse than MEDLINE when we turn our attention to EMBASE, hopefully during 1995. Until the beginning of 1994 the EMBASE vocabulary had no suitable terms to differentiate RCTs from other clinical trials. Following a meeting convened by the UK Cochrane Centre in January 1993, Elsevier has now introduced new indexing terms for clinical trials, including the term RANDOMIZED-CONTROLLED-TRIAL, and has also undertaken to improve the consistency of indexing in this area, as outlined in a recent newsletter[5]. This is important progress, as EMBASE has a strong coverage of both European and pharmaceutical titles.

Despite considerable progress with MEDLINE and EMBASE it will still be necessary to search journals by hand back to c.1950 to identify those reports which have been missed by bibliographic database indexing. A grant of ECU 400,000 (c.£300,000) has been awarded by the European Commission under the BIOMED programme to co-ordinate the searching of general health care journals published throughout Europe. References to reports of trials are being gathered and will ultimately be made available by the NLM through MEDLINE, even for those journals which are not indexed for MEDLINE. The exact mechanism for this is still under discussion, but it will be an extremely important contribution to the identification of RCTs.

The Role of Health Care Librarians and Information Professionals

Medical and health care librarians have a major role to play in three key areas; assisting their clients in preparing systematic reviews based on all the available evidence, helping them to differentiate between good and poor quality reviews when searching for evidence for decision-making, and keeping up-to-date in respect of the availability of good quality reviews.

References

1 Smith R. What's wrong with the BMJ? BMJ 1994;308:69.
2 Last JM (ed). A Dictionary of Epidemiology, 2nd ed. Oxford: OUP, 1988.
3 Dickersin K, Scherer R, Lefebvre C. Identification of relevant studies for systematic reviews. BMJ (in press).
4 Lefebvre C, Kelleher TA, Tihanov G. Identification of randomized controlled trials using MEDLINE: the situation in 1993. Presented at 'An Evidence-Based Health Care System: The Case for Clinical Trial Registries'. National Institutes of Health, Office of Medical Applications of Research, Bethesda, MD, 6 December 1993.
5 Indexing clinical trials in EMBASE. PROFILE: The Excerpta Medica Newsletter 1994;11:2.

NORDIC PSYCHIATRIC LIBRARIES FACING NEW SERVICES AND ROLES AS A RESULT OF PSYCHIATRIC REFORMS IN THE NORDIC COUNTRIES

I.V.Nielsen, Psychiatric Research Library, Psychiatric Hospital in Aarhus, 8240 Risskov, Denmark

Abstract
The psychiatric structure has changed from major institutions to community psychiatric services and small psychiatric hospitals. Psychiatric treatment have changed from purely medical treatment to psychotherapy, environmental therapy and social training combined with medical treatment. Psychiatry is a science with several sub-specialities and auxiliary sciences. A new development in psychiatry is Consumer health information. All these alterations in patterns and structures mean changes in the need of information and supply - and changes in the libraries.

The History of Psychiatry
At all times, in all cultures and in all countries mental illness has existed. The mentally ill has mostly been misunderstood and unappreciated, and the feelings towards them have alternated between pity, sympathy, incomprehensibility, horror and hate. At some ages they were considered ill persons, at others as gods and at others again as possessed by demons. The latter the most long-lasting. If we go back to antiquity, Cicero as well as Homér write that mentally ill are persons deprived of sanity. Socrates also speaks of mentally ill. He makes a distinction between what he calls insanity and foolishness. The madhouses were a new type of institutions which were founded in the Nordic countries in the beginning of the 18th century. At first the general hospitals established a room or two where it was possible to lock up and put away poor, insane people. Later true independent buildings turned up - still to protect the sane from the insane. The conditions in these madhouses were mostly poor, and the treatment not much different from the one in the former prisons.

Not until the 19th century new ideas entered the scene. The humanitarian ideas of the Age of Enlightenment, The French Revolution and the Declaration of the Rights of Man were of importance to the insanes' social position. Especially Philippe Piret, the leader of The Reform Movement in France, became important for the definition of mental illness, and he formed the basis of modern psychiatry. He defined mentally ill as patients with need for medical treatment. In the beginning of the 19th century this led to the foundation of the first psychiatric hospitals. The first one opened in Denmark in 1816 with the founding of Sct. Hans Hospital in Roskilde. Still the psychiatric patients were placed outside the cities - the sane were not constantly to be reminded of the insane. In Finland the first hospital for mentally ill was founded in 1841 (Lappviken Hospital outside Helsinki), in Norway in 1855 (Gaustad). Sweden built its first psychiatric hospital in Stockholm in 1861 and in 1907 Kleppspitalinn was founded in Reykjavik, Iceland. The hospitals rather quickly developed into major institutions, which also became overcrowded. The psychiatric hospitals were run by doctors, who tried to treat the mentally ill. As the treatment-possibilities gradually increased, the crowd grew even bigger. Not until the middle of the 20th century the psychiatric hospitals affiliated with the general hospitals, and gradually psychiatric departments were established at many general hospitals.

Modern Times
In the middle of the 20th century the first attempts with community psychiatry were initiated. Today community psychiatry exists in all the Nordic countries, but is not equally good organized everywhere. The major psychiatric hospitals have either been closed (Sweden), or heavily reduced (Denmark). Generally, the bed-days have decreased to one third of the capacity from the time when the psychiatric hospitals were at their highest (in the middle of the 20th century). In the same period (the decrease of bed-days) the out-patient facilities increased with a factor 2-3, dependent on the Nordic country in question, but the total resources for psychiatry have not increased. Therefore, the money for the out-patient treatment has come from the hospital treatment.

We are all familiar with the results of the decreased hospital psychiatry. It has become more difficult for the mentally ill to be hospitalized and treated, more mentally ill walk the streets, because they cannot get the help necessary, and many places the mentally ill are considered "social cases", and psychiatry has been transferred to the social area. Nils Retterstøl in 1973 stated:

> "*We should consider carefully before we agree to deprive the person identified as a psychiatric patient his status as patient. We might risk to throw out the baby with the bath water*".

Perhaps this is what happened many places.

Library-Service

The library-service of psychiatry in the Nordic countries is distributed to several types of libraries. In all the Nordic countries there are university libraries, which function as a superstructure to the medical field. Apart from that there are libraries for the staff in many hospitals. In the general hospitals psychiatry is only a speciality, and as a such it does not take priority over other specialities (some places it even ranks lower). The structural changes in psychiatry mean that the libraries must change, too. In Sweden, where the major psychiatric hospitals have been closed, the libraries of the psychiatric hospitals have been closed as well. I can tell that one hospital LÅNGBRO had 100 beds in 1978 and 150 in 1994 - the hospital will be closed in 1996. In the other Nordic countries the psychiatric hospitals still exist, but the grants for the libraries are generally small. The only exception is Psychiatric Research Library in Aarhus, where I come from. The library is a hospital library and at the same time it is a department of Institute for Basic Psychiatric Research under Aarhus University. The library is financed via Government funds and has a national function, as we have to service the psychiatric field in all Denmark, the public as well as the private.. The library is big and old, and it is said to be the second largest psychiatric special-library in Europe. The library contains almost 20,000 books and approximately 620 titles of periodicals (of these the 380 are standing subscriptions). The increase in books vary from 1,000-1,200 books annually.

In Denmark and Norway there are some special collections. These are about catastrophe-psychiatry in Norway, special collections on refugees and torture in Norway as well as in Denmark, psychoanalytic special collection in Norway and the Lithium-collection in Denmark. The only collection of which I know the size is the Lithium-collection in Denmark. It is situated at Psychiatric Hospital in Aarhus and contains approximately 17,000 articles and books solely about lithium.

Today there are on-line-catalogues in the major university hospitals. The Nordic countries have also, individually, made national union-catalogues. In some of the countries also the hospital-libraries have affiliated with these national union-catalogues, especially Denmark, Norway and Finland, but not all hospitals in these countries report information about their stock to the union-catalogues. Therefore, the picture is most heterogeneous, and it is not easy to receive exact information on topics that can be found in the individual union-catalogues. Therefore, you cannot trust that materials you want to borrow cannot be found near by. Meanwhile, one can hope that more and more medical libraries will report to the union-catalogues, as the on-line catalogues gradually spread. The interlibrary loan between the Nordic countries is well-functioning. Though, the differences in the grantings charged by each country are still major. In Finland all libraries charge delivery of photo copies as well as loan. In Iceland and Denmark the situation is the opposite - none of the services are charged here. Norway and Sweden is in-between. It is obvious that these different guidelines result in an unbalanced interlibrary loan, but I believe that all the Nordic countries will have equal guidelines in a few years. As the way of handling psychiatry has many facets it is difficult to standardize the library service in the Nordic countries-well even in the individual Nordic country. Decentralization will differentiate the service further, as it is more difficult to co-ordinate things, when grants are de-centralized.

Another thing that has changed in the libraries, or at least in the acquisition structure , is the revised face of psychiatry. Psychiatry has become an extensive science with sub-specialities and auxillary sciences. So, provided that the service of psychiatry has to be optimal, the acquisition profile of the psychiatric special-libraries must innovate. The latest auxiliary science within psychiatry is the neuroscience, meaning acquisition of new periodicals and resulting in cancellation of some of the periodicals already existing, as no one receives increased grants - as well as acquisition of expensive books. The interdisciplinary and intercommunicative co-operation which characterize todays' psychiatry, also enlarges the demands on the libraries. Today the libraries must service all branches, and especially the nursings' utilization of the libraries demand increasingly on better retrieval of material in the on-line catalogues. It is not sufficient to be able to find an exact book anylonger. As regards nursing it is chapters in books, that are interesting, and this increases the demand on cataloguing and indexing.

The entirely changed structure within psychiatry, the changed scientific allocation and the withdrawal from the scientific theoretical viewpoints, create new roles for the librarians, alongside the heavy technological development in the library area, the new databases, bibliographic as well as full-text databases, the different electronic media, and the possibilities of the interlibrary loan. We do not only lend from own collections. We have to be specialists within location and mediation of knowledge. We must be extremely familiar with psychiatry and its terminology, we must be qualified instructors, and we have to be first man on the spot with new products and auxiliary instruments for doctors and researchers. We are the ones who must know:

- which software the doctors can use profitably for handling information retrieval.
- what Internet can be employed for.
- what bases to search in order to get througth to specific topics at a profitable price.

I myself come from the generation of librarians who was taught to catalogue and lend. I think the changed structure within psychiatry and treatment, together with the development within information theory have made my job more inspiring and rich, but also more demanding. To keep up with development you must see to adjust your field of activity all the time .

Patient Libraries/Information Centres

Finally, I will briefly describe the library service for the psychiatric patients. Most places the patients in the psychiatric hospitals are better off than the patients in the general hospitals, as practically all patient libraries in the general hospitals are closed. This is not the case in the psychiatric hospitals, but as these hospitals grow fewer, the conditions for the psychiatric patients will gradually reduce as well. Some places there are combined patient and doctors' libraries, (mainly in Sweden), but most hospitals operate with two libraries, one for the staff and one for the patients. The latest occurrence within the service of patients is the establishment of information centres for patients and relatives. Only one such centre exists in the Nordic countries. It is situated at Psychiatric Hospital in Aarhus, but certainly more will appear gradually. The aim of this centre is:

- to provide people with mental illnesses and their relatives a possibility to fetch information about mental illness, either by loan of literature, or through general personal advise by a nurse or a relative from the national league SIND.

- to spread information about mental illness in order to obtain increased insight in and understanding of these illnesses in the population.

This is effected via public information meetings. Such a centre is an incredible privilege. It has existed for 6 months at Psychiatric Hospital in Aarhus, and there have been many inquiries during this period. More than 60% of these came from patients and relatives, but also from specialists, among others domestic helpers, social workers and others who work with psychiatric patients. A most popular initiative of the centre is the public information meetings, where individual psychiatric topics are discussed. The need for this kind of information is so enormous that more people wish to attend these meetings than the auditorium has accommodation for. Thus we have had to double these meetings. 4 information meetings have been held with the topics: dementia senile, forensic psychiatry - the criminal part - schizophrenia, and manio-depressive psychoses. The topic schizophrenia was so crowded that it was arranged twice within three weeks. More than 500 people participated in these two information meetings qbout schizophrenia. In the autumn information meetings on community psychiatry, anxiety, and eating disorders are arranged as well as manio-depressive psychoses once more.

Working with this part of the mediation of information is exiting, especially because you can feel that the need for information is enourmous, and that you are able to meet this need.

References

Harding, G.: Utvecklingen av svensk psykiatri. Läkartidningen. 76 (10), 1979, 845-848

Odegaard, O.: Perspektiver efter 5 aars psykiatrisk virksomhet. Nordisk Medicin 97 (12), 1982, 310-313

Retterstøl, N.: Trekk av psykiatriens historie i Skandinavia frem til aar 1990. Tidsskrift for den norske laegeforening. No.7, 1973, 429-433

Psykiatriska behandlingssystemet i Finland. (Unpubl.)

Olafsson, P.: Psykiatri og psykiatriske biblioteker i Island. (Unpubl.)

SECTION 6

ELECTRONIC INFORMATION DELIVERY

EXPERIENCES WITH *EXCERPTA MEDICA* ON-LINE VIA BIDS AT UNIVERSITY OF OSLO, FACULTY OF MEDICINE LIBRARY.

Kari Halldal, Det Medisinske Fakultetsbibliotek, Universitet i Oslo, PB 1113 Blindern, N-0317, Oslo, Norway

I am going to talk about searching Excerpta Medica via BIDS, Bath University Information and Data Services. The faculty of medicine at the University of Oslo is spread at different hospitals and institutions all over Oslo, but my experience is limited to the library where I work and to the end users working in the same building. Other institutions may have different patterns of use and different experience. One of the Norwegian librarians, Elisabeth Buntz, director of the Medical Library and Information Center at the National Hospital, spent some time studying in UK a couple of years ago. She was impressed by JANET, the Joint Academic Network, which gave students and faculty at universities all over the country unlimited access to databases like Science Citation Index and Excerpta Medica/Embase for the purpose of study or research. Back in Norway she worked to make the same resources available at the University of Oslo and in January 1993 a 5-year contract was signed which gives access to Embase. The system is operated from Bath University and is searched via Internet. It took some time before the system was operable and practical matters were arranged. Then came the summer and vacation time but since autumn 1993 we have used it regularly.

The faculty of medicine library where I work, is the largest medical library in Norway and resource library for medicine as well. My main job is online searching in biomedical databases for internal and external clients. The end users working in the same building belong to the Institute for Basic Medical Sciences like anatomy, physiology, biochemistry etc. There are 72 university positions for scientific personnel and in addition there are a changing number of researchers paid by external funds. When you turn on your PC in the morning, you will always get a screen with NEWS. When EMBASE got available the NEWS screen had a message about it for approximately two months. In addition information about EMBASE was sent to each department. EMBASE covers 3500 journals from 110 countries and 46 languages. 350000 records are added each year. The database goes back to 1974, the BIDS version to 1980. All major US journals are covered, but the focus is primarily on European biomedical literature. 65% of the records have abstracts, and this number is going to increase as all English abstracts will be included. EMBASE is updated weekly, and they are trying to get the records into the database fully indexed within 15 to 18 days of receipt of the journals.

Searching EMBASE at BIDS is very different from searching EMBASE at DIALOG or EMED at DATASTAR which are the two hosts that are most used here in Norway. On purpose the database interface is made for users with no knowledge of database searching and not for librarians. There is a small search guide, but you literally can sit down and make a search with no instruction at all provided you read the text on the screen. From a menu you can select a T if you want to search for words in the title and will then get prompted to write a title word or expression; if you press an A you will be prompted for an author name and so on.

-- SEARCH MENU --

T - Word(s) In Title
B - Word(s) In Title/Abstract/Keywords
A - Author Name(s)
J - Journal Title
I - Index Terms
R - CAS Registry Number(s)
M - Trade and Manufacturer Names
N - Address
F - Save/retrieve Sets
U - Use Previous Sets
Z - Repeat Current Search for Previous Year

or Display(D) Output(P) Options(O) Thesaurus(H) Issues(E) Order(*) or type HELP or EXIT

As in other databases you can combine words with each other.You use a + instead of AND, a comma instead of OR, and a minus instead of NOT. The + for AND confused me a little. In the early days of online searching, for instance with DIALOG, a + meant OR and you used an asterisk for AND. Here the asterisk is the truncation character. If the search is a little complicated and you need to combine different sets you can select U - Use Previous Sets from the menu and you will get a screen listing the search sets you have got so far and then can combine the different set numbers. In Embase you search only one year at a time. If you need to go farther back you can select Z - Repeat Current Search for Previous Year from the menu and then the search is repeated without you having to write anything. Or at least, that is what it is meant to do. BUT, if the search is a little complicated, for instance a combination of more than 2 words or containing explosions or truncations, I have discovered at several occasions that it doesn't work. When you get 1 hit from 1994 and then get 275 hits from 1993, you ought to get suspicious. And if I do the search from the beginning again in the 1993 segment the 275 hits turn out to be the number of hits for one of the search terms and no combination of terms has been done ! So, when this happens I have to rewrite the search formulation for every year. The database goes back to 1980, so then the search will be very time-consuming ! When you want to display hits you will get prompted for format and number of references to display. You can choose to print all the references or you can mark the ones you want to print. Again you will get prompted for format and which references to print, either marked or the last search. Then you are asked about your E-mail address and the references will be sent by E-mail. It usually takes a couple of hours; once it took less than 10 minutes and sometimes we have had to wait until the next day. Two or three times the references did not arrive at all and we had to do the search once more. So if I am in a hurry, I just download the whole search, but it needs editing afterwards to get rid of all the screens.

For more elaborate searches one can use the online thesaurus and then may be prompted to explode terms and in some cases add subheadings. Synonyms and some MeSH terms will be translated into the official Excerpta Medica-term. This may give some funny results. One day I tried searching for MEDLINE as a thesaurus term. It was translated into Medical Information and gave 45 hits from the 1994 segment. It surprised me that Embase had that many references about a competing system, but when I looked closer it turned out that only 3 of the 45 references mentioned MEDLINE at all. On second thought it was quite logical as the term medical information must be more comprehensive than the term Medline. The BIDS system design is very user-friendly. The screens tell you all the way what you can do and gives you a choice but as mentioned earlier I have found several limitations. Also searching can be very slow, for instance big explosions. To save time and avoid some of the screens you may stack commands provided you remember the letters for each option or command. Part of the slowness may also be due to an overload on Internet. It works best early in the morning. Later in the day I often get the message "node unreachable". Even if the system is self-explanatory I have offered introductory courses. But only one person has been interested and when he came to the course the node was unreachable. Through the years there have been many papers comparing results from EMBASE and MEDLINE. Still I wanted to do my own comparison. Due to lack of time it is not very scientifically done. For instance I suppose I ought to have done all my searches in both databases. But since EMBASE searches are slow and I met a lot of trouble with complicated searches I decided to search EMBASE only when the questions were simple and I thought I might find something valuable. The search profiles to be compared were set up to be identical as far as possible. I have always been told that EMBASE has a very good coverage of drug literature, so I divided my 18 search examples into 11 drug searches and 7 non-drug searches.

	11 DRUG	7 NON-DRUG	18 TOTAL
EMBASE	189 refs	28 refs	217 refs
MEDLINE	139 refs	56 refs	195 refs
OVERLAP	43 refs	11 refs	54 refs
EMBASE UNIQUE	146=77%	17=61%	163=75%
MEDLINE UNIQUE	96=69%	45=80%	141=72%

My conclusion is, not surprisingly, that the two databases complement each other. There were fewer overlaps than I had expected and if you need a comprehensive search you certainly ought to use both databases. The BIDS statistics for the first 5 months of regular use, period monitored 25.10 - 14.03, showed that there had been 325 sessions of which my library had 72 and "my" endusers 21 sessions. 21 sessions in 5 months is not very much. Anyway I wanted to know the users' opinion of EMBASE. Eight people answered a questionnaire. Four had a password but had not used the system. Two of these said they used MEDLINE instead. Among the other four persons three had used EMBASE more than 5 times, one had used it 2-5 times. They all found the system easy but slow and somewhat cumbersome, especially since they could only search one year at a time. Among the different options for searching all had used the common Title/Abstract/Keywords/Author options, whereas only one had tried the thesaurus. One said he preferred EMED on DATASTAR. Even if they had tried EMBASE several times, the other three said they preferred MEDLINE on CDPLUS-OVID which became available for everybody at the University shortly after EMBASE.

And to sum up my experience with the BIDS version :

- it is easy to use for simple searches
- the updating of the database is very good
- searching is rather slow with all the screens to read, but stacking helps
- the E-mail function is convenient when you are not in a hurry
- the database segments ought to contain more than one year's references
- for complicated searches and backsearches you can not trust that you get what you ask for
- for comprehensive searches one ought to search both MEDLINE and EMBASE
- useful for checking references not found in MEDLINE

And I can add the experience of my colleague at the Institute of pharmacology. She tells me that her users are very happy about EMBASE and have found a lot of useful references there.

CD-ROM USED FOR LITERATURE REFERENCE DISTRIBUTION WITHIN A PHARMACEUTICAL COMPANY

Christina Max, Lilian Gustafsson, Elisabet Wijk & Stefan Olsson, Astra Hässle, S-431 83 Mölndal, Sweden

A CD-ROM with about 60 000 references on astra pharmaceutical products is produced for distribution to Astra marketing companies around the world. It has been updated quarterly during more than two years and a version for Windows interface is under construction. Astra is a worldwide pharmaceutical company with its corporate basis in Sweden. Astra includes four research and development daughter companies where the basic research on drugs or drug administration takes place. Astra Arcus is focused on research within the central nervous system related diseases as well as immunology, Astra Pain Control within the area of local anesthetics, Astra Draco on diseases of the respiratory system, and finally, Astra Hässle with research on gastrointestinal and cardiovascular diseases. Production is located both in Sweden and abroad. About 40 marketing companies are spread over the world and in all, Astra has over 12 000 employees. Furthermore there are agreements with more than 50 licensees who market Astra products.

Astra Medical Information Service

In the 1970s, when Astra still was a small company there were different ways of keeping track of medical publications on the different research companies. Then in the middle of the 1970s Astra in Södertälje started a computerized system for literature registration which was managed at the library. The other research companies were invited to use the system. Indexed references were sent to Södertälje for registration. The reference data bases that were built up consist of published literature mainly on marketed products but also research project literature. The corporate language is English and all documentation work is in English. It was during this time that the Astra Medical Information System was named and abbreviated AMIS. A group with representatives from all research companies was initiated and this AMIS-group is still working. The aim of the group was to organize the literature support to the marketing companies in a similiar way for all Astra products.

In 1987 a new Information Retrieval (IR)-system called TRIP was installed at all research companies. In our environment TRIP is a VAX/VMS-based system for large text registers. It is characterized by easy tailoring of the structure and quick retrieval. It is also well suited for literature reference handling, and there are possibilities to use an attached thesaurus which is essential to our files. All the AMIS files were converted to the new system. With this conversion all administration of the inhouse literature databases was transferred to each of the four research companies. The general outline of the structure and contents is similar but local adaptations exist. Today there are 14 databases from the three sites covering six indication areas which together comprise the AMIS service.

Distribution

The computerization of the literature references made it possible for us to provide the marketing companies with different kinds of lists for manual searches. For each product or product group bibliographic lists and index lists for authors and keywords were frequently distributed. However, the files grew rapidly, and manual searches became more and more laborious. In order to simplify the use for the marketing companies, Astra also kept a private file at Dialog during 1984-1991. According to the agreement with Dialog, however, the number of users were limited, which complicated the addition of new marketing companies. A more efficient system was then sought to simplify the literature information supply to the marketing companies and the licensees. CD-ROM was chosen as a fast, easily updated and easily available medium. In collaboration with Optitech (a consultant company in Dalby, Sweden) a CD-ROM system was built. A test disk was evaluated in the beginning of 1991 and the production has been going on since March 1992. The stationary system, TRIP, was not available for PC or in CD-ROM version at the time, so instead CD-Answer which is produced by Dataware Technologies was chosen. The AMIS-CD is updated quarterly, and it has been possible to keep this updating frequency from the start. A user guide with searching instructions and database descriptions was printed, and with each updated disk a couple of pages with release notes are distributed.

Production Steps

Most of the information from the stationary TRIP data bases is transferred to the AMIS-CD. The references amount to about 60 000 in all. An output format has been agreed on that presents the references in a little more condensed form compared to the TRIP bases where separate fields are used for each category of information. Since CD-Answer cannot provide a built-in thesaurus application a conversion program was created to supplement the descriptors with all broader terms. Furthermore, in order to prevent problems with national characters (that is, letters with diacritic marks), the conversion program replaces these with international characters.

This conversion program was created and is held at Astra Draco. Thus, textfiles from all 14 literature files are collected at Astra Draco and the conversion program is run together with their corresponding thesauri before sending the files to Optitech. Optitech then provides the search program and runs program and contents together before transferring the result to the CD production company. There the whole information is run through a mastering process to make the master CD which is used for pressing the AMIS-CD. With this system it is not practical to press less than 100 CD copies. The main cost are on the production of the master CD and the pressing of each CD is not expensive.

Information Availability

Since there are several licensees who market only parts of the Astra portfolio it was necessary to find a way to select material for these companies. This has been done using an encrypted version of the AMIS-CD. To be able to read this version the licensees are provided with a floppy disk allowing the user access to certain parts of the contents. Thus, we have produced two different kinds of CD-s, one for those recipients who are entitled to all the material and the encrypted version for those who only should have limited access.

Comparison of AMIS-CD with Printed Lists

* Searching is much easier and faster
* Production and distribution is simplified
* References from all files are collected in the same physical entity (AMIS-CD)

Comparison of the AMIS-CD with the Private Dialog File

* It is easier to include new users, and it is possible to distribute even to those who have limited access
* Communication problems are avoided
* No time stress for the user
* No extra cost included in the search
* Better control of the production process ---> updates can be better planned

General Properties of CD-ROMs

* The disks are durable
* CD-ROM readers are inexpensive and readily available
* Networking is possible
* The costs are predictable, both for the production and use

However:

* A CD-ROM disk could be used by someone not entitled to the contents

User Response

When we made the AMIS-CD test disk we had a lot of contacts with the companies that were chosen for the test. We wanted to cover different kinds of companies, from the large, technically well equipped ones to small ones, where the medical documentation is handled by persons with responsibility for several products. We made a thorough evaluation of the response to the test disk which took some time. However, when the first regular version was distributed in March 1992 we had few problems. About half a year after the introduction of the CD, a brief questionnaire was sent out. At that time 75% of the Astra companies had a CD-ROM reader installed and were using the CD. A few small licensing companies prefer a printed version, but most contacts are very happy with the AMIS-CD. All spontaneous response has been very positive and we feel proud that most things have worked so well.

Windows Version

However, during the two years that AMIS-CD has been produced suggestions for improvements have appeared. Most of them will be managed in a new version which is run from Windows. A test version is to be ready during summer 1994 for selected users, and the final version is planned to be launched at the next regular release which is in September 1994. This version is also made by Optitech, but the search program is new.

Some Improvements

These are the improvements compared with the original AMIS-CD

* The Windows interface will be more user friendly
* Predefined filters can be used - you see only the part that is filtered out
* When browsing the indexes, these previously included everything on the disk. With the new version only the indexes of selected files will be displayed
* Only one kind of CD will be used - a password will define what parts the user will access. This will reduce the cost and administration
* Output formats suited for certain reference editing programs will be available
* "Selferasing" - after 3 months the user will be informed at login that a new version is available. After 6 months the disk contents will be unavailable
* The user guide can be short and simple - help texts will be available on the screen

Conclusions

In order to serve the marketing and medical information personnel in a worldwide pharmaceutical company with literature references, the CD-ROM has proved to be valuable. The references data bases with added value in the way of indexing and evaluation cover more than 30 products on the market. The CD is easily put in production and distribution and the use of it is simple and unexpensive. To further improve the usage of the CD a Windows interface is preferable and access to selected parts of the contents can be allowed. In view of the time saved by persons all over the company the CD-ROM is a cost-effective way to distribute information.

IMPACT ON PEOPLE OF ELECTRONIC LIBRARIES (IMPEL) PROJECT: its Implications for Health Sciences Librarianship

Graham Walton, Joan M. Day, & Catherine E. Edwards, Department of Information and Library Management, University of Northumbria at Newcastle, Newcastle-upon-Tyne NE1 8ST, UK

Abstract

The paper outlines current developments in both the health service and higher education electronic networks in the United Kingdom. It examines issues in linking the networks together. The relevance of the IMPEL project is identified for health sciences librarianship as well as the outomes.

Introduction

The purpose of this paper is to outline the relevance of the IMpact on People of Electronic Libraries (IMPEL) Project for those librarians working in the health setting. This project is being jointly administered by the Information Services Department and the Department of Information and Library Management at the University of Northumbria at Newcastle. It is primarily concerned with investigating the way in which academic librarians are being affected by delivering services electronically. I will first describe the development of the health service electronic network in the U.K. The higher education network in the UK will also be outlined. Issues concerning the relationship between the health service and the higher education networks will then be investigated. The IMPEL project will then be described in more detail. Finally I will attempt to forecast how electronic networks may impact upon the work of the librarian working in the hospital.

United Kingdom Health Network

In the UK National Health Service (NHS) there have been many initiatives in local area networks (LAN)(High wires and safety nets,1994). This is against the backdrop of the proposed development of the NHS wide network (Nicholls, 1994). The strategy was launched in 1992. The need for this is illustrated by the estimate that a billion pieces of paper pass round the NHS each year. The intention is that it will primarily have a function for the sharing of data. This data will be hospital waiting lists, morbidity data and supplies. It is unlikely that this network will be in place soon. The initial intention was to have the NHS wide network in place by 1996 but the basic contract for the initial work has only just been put out for tender.

There is very little evidence to indicate that librarians have played any role in the planning and developing of the NHS network. In the UK some librarians have succeeded in providing access to CD-ROM databases and the OPAC via the hospital local area network. Various actions are being taken to try to ensure that, at a national level, there is an appreciation that library services can be enhanced through access to a wide area network(wan). Celia Durkin (1994) ,a hospital librarian in Virginia, USA, undertook a survey to establish the justification for hospital access to the INTERNET. The four rough categories she identified were FTP (file transfer capability(the downloading of documentation from remote computers), TELNET capabilities (access to library OPACS, commercial services), E MAIL and resources only available through INTERNET. A valuable forecast about the INTERNET will improve access to information in public health has beem written by Laporte.

UK Higher Education Network

The UK higher education electronic network has been in place since 1984. It is called Joint Academic NETwork (JANET) and links over 50,000 computers across 200 sites. It enables remote access to computing facilities and information services and the transport of data and electronic mail. It is worth mentioning the Bath Information and Data Service (BIDS) experiment. This allows free for the user access to various bibliographic databases via JANET. Recently the Embase databases have become available in this way. A major initiative is the development of SuperJANET which will be a much faster network than JANET. This will allow the handling of multimedia and the transfer of sound and video as well as text and numeric data. Some university libraries have become accustomed to using JANET in delivering information services electronically. In other university libraries electronic networking is only just making an impact.

Linking Health Service and Higher Education Networks

Even though the NHS network is only in the planning stage concern has already been expressed about the implications of linking with JANET. At a recent conference it was said "Joining university and hospital networks is desirable, but dangerous"(Cross,1994). Threats to patient confidentiality were seen as a major stumbling block. This problem could limit significantly the range of applications that the NHS network can be used for. SUPERJANET will have immense potential with ability to transmit sound and visual information. For example in the States there is INTERNET interactive multi- media access to 59,000 prints/photographs from the History of Medicine Division at Lister Hill National Centre for Biomedical Communication (Rogers,1994) Investigations are taking place on the possibility of a single national connection between the NHS and higher education sectors. In the interim, locally arranged agreements between a JANET site and a NHS site are recommended (Wells,1994).

IMPEL Project

A major development in UK higher education libraries has been the publication of the Follett report (1993). This is a far ranging report which sees information technology as a key tool in coping with such issues as increased student numbers, high costs of libraries, changing teaching methods and supporting research. The focus of the IMPEL project is described by the following quote from Follett(para.123): "failure to provide staff with adequate training and deploy them effectively represents one of the single most important constraints on change and development in library and information provision, and can seriously undermine its effectiveness, especially when this depends on the implementation of new practices, or on information technology".

A literature review (Edwards, 1993) is being published which gives the background to the IMPEL project. In UK university libraries there have been extensive development work in information technology and electronic networks. Little has been done to investigate the human issues behind the technology. In some institutions the library and computer units have merged. In others the management structures and traditional hierarchies have changed in order to function effectively. The first stage of the IMPEL project will be to look at the impact on qualified librarians. The emphasis is on developing useful outcomes and knowledge upon which to base future developments. These will be to identify the following:

* the organisational impact of educational and technological change for library management and personnel
* the social impact of education and technological change and the cultural implications on library management and personnel
* the knowledge, skill and training required of academic librarians and implications for initial education and continuing professional development
* factors which influence strategy in implementing electronic networks
* factors contributing to a model of "best Practice" in managing information provision in a networked campus environment

The investigation will be through the case study approach where universities demonstrating good practice will be investigated. The following criteria was used to establish which university libraries should be visited:

* Written IT strategy
* Extensive Library/Computer Unit co-operation
* Special training
* Innovative use
* Student access to JANET

A brief survey of 98 UK academic libraries was undertaken to identify which institutions fulfilled the criteria. There was a response rate of 83% with Aston, Central Lancashire, Cranfield, Cardiff, Stirling and Ulster Universities being selected and agreeing to take part in the IMPEL project. They will each be visited for a week by the Senior Research Assistant who will interview library and other relevant staff and examine key documents. Qualified library staff will be interviewed on how their job has changed, relationships with library and non-library staff and the problems they have resolved. At present the pilot is being undertaken at the University of Northumbria at Newcastle where the research protocol is being tested. The data collection and analysis will take place from September 1994 to November 1995. It is the intention to produce the final report in March 1996.

IMPEL Project and Health Sciences Librarianship

Librarians based in the health sector should benefit from the findings of the IMPEL. This is especially the case with the health service networks being at early stages of development. With the current rate of change the future is difficult to predict but the following developments may occur:

* Hospital libraries and computer departments become amalgamated into single units
* Information has to be delivered to health sciences professionals who are working more in the community, remote from hospital libraries
* Librarians in the health service have to work closer with higher education libraries and become involved in supplying information electronically
* Health service managers recognise the need for staff who can help clinicians find there way around the electronic network
* Health service trainers start to use teaching methods which are electronically based.

In all of these the health sciences librarian could have a major role and function. It is important that they are prepared to both realise the opportunity and also cope with the situations. The IMPEL project should help librarians in the health sector learn from higher education libraries. Important lessons will be gained from those university libraries which have already faced the issues that may be just around the corner for the health sector. I will leave you with a dramatic quote from Cecilia Parkin the hospital librarian from Virginia

The Information Highway is already in place; we can either get on the road and move with the traffic, or sit by the roadside and watch our competitors whiz by. Or, as our Information Systems expert suggested-we can get on the road or be paved over.

Citations

Cross,C.(1994) Bill plays with JANET Health Service Journal 21st April 104(5399), p13.

Durkin,C. (1994) INTERNET justification for hospitals 17th May MEDIAL E mail communication

Edwards,C.E.,Day,J.M.,Walton,G.(1993) Key areas in the management of change in higher education libraries in the 1990s:relevance of the IMPEL project British Journal of Academic Librarianship (forthcoming)

Follett report(1993) Joint Funding Council's Libraries Review Group (1994) High wires and safety nets Health Service Journal, 104(5395) 17th March pp6-11.

Laporte,R.E.(1994) Global public health and the information superhighway British Medical Journal 25th June pp1651-2

Nicholls,I.(1994) Making the most of the network. In Managing the Knowledge base of Health Care: report of a seminar. British Library R&D Report 6133. British Library Research and Development Department, pp13-25.

Rogers,R.P.C.(1994) On-line images for the history of medicine 8th June MEDIAL E mail communication

Wells,M.(1994) Linking NHS sites to JANET (unpublished)

MEDLINE PROMOTION

L Locche, A Stanzani & L Loiacono Biblioteca Centralizzata USL 28 - Bologna Italia

The CD-ROM bibliographic research service of the Library of the USL 28 of Bologna (Italy) is staffed by a full-time librarian (37 hours a week) and is equipped with several SilverPlatter CD-ROM databases (Medline since 1966, ISPlus, Excerpta Medica Psychiatry, Excerpta Medica Neurosciences, Psychlit, and other "try and buy" discs). Its potential users are about 950, subdivided among hospital staff doctors and staff of the Faculty of Medicine. Research is done by the librarian in presence of the doctor on an appointment basis. The starting point for the investigation was to provide an answer to the question why the service should be utlied only up to one third of its capacity, and to encourage access to the service, as well as to optimize the yield of the librarian's work hours.

In order to fulfill this aim, a form was sent to all 950 doctors, through which they were allowed to request by internal mail a certain bibliographic research, which the librarian was supposed to carry out himself, without any need for the doctor to go to the library, nor for the librarian to wait for him, thus allowing a better planning to the latter for his work routine. The form contained 5 simple questions: Title, MESH, Free words, Articles already seen, and Quantitative expectation (Table 1). A table was also set up in order to verify from the correctness in form filling whether its formalution was to the point or not (Table 2). The results of the research were finally transmitted to the doctor along with a questionnaire meant to obtain:

1. Information of the user's attitude toward the service (Table 3);
2. Information on the quality of the research (Table 4);
3. Information as to the future usage of the library (Table 5).

The answers to the questionnare are reported. Three months after the start of the initiative a positibe result is already shown by the 100% increase in the utlization of tyhe service, with respect to the corresponding period of 1992.

Fill the following fields:

1. Topic of the research
2. MESH terms
3. Free words
4. Articles already seen
5. Quantitative expectation

Send to the Library

TABLE 1: FORM FOR CD-ROM MEDLINE RESEARCH

TABLE 2: EVALUATION OF THE EFFICACY OF THE FORM

1.	Clearness of topic	100.0%
	Fulfilled fields:	
2.	MESH term	50.0%
3.	Free words	87.5%
4.	Already found articles	65.0%
5.	Quantative expectation	64.0%

	How the research was performed	
a.	Directly by the Librarian	94.5%
b.	Need of explanations (telephone call)	4.0%
c.	Need of presence of the User	1.5%

72 FORMS RETURNED = 100%

TABLE 3: CUSTOMER'S ATTITUDE TOWARD THE SERVICE

How do you usually find references?		How the User prefer to access CD-ROM databases?	
41%	Bibliographic directories	43%	Together with the Librarian
38%	Journal contents	38%	Sending a form to the Librarian
21%	Databases	19%	The User by himself

Have you ever used MEDLINE before?	
77% Yes	23% No

TABLE 4: QUALITY OF THE RESEARCH

WELL PLANNED FORM = 97.5%

Outcome of the research		Number of records retrieved	
54%	OK, pertinent	67%	As expected
42%	OK, but ... information noise	24%	Too few
4%	Not pertinent	9%	Too many

Comparison between MEDLINE and other sources		
85% Faster	10% Similar	5% Slower

TABLE 5: FUTURE USAGE OF THE LIBRARY

WILL CONSULT A LIBRARY FOR FURTHER INQUIRIES = 90.5%

Which services of the library will be used	
50%	CD-ROM
40%	Consultation of the library journal holding and photocopying
10%	Interlibrary loan

BECOMING AN ONLINE MICRO-HOST

Jane Rowlands, William Forrester & Tony McSeán. British Medical Association Library, Tavistock Square, London WC1H 9JP, UK .

My paper will begin with a very brief introduction to the BMA Library. I shall go on to discuss the initial decision and installation stages of the Library's PlusNet2 Medline system and the pilot scheme with which we first began the Free Medline Service. I will next consider the rapid development of the service since its official launch in June 1993, reflecting upon the experience of supporting a large number of physicians, who were, to a great extent, inexperienced and untrained in both information retrieval and PC communications. I will conclude by looking forward to future developments in the service and explain steps being taken to further develop complementary Library services in conjunction with the Medline service.

The BMA is the professional association for doctors throughout the UK. It has 100,000 members representing over 80% of UK doctors. The BMA Library is very much a Library for the working doctor, concentrating on current clinical practice, medico-political issues and medical ethics. The main purpose of the Library is to provide members with access to published information in a way that is most convenient for them. In order to best cater for a widely dispersed membership, the Library has specialised in providing services at a distance and in using new technology to improve and extend these services. The PlusNet2 system, allowing simultaneous access to up to 24 remote users to the entire Medline database from 1966 to date, fits exactly with this overall aim.

Plans to purchase the Plusnet2 system began back in 1991. Four important factors influencing the final decision were:

1. Medline's position as one of the largest, most widely used and recognised of available medical databases.

2. The opportunity to develop an exclusive service for BMA members and one that is, in many ways, a world's first.

3. The technology was at an ideal stage of development in that it was still exciting and innovatory, but we could also contact a number of campus sites in the USA, where similar systems had been already installed, to hear their own experiences and evaluations.

4. CDPlus were eager to make their first sale outside of the USA of an application of this particular type. We were confident of at least baseline support.

The system was purchased using funds from members subscriptions, contracts having been negotiated with both the National Library of Medicine and CD Plus. The equipment was installed in October 1992.

PlusNet2 is a Novell-based Local Area Network (LAN) system incorporating Norton pcAnywhere host software. The BMA system comprises a 9.2 gigabyte hard disk server, 8 diskless PCs with modems (known as random access units) and importantly an uninterruptable power supply. Additional PC's are attached in order to monitor the system. A CD ROM drive is attached for carrying out monthly updates to the database. The system runs in VT100 mode. Files can be downloaded using the X-Modem and more recently Kermit file transfer protocols. Access is restricted by login names, issued by the Library to BMA staff and members. Dial up users are also required to select, for themselves, a unique password every 90 days. We began with the CD Plus 2.0 (DOS) interface and in February 1994 upgraded to the 2.1 (DOS) interface. With the installation of the Library's own network during 1993, including a link to the Joint Academic Network (JANET), the number of possible simultaneous users via dial-up is now 20. In brief, 8 lines connect directly to the Medline system, 6 lines connect to Medline via the Library network and another 6 via JANET. Terminals throughout the Library itself have direct ethernet links to the system.

A pilot scheme operated from October 1992 until May 1993. BMA members alerted by a planned press release and having the necessary equipment (that is a PC or Macintosh, modem and relevant communications software) were able to dial into the service, carry out their own searches and download or print results. The system was made available 24 hours a day, 7 days a week. An information pack was sent to each member requesting access to the service. This contained the telephone number, details of the logging in procedure, communications software settings for recommended packages, general settings to try for non-recommended packages and a guide to searching. Also enclosed was an application form for the member to return in order to receive their login name. A help desk operated between 9.00am and 5.00pm each weekday. On entering the system users were warned of the potential limitations of the database and, as new searchers, their own ability to retrieve all available information from it. The pilot scheme gave us the opportunity to streamline administrative procedures, to ensure that the system would operate smoothly, and to update and improve the original information pack.

A questionnaire was sent to the first 108 members to join the pilot scheme. Results from 61 users provided valuable feedback on all aspects of the service with details relating to the users themselves, their equipment, their use of the service and their comments and suggestions for further improvements. Results showed that the three most popular features of the PlusNet2 system were the mapping of the users own words to MeSH headings (standard keyword terms with which the Medline database is indexed), the speed of operation and the ability to download search results.

The Medline service was officially launched, at a ceremony on 2 June 1993 by Sir Duncan Nichol, Chief Executive of the National Health Service Management Executive, coinciding with a wave of publicity in the medical and information press including the BMJ and BMA News Review. Updated and improved information packs, in brand new wallets and bearing the chosen name "BMA Library Free Medline Service" were sent to members requesting access. Continuous access, our warning message for novice searchers, registration and logging on procedures remained as they had been throughout the pilot scheme. The response was overwhelming. Secretarial support for the Library was reduced to practically nil during the first hectic weeks as it was spent sending out information packs and registering new users. The original target of 1000 registered users by the end of 1993 was soon passed, the graphs having to be completely re-drawn. Additional publicity followed. For example, the registering of the 1000th user; letters in the BMJ; a feature article in BMA News Review and an article written by one of the early users of the system published in the Bulletin of the Royal College of Psychiatrists. We now have over 4000 registered users.

However, the rapid increase in the number of users meant that more and more of the members registering for access to the Medline service were inexperienced in information retrieval and communications. We have developed a range of facilities in order to support these members.

1. In addition to the information provided previously the revised information pack includes the new network telephone number and JANET address, details on the purchase of hardware/software, and some basic facts and figures about the Medline database itself.

2. A help desk continues to operate between 9.00am and 5.00pm each week day. William Forrester and I daily deal with questions including re-instating users' passwords; the purchase of equipment; the setting up of communications software; search technique; the printing or downloading of search results and the importing of downloaded results into personal bibliographic software packages such as Reference Manager or Pro-cite. As an aid to the help desk, we have set up an ever growing number of communications packages to access the service. We can, therefore, provide direct assistance in using these packages or send printed copies of correct settings. We also have screens for viewing activity on the lines connected to the Medline system and can see what is happening at the user's end of the connection. In April this year we acquired the Library's first Macintosh machine and so are now in a much better position to help Mac users with their communications problems. We have obtained demonstration copies of the major personal bibliographic software packages which we have loaded to help assist with importing downloaded results into these packages. Particular difficulties have been experienced with Windows Terminal communications software. Results will not print due to a conflict with Widows print manager and screen refresh facilities are very poor. We would certainly advise the use of a more comprehensive communications software package. The cleanest connection of all can be made with Norton pcAnywhere, remote version, for DOS, as the PlusNet2 system actually incorporates the host version of this software.

3. We maintain a database of registered users, including software communications packages used, as noted on the application form. We can put members in contact with others using the same communications software, particularly

non-recommended packages, for mutual help and advice. Members reporting that they have accessed the system successfully using non-recommended packages have been encouraged to send in details of the appropriate settings. These are kept on file and can be sent out to other members requesting help.

4. Beginners and advanced Medline courses have been arranged to run during 1994 using BMA facilities and with the help of senior members of Library staff. It is hoped also, in the near future, to arrange Medline demonstrations in conjunction with BMA local offices throughout the UK.

In the future we hope to upgrade to the new OVID 3.0 (DOS) interface for dial-up users. The information pack is being re-written and will be sent out to all users of the service in preparation for this. We are currently negotiating a special hardware/software, support and installation deal for Medline users with a small group of computer suppliers. Users dialling into the Library network, either directly or via JANET may also search the Library catalogue and we hope in the future to make further information sources available. For example, the UK Cochrane Centre database of clinical trials relating to pregnancy and childbirth. It is hoped that the users dialling into the Library network will soon have access to bulletin boards provided by other BMA departments. For example, those dealing with fees or pay and conditions, plus the Association's new medical informatics and clinical audit services. We plan to have e-mail facilities available for those dialling into the Library network, for enquiries and for users to request Library document delivery or loan services.

To conclude, the Medline service has proved extremely popular with members, and has even been reported by one as changing the nature of their working week. Doctors have joined the Association in order to use the service. The service has played an important role is raising the profile of the library within the organisation, a vital concern for any special library. We hope in the future that the service will continue to expand and to diversify in helping to fulfil the Library's primary function in bringing up-to-date clinical information to the desk-top of the busy working doctor, throughout the UK. In doing so we hope to continue to play an important part in helping them to access and manage the ever growing volume of information within medicine and the health sciences.

References

1. MCSÉAN T, LAW D. Buying databases: many problems, many solutions. In: Bakker S, Cleland M, eds. Information transfer: new age - new ways, proceedings of the 3rd European conference of medical libraries. Dordrect: Kluwer Academic Publishers, 1992 23-26.
2. MCSÉAN T, ROWLANDS J, FORRESTER W. Becoming a micro-host : using desktop computers to run an online retrieval service. In: Raitt D I, Jeapes B, eds. Online information 93, proceedings of the 17th international online information meeting 7-9 December, London, England. Oxford: Learned Information Ltd, 1993 367-376.

TOWARDS ELECTRONIC INFORMATION: the example of the Multimedia library of the University LYON I (France)

Pierre Marie Belbenoit-Avich, Bibliothèque universitaire de l' Université LYON I, section Santé
8 avenue Rockefeller 69373 LYON cedex 03, France

Abstract
The multimedia library of the University LYON I (health part) is going to be opened in a few months. It will contain several departments. In the very fields of documentation, it will offer in particular CD I or multimedia. This paper deals with all the difficulties we have met to develop this specific section : lack of information about the contents and the media of the new products and problems to get them on demo; prerequisites however essential before any purchase. It is important for us to be kept informed of new technologies, as this aspect of consulting will be a major part of our job in the next future.

L' Université de Lyon I est dans le domaine scientifique et médical une des plus importantes en France après celles de Paris. Un des événements intéressants de cette année y aura peut-être été sur le plan du transfert de l' information, la mise en chantier -au sens large- d' une médiathèque qui doit ouvrir ses portes en septembre prochain . Elle comprendra plusieurs départements : audiovisuel, micro-informatique, accès aux réseaux extérieurs et une partie nouvelle consacrée aux nouveaux supports en particulier les CD Interactifs et les multimedia. Mon rôle a été de proposer l 'acquisition de ces produits, c'est à dire de les recenser, de me tenir informé régulièrement des nouvelles publications, d' obtenir toutes les informations nécessaires et enfin d' essayer de les obtenir en démonstration.

Lorsqu' on veut commander un livre, on peut facilement obtenir de l' éditeur un résumé qui figure du reste sur les publicités ou en lire une critique. Pour les périodiques, on peut se faire une idée assez précise en demandant un spécimen ou en étudiant le classement des titres de SCIENCES CITATION INDEX. En ce qui concerne les multimedias ou autres compact disques interactifs, les difficultés sont beaucoup plus grandes. La première tient à l' information sur les nouveaux titres. Mis à part certaines sociétés importantes, la majorité des CD interactifs ou des multimedia est produite par des fabricants qui en font peu, sont donc assez peu connus et ne font pas de publicité ou de campagnes d' information assez importantes. Il faut vraiment lire régulièrement plusieurs titres internationaux spécialisés pour se tenir informé de ce qui sort. La conséquence en est fâcheuse, et j'en ai souvent fait l'expérience :en particulier nous avions vu dans le JAMA (Journal of the american medical association) l' annonce de deux ou trois nouveaux titres de CD Interactifs très connus produits par un éditeur américain très connu. Lorsque nous avons voulu plus d'informations, le service marketing de cet éditeur nous a fait dire qu' il n' était pas au courant de la commercialisation de ces titres et il a fallu leur envoyer les photocopies des pages correspondantes du JAMA pour obtenir relative satisfaction.

On retrouve ici ce qui s' est passé il y a encore peu de temps encore avec certains CD ROM aujourd' hui bien connus, à savoir une annonce de mise sur le marché bien antérieure à la commercialisation réelle, comme si -là aussi-les éditeurs voulaient connaître la demande potentielle avant de fixer leurs prix. Et de combien de titres n' entend-on plus parler après une annonce trop précipitée. Si on manque d' informations sur les nouveaux titres, on n' en n' a guère plus sur le support lui-même. Pour paraître "à la mode", plusieurs produits se parent du terme de multimedia pour se révéler n' être en fait que des disquettes ou des bandes magnétiques. Les choses se compliquent quand vous demandez à l' éditeur comment mettre ces produits en réseaux et quel serait alors le droit en multi-utilisateurs. Et vous sentez très vite alors que vous allez plus vite et plus loin que le producteur lui même.

Une autre difficulté est encore plus importante. Et elle nous gêne beaucoup dans notre travail d' acquisitions de CD Interactifs ou de multimedia. C' est la quasi-impossibilité ou à tout le moins la très grande difficulté d' obtenir ces documents en démonstration gratuite ou payante. Dans le cas où un nouveau produit est commercialisé sous forme de disquettes ou de bandes magnétiques, on se heurte immédiatement à un refus de fournir en prêt même une disquette de démonstration, de peur que vous la copiez. En ce qui concerne les CD Interactifs ou les multimedias, nous avons rencontré deux types d' attitudes : l'une venant d' un éditeur de CD bien connu. Il n' a pas été possible d' obtenir ces titres en prêt, alors même que leur prix (10.000 F.F.) justifiait une réflexion préalable à l' achat. Pour les tester, nous avons du passer par les bons services d'une agence d' abonnements qui nous a prêté leur exemplaire de démonstration. Par contre, dans un autre cas, un éditeur scientifique des plus importants en Europe nous a envoyé fort aimablement son produit sans l' ombre d' une hésitation.

Les producteurs de nouveaux supports électroniques doivent offrir plus de transparence s' ils veulent faciliter l' accès à leur produit. A l' heure où les multimedia deviennent de plus en plus nombreux puisqu' ils représentent aujourd' hui un CD sur quatre ou cinq, une attitude aussi frileuse et réservée n' est pas concevable. Il est nécessaire que l' acquéreur -bibliothèque ou centre de documentation- bénéficie d' une information plus rapide et plus importante sur le prix, sur le contenu, sur le support enfin du produit. Les producteurs ne sont pas le seul maillon de la chaîne. Les bibliothèques en sont un autre, tout autant nécessaire pour le transfert de l' information, et à ce titre elles doivent connaître les nouveaux produits. Dans ce domaine, comme dans l' ensemble du transfert de l' information nous avons un rôle actif à jouer. Nous, bibliothécaires ou responsables de documentation, nous ne devons pas assister passifs à l' arrivée des nouvelles technologies. Nous avons à exercer un rôle critique vis à vis des outils qui nous sont proposés.

Les producteurs doivent nous considérer comme un partenaire valable et qui veut tenir sa place dans l' ensemble du transfert de l' information. Ils doivent donc nous fournir toutes les informations qui nous sont nécessaires pour exercer notre fonction de conseil. Car cette fonction est peut-être bien une des nouvelles facettes de notre métier. Il est bien possible qu' un de nos nouveaux rôles soit celui de consultant en information. Pour cela nous avons besoin de bien connaître les nouveaux produits.

THE IMPACT OF LOCAL CD-ROM NETWORKS ON USER AND LIBRARY: A Study in Eleven German-Speaking Libraries

Oliver Obst, University and State Library Münster, Germany

Abstract
An inquiry in twelve German-speaking academic libraries was undertaken to determine the changes associated with the unlimited enduser access to MEDLINE on CD-ROM. Eleven libraries and 287 users responded. The inquiry shows that almost all of the users not only accepted MEDLINE on a CD-ROM LAN but liked it very much. 54% of the inquired CD-ROM users never before performed a search in the MEDLINE database, either in printed, online or CD-ROM form, thus demonstrating the powerful attraction by this new medium. MEDLINE on a CD-ROM LAN offered an unlimited and easy access to this important bibliographic database and thereby fitted very well to the information needs of both physicians and students of medicine. The introduction of MEDLINE on a CD-ROM LAN enhanced not only the work load of the librarians but also the work quality. The staff has to be well prepared to keep pace with the changes, and new skills have to be developed. The library management has to make that change palatable to the staff, because work load seems to grow in every department, and because some librarians became frustrated in front of a changing environment.

Introduction
In 1992 twelve academic libraries in German-speaking countries offered for the first time unlimited access to the database MEDLINE via a CD-ROM LAN. It was to be expected that this did not only lead to the widespread use of this database but also to a changing relationship between the user and the library. This led me to start an inquiry, to which eleven of the twelve libraries and 287 of 600 users responded. Ten of the eleven responding libraries are located in Germany, one in Austria. In Switzerland no academic library at that time offered MEDLINE via a CD-ROM LAN. Six of the ten German libraries are located in one German federal state, in Northrhine-Westfalia because of a special fund of the state ministry. Three of the remaining four libraries are located in the former German Democratic Republic. They received grants to build up CD-ROM LANs too. This strongly confirmed that at least in Germany the financial background is most important for the development of this new library service.

Results
The inquired libraries subscribed to 150 to 7000 journals, the number of staff ranged from 3 to 80, and of students of medicine from 50 to 5000. The size of the CD-ROM LANs varied too. Two libraries (not the biggest ones) offered 200 and 300 terminals for MEDLINE access, the LANs of the remaining nine has only 2 to 10 terminals. 57% of the responding users were physicians, 38% were students, and the remaining 5% of different professions or faculties.

User
Only 2% of the students were in the first two years of their studies, but over $^2/_3$ were performing their MEDLINE search close to the end of their studies, i.e. beyond the 9th semester. This is obvious due to the fact that they used MEDLINE first of all for their dissertations (Fig.1), which usually fall in line with the end of their studies. Every other reason was not true for more then 10%. The physicians were using the MEDLINE system primary for research (36%), dissertations (27%), and publications (20%). The high level of 'dissertations' was obvious due to the fact that many students were finishing their dissertations only after having become a physi-cian. Only 2.5% of them used MEDLINE for the purpose of therapy or diagnosis, which looks quite astonishing.

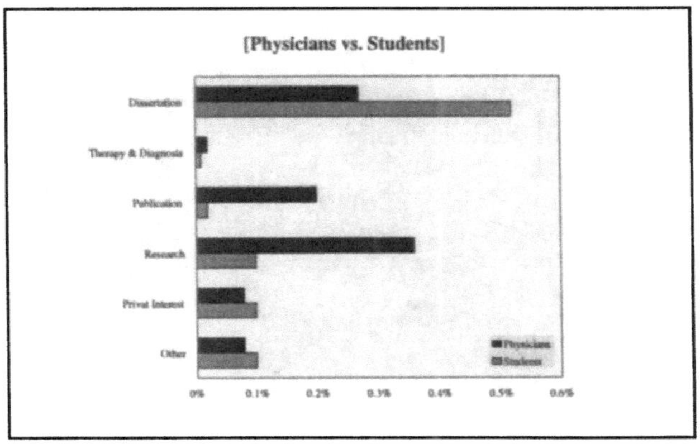

The acceptance of the database was enormous. Only one fifth of the users declared themselves as beginners. The average of searches amounted to 13 per year, and so it seemed that for the majority of the users a MEDLINE search has become a routine. Every twelfth user accessed the MEDLINE system for 40 times a year and even more! So it is save to suggest that the users fall in two categories: Two thirds of the users seemed to perform a MEDLINE search on occasion, whereas one third seemed to be periodical searchers. Most users were searching only the latest years of MEDLINE, only one third of the physicians and one fifth of the students was looking for articles older than seven years.

Search Results

More than one half of the users retrieved 1 to 20 documents per search, and further 30% 21 to 50 ones. Interestingly their existed a second peak of the distribution curve at 100 and more documents, which was retrieved by about 15% of the users. The overall mean amounts to 50.1 . This two-peaked distribution curve reminds us of the two major problems connected with enduser database searching well known in literature: First, that the search result is zero, because the users do not know how to perform a complete search, and second, that the users get too many documents and do not know how to select the relevant ones. The last statement matches closely with another result of the inquiry, i.e. more than one half of the users (57%) considered 40% or less of the retrieved documents as relevant. Nevertheless, they were very pleased with their search results, indicating that they did not put the blame on the system. The inquired users retrieved a total of 12.210 documents, of which they regarded 29% as relevant, 25% as read, and 5.2%, i.e. 633, as requested per interlibrary loan. 79% of the read ones could easily be accessed in the local library, indicating a quite satisfying coverage ratio of the local library holdings.

Satisfaction Rate

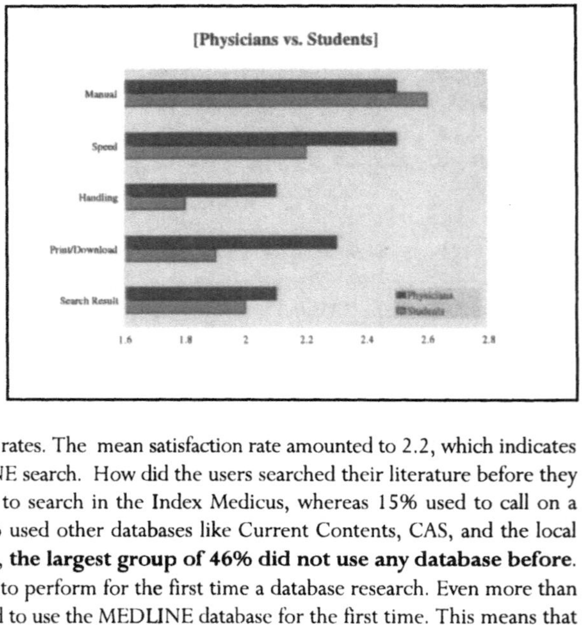

One of the most important questions for librarians is, if their users were content with the services they offer. Fig.2 shows to which extent the users were pleased with the MEDLINE system. The users could specify their satisfaction with five characteristics of the system on a one-to-six scale, on which one means very satisfied and six very unsatisfied. The Physicians (black columns) were almost more critical than the students with the exception of the manual, which they jugded a little bit better. The users, if physicians or students, were most of all pleased with the handling of the system, and the physicians with the search result, too. The option to print or download the search result was welcomed. Speed of search and the manual got higher rates, indicating lower satisfaction rates. The mean satisfaction rate amounted to 2.2, which indicates that by far most users enjoyed to perform a MEDLINE search. How did the users searched their literature before they knew about MEDLINE on CD-ROM? 31% used to search in the Index Medicus, whereas 15% used to call on a mediated online search in MEDLARS. Further 8% used other databases like Current Contents, CAS, and the local OPAC. However, what seems most important to me, **the largest group of 46% did not use any database before**. This group was attracted by the MEDLINE system to perform for the first time a database research. Even more than one half of the inquired users, i.e. 54%, was attracted to use the MEDLINE database for the first time. This means that this single CD-ROM database was capable of attracting a lot of fairly new users not only to the MEDLINE database but apparently also to the library.

Library

Every library reported about additional work load due to the CD-ROM LAN. They complained about user education (8), writing manuals (7), installation and trouble shooting of the CD-ROM LAN (6), as well as reference service (5), and staff education (4). Although not inquired, the ILL was increasing, too, as well known from literature. One important consequence of unlimited enduser access is the decrease of a traditional library service like mediated online searches. In all libraries responding to that question (7) the number of mediated online searches decreased to at least one half or even to one fifth of the level before CD-ROM LAN installation, showing an immediate and strong impact of CD-ROM on online. Only one library declared that they benefited from this decrease, but in the remaining libraries the additional work load caused by the LAN was not outweighed by the gain due to the decrease of the mediated online searches. Because in the meantime every single of the inquired libraries offers more terminals and databases, the tendency of increase of the overall work load is becoming even stronger.

Who Has to Cope with the Additional Work Load ?

In five of the eleven libraries the library manager itself took care of the LAN, in further three libraries another librarian. In five libraries the library computer department was responsible for the LAN or supported the responsible librarian. In three libraries the task of maintaining the LAN was not within the library itself, but was transfered to a commercial company or the university computer center. This very heterogenous method of handling the CD-ROM LAN strongly suggests that at once there did not exist a common mode to integrate this new and surprisingly successful medium into the libraries organization structure. The future will show if a special way of administration will take shape as the common way or if libraries will go on to implement the LAN in their organization structure where it fits best.

Conclusion

MEDLINE on a CD-ROM LAN attracted both students and physicians very well. They were delighted about that new medium. Obviously this was because it combines most of the advantages of the online- as well as the print-version. Like the print-version it can be used from many users at the same time; it has a fixed price, no matter how often it will be used; it is free of charge for the user, if the library does not charge him; and perhaps most important for the great success of MEDLINE on CD-ROM: the user is independent of any intermediary. He can search by his own. He can do or leave as he likes. MEDLINE on a CD-ROM LAN offeres multiple search options like the online-version; the user can perform a comprehensive search in a fraction of the time he would need to do the same search in the Index Medicus; he can get abstracts with a lot of additional information he does not find in the print-version; he can print his search results, walk away with them, and study them wherever and whenever he liked. In summary: **MEDLINE on a CD-ROM LAN fits very well for the information needs of physicians as well as of students of medicine**. But the library has to take care, because the expectations of their users will grow after the first enthusiasm fades away. But there are also some disadvantages. If the user performs his own search, the librarians have to teach him the right way to use the system. The library has to make space available either for the printed books or for many terminals. Until now the user cannot perform a search in more than one database at a time. Like online the user has no browsing facility, he cannot find something in the way of serendipity. An further important drawback of the CD-ROM is that in most cases it cannot be owned by the library. Even if a producer sells it, nobody knows anything about the stability of the CD-ROM, apart from technical problems to run it in the future, when hardware has changed to incompability. In most cases databases on CD-ROM are more expensive than the printed analogues, and the library cannot buy everything which might be useful. On the opposite the economic analyses in the literature suggested that some databases have to keep in printed form, some as online version and only a minor part could migrate to CD-ROM. However, as the inquiry shows clearly, each CD-ROM the library buys, means more work, and in special more sophisticated work, for which the library staff has to be well prepared to keep pace. But after all, almost all of the librarians welcomed the CD-ROM, because they knew that there was not any such extraordinary publicity for the library before.

THE DEVELOPMENT AND USE OF DRUGLINE: a full text drug information database

Birgitta Öhman, DRIC, Department of Clinical Pharmacology, Karolinska Institute, Huddinge Hospital, S-141 86 Huddinge, Sweden

Abstract

Drugline is a fulltext,Question and Answer (Q&A) database offering drug information that has been evaluated as a result of consultations in a drug information centre, run jointly by clinical pharmacologists and pharmacists. A problem-oriented database such as Drugline can be an efficient way to meet the increasing need among health care professionals for timely and accurate drug information. Physicians as well as other health professionals have increasing difficulties in finding the information necessary for carrying out their daily work. Relevant information has to be available when needed. When it comes to drug information textbooks, medical journals, printed information from health authorities, local drug bulletins, drug compendias are traditional aids. The importance of having access to online databases such as Medline has increased in parallel with the accumulation of knowledge in medicine. The development of more efficient and potent drugs has increased the demand for patient-oriented drug information by clinicians. Drugline is an example on how this need can be met.

Development

Drugline is a fulltext, Question and Answer (Q&A) database, available online. It contains problem-oriented and patient-related drug information, based on evaluation of the scientific literature. The database was developed within the Drug Research and Information Centre (DRIC) run jointly by clinical pharmacologists and pharmacists at the Department of Clinical Pharmacology, Huddinge University Hospital, Sweden. The information available in Drugline corresponds to more than 6500 questions and answers dealt with since 1982 when the computerization started. Drugline is updated ten times a year involving an annual growth of 600 documents. The language in the text fields is mainly Swedish, but 10 percent of the documents so far have been written in English, as have all the key words and field descriptors. Since 1992 a majority of the documents are written in English, which means that the number of English written documents is increasing. All documents in Drugline are indexed with key-words according to the MeSH vocabulary used for Medline. The database is today produced by a network of Swedish Regional Drug Information Centres. Drugline is hosted by MIC at the Karolinska Institute Library and Information Centre on the same computer as Medline using the Elhill program for searching. This means that a person who knows how to search Medline at MIC also knows how to search Drugline. The same user identification code as for Medline is used and Drugline is available via Medline by the command: file Drugline.

Network of DICs

Drugline has been available for online searching since 1984. Two years later a cooperation project was started between the National Corporation of Swedish Pharmacies (Apoteksbolaget) and the departments of clinical pharmacology at the university hospitals. The aim of this project was to establish DICs at the university hospitals and today there are seven Regional DICs in Sweden all organized according to the model developed at Huddinge DRIC (1,2). All DICs have access to Drugline for both searching and storage of questions and answers. The result of this cooperation project shows that, during 1993, 62% of the questions entered into Drugline were answered by DICs other than Huddinge.

Working Method

To better understand the content of Drugline the working method in a Regional DIC has to be described: A question is asked to the DIC, a literature search is performed, the information in available sources is evaluated, a preliminary telephone answer is given if needed and a referenced written answer is sent to the requester after internal review and approval at a weekly staff meeting. A standard form is used together with a check list of literature sources (available on request). Simultaneously the document is transformed to a database format and indexed with keywords according to the MeSH vocabulary used for Medline.

Quality Assurance

To assure the quality of Drugline I want to emphasize these five objectives:

1 Drugline contains evaluated drug information. The evaluation has been done by clinical pharmacologists and pharmacist.
2 The answers have been discussed and approved at a weekly "round-table" meeting.
3 When the answer is written by a junior physician or a pharmacist the medical responsibility is shared by a senior colleague.
4 If possible the answers are based on original references and not only referring to secondary sources such as textbooks.
5 Inclusion/exlusion criteria have been developed.

Types of Questions

The types of questions asked to a DIC, and consequently the profile of the Drugline content has been similar over the years: A majority of the questions concern adverse effects including risk of drug treatment during pregnancy or breast feeding, pharmacokinetic problems, choice of drug therapy and drug interactions.

Drugline Users

The utilization of Drugline has increased steadily since its introduction in 1984. Presently about 150 users access Drugline during a three-month-period and the total amount of access time in 1993 was 261 hours. The use of Drugline has been investigated (3). Questionnaires concerning the use during 1988 and 1990 were sent out on two occasions to all users having access to Drugline. The number of Drugline users increased among all professional groups studied: physicians, medical librarians and pharmacists. The pharmacists are the largest user group. During the last two years, 1992-1993, the use of Drugline has increased markedly by physicians and among these mainly clinical pharmacologists. A major user group is pharmacists and physicians working in DICs. Other user groups by branches are drug industry and education. The use of Drugline by medical librarians has been fairly constant during the last years (Figure 1).

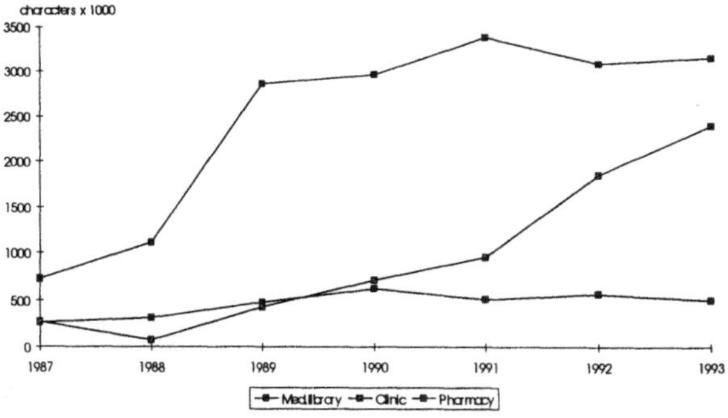

Figure 1. Drugline use by pharmacists, physicians and medical librarians 1987-1993.

Fields of A Drugline Document

One document in Drugline corresponds to one question and answer: One document contains 17 fields:

SI = Drugline
LO = location (DIC)
ED = entry date
QD = query date
QN = query number
GN = generic name
TN = trade name
ATC = ATC code
RN = CAS number
MH = MeSH (Medical Subject Heading)
QT = query text
AT = answer text
AC = answer conclusion
SO = references
IR = signature(s)
LC = literature search
FN = follow-up note

Norfloxacin - breast feeding (Question nr 09904): To illustrate this an example of a Drugline question was reviewed concerning a woman who was currently treated with Lexinor (norfloxacin) in ordinary doses and was breast-feeding her five-days-old infant. Should she continue breast feeding? The conclusion of this answer is: Avoidance of long-term treatment with norfloxacin during breast-feeding is our general recommendation. Treatment for a short period of time would probably result in only minute amounts of norfloxacin reaching the infant.

Further examples of English written questions and answers entered into Drugline in april 1994:

Can lisinopril or felodipin cause vision disorders?

Is it safe to reintroduce salazopyrine or azathioprine in a patient who has developed leukopenia?

Is there any documentation of peripheral paresis as a side-effect to oxybutynin?

Clenbuterol is misused extensively among athletes. Information is requested, especially about side-effects.

Are there any restrictions in taking ibuprofen before surgery?

Is carbamazepine teratogenic? The patient wishes to know about the risk posed to the baby in the event she becomes pregnant.

A printed collection of these documents is available on request.

Future Directions

In conclusion, I would like to point out that this model of a Drug Information Centre Network producing a database containing rather complex and time consuming pharmacotherapeutic problems has the potential to be expanded throughout Europe. It is our experience that a Question and Answer database has great potential to help problem solving in medical care. During a workshop in Italy one month ago on Health Information Services in Europe, arranged by The Mario Negri Institute and supported by the Commission of the European Communities, it was agreed upon to start a pilot cooperation project between DICs with a similar structure, aiming at producing a European Drugline. A working group was established with members from 5-6 European countries.

Finally, I would like to end my presentation of Drugline with a citation : "Where is the knowledge we have lost in information?" This was written by T.S Eliot already in 1934 and with these words I want to emphasize that medical librarians have an important role to help find the existing knowledge and of course I hope that you will add Drugline to the list of literature sources you use when you look for evaluated drug information

1 Alván G, Öhman B, Sjöqvist F: Problem oriented drug information - a clinical pharmacological service. Lancet 1983; II: 1410-1412

2 Öhman, B., Lyrvall, H., Törnqvist, E., Alvàn, G., Sjöqvist, F.: Clinical pharmacology and the provision of drug information. Eur J Clin Pharmacol 1992; 42:563-568

3 Öhman B, Lyrvall H, Alván G.: The use of Drugline - a question and answer (Q/A) database. DICP, Annals of Pharmacotherapy 1993; 27:278-284

SECTION 7

INFORMATION IN THE PHARMACEUTICAL INDUSTRY

HOW MANY PHARMACEUTICAL PERIODICALS IN EUROPE TODAY?

P Bador, A Picard, F Locher, Centre de Documentation Pharmaceutique, ISPB Faculté de Pharmacie de Lyon, 8 ave Rockefeller, 69373 Lyon Cedex 8, France

Introduction

Pharmaceutical periodicals represent a very important and invaluable source of information to pharmacists. To facilitate access to this information and because no recent work has been made on this subject, we though that it might be interesting to make an exhaustive list of the pharmaceutical periodicals published in Europe to help pharmacists locate international information.

What is A "European Pharmaceutical Periodical"

After consulting dictionaries and discussing with editors of pharmaceutical periodicals, the followed definition was retained: "A European Pharmaceutical Periodical is (i) a periodical in circulation today, published in Europe at least twice a year, and (ii) a periodical published by pharmacists or non pharmacists, carrying articles intended to help, inform, train different categories of pharmacists: community, industrial, hospital or research pharmacists, and/or (iii) a periodical dealing with pharmacology". Single-subject periodicals dealing with homeopathy, cosmetology, toxicology, pharmacognosy and those exclusively dedicated to drug monographs were not taken into account. The number of these periodicals is exceedingly high and information on them often piecemeal. Taking them into account would have made the result of the survey too hereogenous and inconsistent. We also wanted to be as comprehensive as possible in the geographical coverage of our European periodical count. So, our survey was carried out in the whole of geographical Europe and not just in the European Community. It seemed to us it was important to encourage the dissemination of pharmaceutical information in all European countries.

Methodology

1) Collection of information on European Pharmaceutical periodicals

(a) Consultation of books and lists of scientific periodicals

- 2 international directories:
  - The Ulrich's International Periodical Directory
  - The Serial Directory EBSCO

- The list of the database Serline from the US National Library of Medicine
- The list of ASHP (American Society of Hospital Pharmacists)
- The list of the international subscription agency Dawson.
- The lists of periodicals abstracted in Index Medicus, Biological Abstracts, Chemical Abstracts, Excerpta Medica, International Pharmaceutical Abstracts, Current Contents.
- The list of the current periodicals of the Health Department of the University of Lyon Library.
- The list of the French CD-ROM Myriade which provide information on two hundred and ten thousand (210,000) periodicals from two thousand and eight hundred (2,800) documentation centres in France.
- the book "La Presse du Pharmacien Francophone" by F. Locher (1985)

(b) Questionnaire

In addition, a questionnaire was addressed to publishers of periodicals and Drug Information Centres about the periodicals to which they were subscribed, especially national periodicals which were often not recorded in international indexes.

2) Data Processing

Finally, the data collected was processed on a Macintosh computer using the database management system "Quatrième Dimension". The advantage of a computerized processing is that makes for rapid and complete analysis of information using multicriterion access. Furthermore, it should be possible to permanently maintain an up-to-date list of European pharmaceutical periodicals.

Results and Discussion

Austria	3
Belgium	7
Bosnia	1
Bulgaria	5
Croatia	5
Czech Rep	3
Denmark	6
Finland	1
France	60
Germany	44
Greece	4
Hungary	2
Iceland	1
Ireland	3
Italy	17
Netherlands	12
Norway	2
Poland	10
Portugal	2
Romania	1
Russia	4
Serbia	2
Slovenia	1
Spain	28
Sweden	12
Switzerland	19
Turkey	3
Ukraine	1
UK	62

Fig. 1

1930-34	6
1935-39	2
1940-44	5
1945-49	14
1950-54	20
1955-59	15
1960-64	13
1965-69	18
1970-74	21
1975-79	40
1980-84	34
1985-89	40
1990-93	25

ʼig 2

The survey resulted in a list of three hundred and eighteen (318) European Pharmaceutical Periodicals distributed in twenty nine (29) countries. The address, country, date of first publication, frequency and language were known for more than eighty five percent (85%) of the periodicals. Other categories of information were more difficult to obtain. The creation of European pharmaceutical periodicals from 1930 to 1993 is reported in figure 2. Three (3) periods can be distinguished:

- period I from 1930 to 1944 for which less than six (6) periodicals were created every five years
- period II from 1945 to 1974 for which between thirteen (13) and twenty one (21) periodicals were created every five years.
- period III from 1975 to 1993 for which thirty four (34) to forty (40) periodicals were created every five years, twenty five (25) of which were created between 1990 and 1993.

We notice that there was a considerable increase in the number of new periodicals but we also know that many periodicals whose number is very difficult to determine, also went out of circulation.

The number of pharmaceutical periodicals published in European countries is reported in Fig 1. Three groups can be distinguished. Group I comprises periodicals published in the United Kingdom, France and Germany, each of these countries publishing more than 40 periodicals. It should, however be noted that it was easier for us to obtain information on French and West European periodicals than on periodicals published in other countries. Group II is made up of periodicals published in Italy, the Netherlands, Spain, Sweden and Switzerland, each with 12 to 28 journals. Group III comprises those published in other European countries and their number is generally less than 10 for each country. Periodical type was known for two hundred and fifty four (254) of them - eighty percent (80%). The periodicals were classified into three types: scientific periodicals, professional periodicals, scientific and professional or education periodicals :

- Scientific periodicals were the most numerous: a hundred and thirty eight (138). They maintain a high scientific level and are very specialised; their circulation is generally international.
- We see that professional periodicals are less numerous: forty five (45), their circulation is generally national.
- Sixty-six (66) scientific and professional or educational periodicals which are generally national in circulation

We can also distinguish the special group of thirty (30) independent periodicals belonging to the ISDB (International Society of Drug Bulletins). These bulletins provide reliable and impartial information assessed by an independent editorial board comprising experts who are neither of the industry nor of the governing body. Information published in such independent bulletins is given in the interest of patients and public health. They do not accept advertisements and are therefore completely independent of the pharmaceutical industry. They depend entirely on their subscribers. We can see that English is the main language of publication, a long way ahead of French, German, Spanish and Italian.

Now, we can see the number of European Pharmaceutical Periodicals indexed in six (6) international bibliographic indexes. International Pharmaceutical Abstracts, Chemical Abstracts and Excerpta Medica index the greatest number of European pharmaceutical periodicals: about one hundred and twenty (120) or forty percent (40%) of all periodicals for each of them. It is interesting to note that of these three indexes, International Pharmaceutical Abstracts has the least number of periodicals in common with the others. This means that International Pharmaceutical Abstracts indexes many pharmaceutical periodicals exclusively and this should be taken into account when searching for literature. An important part of European pharmaceutical periodicals - one hundred and twenty seven (127) or forty percent (40%) does not appear in any international index. Most of these are professional and educational periodicals which have no vocation to be international.

Conclusion

In conclusion, I think that although the electronic media is gaining in importance, periodicals are still one of the basic sources of information and are likely to remain so for a long time to come, especially in the field of pharmacy. It is very difficult in fifteen (15) minutes to present the main characteristics of European Pharmaceutical Periodicals and I will only be too pleased to provide the list and possibly more information to anyone who is interested.

References

P Bador, A Picard, F Locher Survey of European Pharmaceutical Journals in Circulation in 1993 (Part I) J. Pharm. Belg., 1994. In press.

P Bador, A Picard, F Locher Survey of European Pharmaceutical Journals in Circulation in 1993 (Part II) J. Pharm. Belg., 1994. In press

CONFRONTING THE 21ST CENTURY: Reassessing Our Value As Vital Health Information Professionals

Josephine M Marshall, The Walter and Eliza Hall Institute of Medical Research, Post Office, Royal Melbourne Hospital 3050, Victoria, Australia

As we race down the information superhighway towards the 21st Century we must ask the question are librarians valuable? The answer to that question must lie not in our perception, but who we ask. We know the value of our experience, ability and services, but is this the correct criteria? We must look at our clients or customers for the answer as the problem could be we do not value them enough. We must not make the mistake of only articulating our value within the confines of our profession.

In 1971 the Council of the National Library of Australia established the Scientific and Technological Information Services Enquiry Committee. In 1973 it reported its findings concluding that evidence gathered leaves no doubt that there is immediate need in Australia for a greatly improved and more closely co-ordinated system to collect scientific and technical information and to disseminate it to those who need it with the minimum of delay. A random sample of 4,000 scientists and technologists in areas including medicine was surveyed for information usage and needs. Amongst the myriad of survey figures and interpretations there is much mention of library services but no mention of the value of librarians in relation to information service. Some alarming figures were tabulated as a result of the survey including: 25% did not consider they had ready access to a library, 33% could not obtain literature searches when required, 45% could not acquire the journal literature with satisfactory speed, 97% of users had no formal selective dissemination of information service, over 50% stated they would be prepared to spend 6 hours of their time learning to search effectively for scientific and technical information.[7]

In 1991 in a paper by King & Griffiths tables rating importance of information resources in 2 surveys used by scientists and engineers in the US in the late 1980's rates the value of information staff in one survey as 3.05 on a scale of 1-5 (1 not important, 5 absolutely essential) and librarians as being used 14% as a source of problem solving for technical information queries.[8] Is the situation any different in medicine?

In 1988/89 the US National Library of Medicine commissioned a survey to assess the information needs of researchers in the developing field of biotechnology. What is reassuring in the case of this survey is that it was in 2 parts, where the scientists get their information and meeting the information needs of biotechnologists in which health sciences libraries were surveyed. This survey had important conclusions for librarians. Although most of all the scientists interviewed indicated that the local health sciences library was becoming increasingly tangential to the scientific process there was also a plea for help in wading thorough the flood of information. When asked what should be the purpose of the library all responded they needed someone to train them in how to identify, use and organise the information more effectively. In particular scientists thought that librarians might be the proper agents to impose some sort of standardization on the myriad of software packages and databases available. In relation to the conclusions of the researchers the conclusions of the study of librarians showed that they felt libraries were not being sought by researchers to assist with biotechnology information needs. It was interesting that librarians also saw a desperate need for help in more effective information provision in the subject field.[9] [10]

---

7 The STISEC report. Volume 1 - scientific and technological information services in Australia. Canberra: National Library of Australia, 1973: 6-7.

8 King DW, Griffiths JM. Indicators of the use, usefulness and value of scientific and technical information. In: Raitt DI, ed. Online information 91. Proceedings of the 15th International Online Information Meeting. Oxford: Learned Information, 1991: 361-77.

9 Grefsheim S, Franklin J, Cunningham D. Biotechnology awareness study. Part 1. Where scientists get their information. Bull Med Libr Assoc 1991: 79: 36-44.

10 Cunningham D, Grefsheim S, Simon M, Lausing PS. Biotechnology awareness study. Part 2. Meeting the information needs of biotechnologists. Bull Med Libr Assoc 1991; 79: 45-52.

In a study by Marshall in 1992 hospital librarians surveyed physicians as to the impact of the hospital library on clinical decision making. By involving the clinicians on a specific patient care request librarians were able to show their value and results were very positive for libraries and librarians. The library appeared as the highest rating source of information for patient care.[11] In a 1993 paper by Curtis and others were information-seeking behaviour of the health sciences faculty at the University of Chicago at Illinois was surveyed, results reflected a wide variation in results and concluded there was a need for the availability of local resources and their use to be better understood and much better training was required. Faculty still relied heavily on traditional methods of accessing information. The authors suggest that the goal of health librarians should be not only to increase awareness of resources but also to alter the faculty's information seeking behaviour.[12]

Whilst the outcomes of the Biotechnology study and Rochester study are a great leap forward from the Australian STISEC report the 1993 Chicago study still shows concerns and I would like to see librarians all over the world take up the challenge and work more closely with user groups. What is evident for librarians from all these studies is the need to develop additional skills in information gathering and information management and to aggressively promote this expertise to the users we serve. We are experts on accessing the huge body of information from the libraries and information databases of the world. It seems as if we have assumed the traditional values of the librarian could simply be taken for granted.

In medicine the new field of medical informatics converging the areas of life sciences and computer science has been developed totally divorced from libraries and there is no clear definition of the role of the librarian in this field. A 1992 US study by Forsythe and others on physicians information needs looked at information from the perspective of medical informatics and computer science. Librarians were not involved at all in the research process.[13] In Australia societies of medical informatics have been formed totally outside our profession, in fact it has been made very clear they as a group do not value our input as librarians. The fact that information services are escaping the hands of the librarian is not something new. As Cleland stated in 1993 to a degree we have been instruments of our own fate. In medical and scientific areas we have quickly forsaken the advantage and aura we developed with arcane classification systems and skilled on-line searching and rushed to put information directly into the hands of the user at its point of use. The CD-ROM experience in medicine has in particular transformed the relationship between the librarian and the user in search of information.[14]

The low value of the librarian and library in medical information provision is also not new. Over the past 20 years the survey data has been available and we, as a profession are guilty of not taking up the challenge to increase our value and perception. Many of use could give examples within our own institutions of the ease of which information systems receive support and forums, while information services, working with the new technological systems, struggle with new issues and new roles without adequate forums for discussion and support. The role of the librarian - the information services professional within the area of information technology is not being given the professional attention it requires. There is a grave danger that information services roles will become sublimated by information system roles.

It is our duty to give the service role more attention. If we do not it will not be developed effectively. In general services are not as pressing as systems, they are not as visible as systems. Many of us would have experienced how much easier it is to acquire funds to set up a CD-ROM subscription and work station or network a system than to add a librarian to the staff to handle service needs.

---

11 Marshall JG. The impact of the hospital library on clinical decision making: The Rochester study. Bull Med Libr Assoc 1992; 80: 169-78.

12 Curtis KL, Weller AC, Hord JM. Information - seeking behaviour: a survey of health sciences faculty use of indexes and databases. Bull Med Libr Assoc 1993; 81: 383-392.

13 Forsythe DE, Buchanan B, Osheroff JA, Miller RA. Expanding the concept of medical information: an observational study of physicians' information needs. Comput Biomed Res 1992; 25: 181-200.

14 Cleland MC. The role of the librarian: today and tomorrow. In: Bakker S, Cleland MC eds. Information transfer: new age - new ways. Dordrecht: Kluwer, 1993: 119-122.

In the case of Internet, in the area of health science resources there is a vast amount of data available direct to users. As at March 1994 in the Internet/Bitnet Health Sciences Resources List there were: 359 Lists; 44 Usernet groups; 38 Freenets; 22 FTP sites; 60 Electronic publications; 24 Databases; 118 Gophers.[15] The system is available but who provides education for easy access? Librarians in a large number of Australian medical libraries still do not have access to the Internet. It is vital that all librarians are aware of the resources and their relevance to their users. Information systems professionals in my experience want to control the system but do not ultimately want to promote the educational and information service role in relation to access. Librarians should see their value as bringing a cohesiveness to the information capabilities and possibilities. We must be network literate in order to be of value and promote our role as being unique in the professions.

The great challenge we all face is how to increase the perception of our value to our user group and our institutions. The reality is that we now have an opportunity to exploit these areas. To some degree in the area of medical research recent examples show that researchers are in fact being disadvantaged by by-passing the information expert, that is, the librarian. In as recent case in the world's most eminent scientific journal the Proceedings of the National Academy of Science a researcher had to publish an erratum admitting that the way in which he had searched the information data-base had been unsatisfactory in finding a key paper relevant to his discovery.[16] Anecdotal evidence is available from any number of librarians regarding problems and in all cases librarians suggested they would have provided more effective access to relevant information.

Librarians should use these bad examples to show their value in a positive light. We must not be negative. The constant problem we all have faced in recent years is that in the rush to keep ourselves up to date with the technology we have left our users wanting in instruction. Electronic information changes not only the way in which information can be used but also the nature of librarianship. We need to educate not only ourselves, but also our users. To increase our value we must show commitment to excellence in information services. In medical areas we must function as an integral part of the research team by translating protocols into simpler language for the researcher and developing programs to train our users. The better librarians are at doing this the more their services are going to be in demand. We must ensure we are proactive managers in the information chain. We must market our information services and integrate the successful delivery into our parent organizations by taking the following measures.

We should establish and maintain liaison with administrators and keep them aware of services relevant specifically to their area as well as our specialised user groups. We can offer current awareness searches and requests on demand in areas such as management, training, occupational health and safety issues. We must take time to evaluate measures to demonstrate quantitative elements of information services. Anecdotal evidence of the value of our services is easy to come by and is therefore unconvincing on its own to non-information personnel, especially those who provide our funding demand harder evidence, preferably in money terms. We can establish direct channels of communication to current and potential user groups and continually evaluate trends in information needs by surveys of users. We should give presentations on new information resources as they become available and provide regular user education seminars. We must make it our priority to keep up to date with current and future research projects and ask to be included in unit and research project meetings and ensure we are involved in clinical decision making processes. We can use newsletters and computer bulletin boards to provide a higher profile and importantly establish close contact with information systems professionals, and work together to promote available data bases, including Internet access and resources.

By actively supporting our professional groups in each country and on a wider scale in groups such as this we have an opportunity to be more valuable than ever before in the information transfer process. Librarians continue to watch the product side of information and have willingly taken must of the developments into our libraries. Together we must establish close relationships with information creators, database providers, publishers, suppliers and telecommunications carriers and take a definite intermediary role in information services.

---

[15] Hancock L. Internet/Bitnet health science resource list. March 1994. Internet via ftp:ftp.sura.net.

[16] Troutt AB, et al. Correction. Proc. Natl. Acad. Sci. USA 1993; 90: 3775.

We must increase our research activity to develop our knowledge base and publish our results. Ensure that library schools include health librarianships as a component. We should attend conferences and seminars. We must articulate our knowledge base more effectively and elevate our authority as a high profile profession. We should look at our role in relation to the ethics of information management. In all areas of research, but particularly in medicine we must work with scientists to ensure the integrity and the quality of the information we are communicating and show we are aware of concerns in relation to fraud and bad research. We should also establish codes of ethics for our own groups within the profession. The 1993 Draft Code of Ethics of the Medical Library Association includes "demonstrating the essential value of library services in meeting the information needs of the institution" amongst its goals.

We must voice our concerns and have input on decisions relating to intellectual property and copyright issues concerning information services. As a profession we should reconsider our education and service roles within the wider information environment, clarify them, strengthen them and make known what is our special value and how we want to be identified. At this moment we are facing a delicate balancing act balancing the technology and personal services. We must become what John Naisbitt terms a high tech/high touch profession. To quote Nancy Lorenzi in an address to the Medical Library Association in the US, in an article by Bastille, "tomorrows libraries will be information central and librarians will be information counsellors who act as human quality filters."[17] We should feel confident that our expertise combines high-tech skills with our understanding or our clients.

When we read in the New Scientist in December 1992, an article headlined "who needs libraries now that the world's information is accessible though computer networks"[18] we can reply - as we approach the 21st century nobody needs a library, but everyone needs a librarian the vital link in the information chain.

---

17 Bastille JD. Articulating our professional authority. MLA News 1993; 257: 12-13.

18 Holderness M. Times to shelve the library? New Scientist 1992; 136 (1850): 22-3

LIDOK: A Group Of Information Professionals in the Swedish Drug Research Industry

Hans I. Holm, Library director Astra Hässle AB, S-431 83 Mölndal, Sweden

Abstract
A short presentation of LIDOK, Läkemedelsindustrins samarbetsgrupp för I & D-frågor, established in 1972 is given. Its aims and activities are briefly described. Examples are mentioned of topics discussed at its meetings. Some of the group's projects are outlined.

Introduction
At the first EAHIL conference in Brussels 1986 (ref. 1) my colleagues Mrs. Kerstin Lindelöf and Dr. Erik Helmer gave a poster presentation of LIDOK, Läkemedelsindustrins samarbetsgrupp för I & D-frågor. It is a privilege and pleasure for me to give a full presentation at this EAHIL conference.

History
In autumn of 1972 a group of directors of libraries and information services in the Swedish pharmaceutical industry decided upon to establish a branch group within Tekniska litteratursällskapet, TLS (Swedish Society for Technical Documentation) representing the industry. Similar branch-wise groups had been established earlier, e.g. a group representing the automobile industry formed in 1968. Special interest groups were established several years later, e.g. the Swedish Online User Group, SOLUG, that was formed in 1978. The first formal meeting was held in February 1973 at AB Astra, Dr. Sixten Ljungberg of Astra was elected chairman and held that position through 1984.

Aims and Activities
The major aims of the group from the beginning were - and still are - to:

* Strengthen the professional competence of the members

* Communicate with providers of drug information in the broadest sense

The leading principles set from the start have proved to be very robust and much efficient. In short they are:

* Active participation by the members

* Generous information exchange between the members

* Minimal management and no bureaucracy

* Minutes from the meetings

Quite soon a meeting pattern developed implying:

* Two meetings a year, one in spring and one in autumn

* Routing the program-making and hostship between the group members

* The meetings lasting 1.5 days and having three modules
  : a study visit
  : a thematic session with invited lecturers
  : a reports and discussions part

The study visits reflect the wide range of interests among information professionals. Examples are:

* University libraries
* Library and information science school
* Governmental bodies, like Läkemedelsverket (the Swedish Medical Products Agency)
* Pharmaceutical production plants
* Compact disc production plant

Already from the start LIDOK took an active part in the debate of contemporary issues in the library and information service field, e.g. a Swedish National Lending Library (mainly a document supply centre) and education and training of librarians and information scientists. Contacts were made with the AIOPI of United Kingdom and later with the Italian group GIDIF-RBM.

Projects

Document supply is a major task in research industry libraries, a supply that comply with high standards on timeliness, reliability, continuity etc. The Karolinska Institute Library is the major external supplier of documents to the Swedish pharmaceutical industry. But a shared opinion from the establishment of the group was and has been through all years that the libraries among themselves should supply photocopies of journal articles. So the group started a project on documentation of periodical holdings. The results is a publication named L i s t P h a r m (ref. 2). In January 1978 an international group of editors of medical journal started work on bibliographical standards for medicine. The rules known as The Vancouver Rules were published in May 1978. Revisions have then been published in 1979, 1982, 1988 and 1991. The rules have been widely accepted and in 1994 some 400 journals have adopted them. The rules are generally brief. LIDOK formed a group for interpretation and application of the rules. The group published its report last year (ref. 3).

The Thematic Sessions

A broad area of topics have been presented at our meetings. The topics reflect the very fast development of drug information - its generation, recording, transfer, dissemination, storage and retrieval. They are also indicative for the rapid changes in our roles as information professionals.Let me give some examples of topics:

1973-74 Coverage and comparisons of databases
"""""""" Product documentation files
Watch for conferences, meetings and symposia
Tracking conference proceedings

1977-78 Education and training of medical information officers
"""""""""" User education
Copyright
Cost/benefit of information centers

1982-83 Regulatory affairs
"""""""""" Drug surveillance
The information officer as an intermediary
The information counselor
Searching chemical structures

1989-90 AI and knowledge systems
"""""""" The Swedish drug industry after 1992
Information quality
CD-ROM and multimedia
Copyright of new media

1993-94 CANDA/CAPLA/CF
"""""""" GLP/GCP/GMP
Internet
CADD

Cooperation with the Karolinska Institute Library and Information Center, KIBIC

The Karolinska Institute Library, KIB is the largest medical library in Sweden and the Medical Information Center, MIC is online host for some 25 databases. The library has very large collections of journals and monographs. It is the main national resource library in medicine in Sweden (in Swedish - Ansvarsbibliotek i medicin). Its role as document supplier to the pharmaceutical industry is very important. LIDOK made a study in 1990 on document supply. It showed that our libraries delivered 50% of the requested copies from our own holdings. For the rest external sources were used. KIB ranked first among those sources. Other major suppliers were the library at Biomedicinskt Centrum, Uppsala University, the Lund University Library and the Biomedical Library of Göteborgs University Library.

The pharmaceutical industry in Sweden is the second largest user group at the MIC. The direct connection between reference searching - MIC - and document delivery - KIB - offers a synergetic effect to the full service to the customers of our libraries. For many years LIDOK has been represented in the Board of Directors of KIBIC and in the advisory group for resource libraries in medicine. Our representatives have had excellent opportunities to express our views on the operations of KIBIC and its important role in the information supply to research on pharmaceuticals. It has turned out to be very beneficial to both LIDOK and KIBIC.

The Future

The structure of the Swedish pharmaceutical industry has changed drastically since LIDOK was founded. There are today to major groups - Astra and Pharmacia and two smaller companies. Pharmacia last year acquired the Italian company Farmitalia Carlo Erba, FICE with a research centre and library in Milano. The Astra group is establishing research sites in Europe - with fine libraries I hope. So in a near future LIDOK eventually will become an international organisation. To describe the situation let me use this metaphor:

> A Swedish graduate student, 22 years old, looking into the possibilities provided by Sweden's membership in the European Union.

References

1. Medical libraries: Cooperation and new technologies. First European Conference on Medical Libraries Brussels, Belgium 22-25 October 1986. Edited by Christine Deschamps and Marc Walckiers. (Contemporary topics in information transfer, volume 5) Amsterdam: Elsevier, 1987
2. List Pharm. Förteckning över löpande farmaceutiska tidskrifter vid Ansvarsbibliotek i farmaci, BMC i Uppsala samt biblioteken vid läkemedelsindustrier i Sverige. Upprättad av Ragna de Flon och Åke Tullgren. Stockholm: LIDOK, 1993
3. Referenser enligt Vancouver-modellen: Råd och kommentarer. Inger Falk, Lilian Gustafsson and Ros-Mari Kristiansson. Lund: LIDOK, 1993.

Acknowledgements

I express my gratitude to Dr. Erik Helmer, Pharmacia for valuable discussions on this paper.

PATIENT INFORMATION IN A COUNTRY IN TRANSITION: The Case of Croatia

Anamarija Bekavac and Zoran Buneta, Zagreb University School of Medicine, 41000 Zagreb,Šalata 3, Croatia

Abstract

Aim: To identify patient information needs and sources.

Methods: A survey of 178 patients in 6 Zagreb university hospitals.

Results: Hospital libraries have no role in patient information. There is a gap in the provision of patient-oriented publications. Physicians are still the most important and almost exclusive source of information.

Discussion: Elements affecting patient information are not only inherent to medicine but to the society as a whole. Croatian national health system did not encourage information-seeking behavior at all.

Conclusion: Patient education should be based on a multidisciplinary approach involving physicians, librarians and book-editors.

Introduction

Dissemination of medical information for non-professionals, if measured by number of popular literature or patient-oriented data bases is increasingly growing. The current interest in consumer/patient education and information is of a recent origin although patient education is not an entirely new entity (1). It has always existed but not as an organized approach to health care. In fact, according to E. Bartlett (2), the significant change in the attitude of health professionals to patient information was due to the spreading of tuberculosis in the 19th century. In a Croatian medical journal published exactly 100 years ago we found a formal recommendation for establishing of patient-oriented hospital libraries (3). The arguments quoted are the same as today: patient education and information influences recovery process and reduces risk factors. However, the growing importance of patient information is not related to medicine only but also to social change and development. There are several elements affecting the present patient information. Firstly, current emphasis on preventive medicine as opposed to curative medicine which has been a dominant orientation in the Western medical heritage. The fact that health is a recognized social priority promotes individual responsibility for personal attitude to health and consequently for health choices. A good health choice requires consumer and/or patient health education, i.e. information for lay persons.

Secondly, physician-patient communication has changed. Due to the increased use of technology, "a rigid dichotomy is maintained between a patient and a patient's illness" (4). Physicians rely on scientifically verified diagnostic methods and spend less time with their patients. Besides, there is no consensus on many health problems and patients are expected to make an informed choice (5). Superficial contact with their personal physician forces them to look for other information sources before reaching a decision. Obviously, patient dependence has been gradually declining. There are other choices to be made: why is a surgical procedure more expensive in one hospital than in another? What about the quality standards, mortality rates, waiting times, physicians? Consumer evaluation of health services is very important. Therefore, lots of information sources are available: physicians' directories with information on their specialties and subspecialties, data bases and publications with statistical data on hospital mortality rates, frequencies of certain therapeutic procedures in different hospitals, etc. It is even possible to verify physicians' credentials (6). An educated, well-informed patient is a must. Naturally, the above mentioned affects libraries, especially hospital libraries. They play an important role in patient education and provision of patient information. How do we cope with it in Croatia? Is patient information in the same focus of interest? Our paper investigates the state of patient information in Croatia. It is aimed to identify patient information needs and sources, the reasons of possible insufficient information and the role of hospital library in the provision of patient information.

Methods

In October 1993 a survey was carried out in 6 Zagreb university hospitals, all with a hospital library. It included the following departments: internal medicine, gynecology, neurosurgery, orthopedics, infectious diseases and metabolic diseases (diabetes). The survey was carried out with previous agreement and verification of head physicians. In order to eliminate the effect of possible ethical dilemmas related to patient information, terminal patients and patients with bad prognosis were not included. The questionnaire was distributed to patients during the hospital rounds and later collected by nurses. It consisted of 14 questions grouped in 2 subject areas: 1. patients' own evaluation of their information needs and sources, sufficiency of one's own medical knowledge and communication with personal physician; 2. objective data relating to published sources of medical information received and the use of hospital library.

Results and Discussion

The structure of surveyed patients (no. =178) is shown in Table 1.

Table 1. Clinical departments and number of surveyed patients

CLINICAL DEPARTMENTS	NUMBER OF PATIENTS	%
internal medicine	16	9%
metabolic diseases (diabetes)	38	21%
orthopedics	25	15%
gynecology	38	21%
neurosurgery	42	24%
infectious diseases	19	11%

The treatment of disease started a year ago (or more) for 49% patients. Subjective evaluation of their personal physician and medical knowledge shows that the majority of patients (63%) believe that their physician has given them enough information on their illness, while 37% thinks that he should have given them more information. Consequently, most patients seem to get information they need from their physicians. Still, 44% of surveyed patients consider their medical knowledge NOT being sufficient. The main reason for insufficient knowledge is superficial patient- physician communication. In their own words, physicians "never have time", "are aloof and too busy". According to these results the practice of withholding information is still existent. Patients generally know their diagnosis (80%), but the majority (88%) of patients want to get more information on their illness. Basically patients want to know. In order to obtain more information on their illness, the majority of patients would ask their physician again (64%). Other information sources are shown in figure 1.

It is obvious that patients have a preference for verbal information. Not surprisingly, physicians provide most information (7). What surprises is that other sources of information are unimportant. This is a considerable difference in patient's attitude if compared with the results in other countries. For example, alternative therapy approaches are not listed while in the USA, 34% of patients use alternative therapy approaches (8). The role of a nurse in information is also unimportant unlike Great Britain where 56% of patient information is provided by nurses (7). Actually, patients would not try to find information elsewhere. Their attitude towards their own medical care is passive. Even those patients who were not satisfied with their communication with a physician list their physician as a main source of information. Obviously a physician is a person of high authority. His authority does not even become questionable -

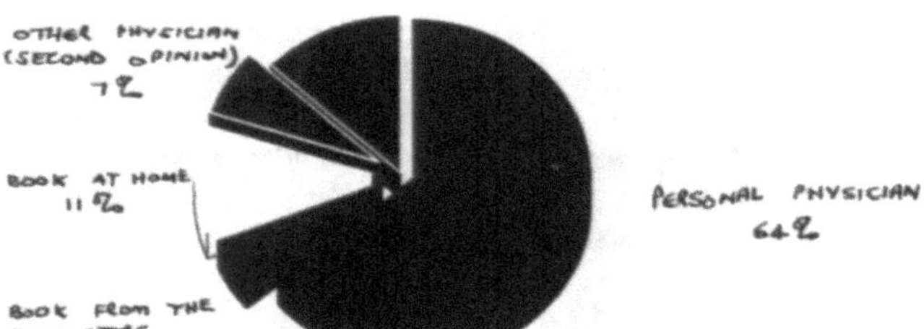

Figure 1. Information sources listed by patients

there is very little demand for "second opinion". This is also a difference from other countries (5). It seems that patients are very dependent on their physicians, and consequently inferior and submitting.
The vast majority of patients (92%) were not advised or referred to use hospital library. They were not encouraged by their physicians to seek information and consequently learn about their illness. A possible explanation lies in the fact that academic medical education emphasizes curative medicine in which physician involvement is much more important than the patient one. The majority of surveyed patients (96%) DID NOT use the hospital library. The libraries included in our survey are not small libraries, on the contrary, they play an important role in the Croatian library system. Currently, all libraries allow patient access. The provision of patient information indicates considerable gaps: 80% of patients did not get any published information like leaflets, booklets or A4 fact sheets. Those who did get it are diabetic patients (54%) and orthopedic patients undergoing total hip replacement (40%). Consequently, a better patient-education approach is related to chronic illness which is not surprising: patients with chronic illness have to participate in their treatment.

Elements affecting patient information are not only inherent to medicine but to the society as a whole. Our results are discouraging: hospital libraries have no role in patient information and there is a gap in providing patient-oriented written and published material. Moreover, physicians are still the most important and almost exclusive sources of information. Why? Croatia is a country in transition. National health system is undergoing change but consequences of the former health system are still present. How has it affected patient education and information? Patients could not make choices within health services. There were only state health services which were free of charge. Private practice was not existent. A patient was assigned to a certain health institution according to the place of living or working. It was not up to the patient to choose a health service because everything was pre-determined. If the waiting lists were too long you could just wait. There was no choice of physician, no directory of physicians. There were no quality indicators available to general public. There was no competitiveness between health institutions (number of patients was established in advance, and so were salaries etc.), there was no way of identifying medical elite or centers of excellence. Patients were not expected to choose (but to obey). Information-seeking behavior was not encouraged at all.

Conclusion

Patients need to be informed. There are many papers verifying the positive effect of patient education on disease outcome (9, 10). There is a positive correlation between quality and cost of medical care and patient education. It should be a starting point in planning and organizing patient education. Patient education should be based on a multidisciplinary approach involving physicians, librarians and book editors. An educational environment should be established offering different resources (11). Physicians should encourage patient information seeking, knowing it contributes directly to patient care. They should improve standards of patient communication by publishing patient-oriented (popular) books and papers, leaflets of simple clinical guides. Publishers should encourage it. Librarians should actively support patient access to medical libraries and promote it. Integrated professional and health collections have to be developed, but till then textbooks or nursing literature can be used for patient education. Libraries could be places where patient education programs are performed. Clinical medical librarian program looks like science fiction at present, but rapid social changes will eventually affect medical librarianship. The more patients will seek information, the greater will be the role of medical library. Becoming a member of the health care delivery team is not entirely beyond reach of the library. Therefore, let us provide information before it is requested, let us anticipate changes to come.

References

1. Gann R. The people their own physicians: 2000 years of patient information. Health Libraries Review 1987;4:151-5.
2. Bartlett E. Historical glimpses of patient education in the United States. Patient Education Counseling 1986;8:135-49.
3. Osnutak knji` nica u bolnicama (Foundation of hospital libraries). Lijec Vjesn 1905;26:82.
4. Rees A.M. Communication in the physician-patient relationship. Bull Med Libr Assoc 1993;81(1):1-10.
5. Rees A.M. Characteristics, content, and significance of the popular health periodicals literature. Bull Med Libr Assoc 1987;75(4):317-22.
6. La Rocco A. The role of the medical school-based consumer health information service. Bull Med Libr Assoc 1994;82(1):46-51.

7. Cameron P, Corbett K, Duncan C, Hegyi K, Maxwell H, Burton P.F. Information needs of hospital patients: a survey of satisfaction levels in a large city hospital. Journal of Documentation 1994;50(1):10-23.
8. Eisenberg D, Kessler RC, Foster C, Norlock FE et al. Unconventional medicine in the United States: prevalence, costs, and patterns of use. N Engl J Med 1993;328(4):246-56.
9. Bertel O. Der Einfluss von Patienteninformation, Compliance und arztlicher Fuhrung auf die Prognose bei chronischer Herzinsuffizienz (Effects of patient information, compliance and medical control on prognosis in chronic heart failure). HERZ 1991;16(1):294-7.
10. Rost KM, Flavin KS, Cole K, Mc Gill JB. Change in metabolic control and functional status after hospitalization. Impact of patient activation intervention in diabetic patients. Diabetes Care 1991;14(19):881-9.
11. Gilpin L. Creating an educational environment in a hospital setting. In: Giloth B, ed. Managing hospital-based patient education. Chicago: American Hospital Association, 1993:55-75.

Section 8

Consumer Health Information

CONSUMER HEALTH INFORMATION IN THE COUNTY OF DALARNA, SWEDEN

Ingrid Helander och **Bengt Holmquist**, The Hospital Library and Information Centre of Falun, Sweden.

Abstract
In The Hospital Library and Information Centre of Falun in Sweden work is going on since 1993 to build up a collection of material for patients and their relatives and to put it into a database, where it will be easily accessible.

We are working in the Hospital Library and Information Centre of Falun in Sweden. Our library is a combined and integrated library consisting of a medical library and a general library for patients and staff. Since spring 1993 we are working to build up a collection of material for information to patients and their relatives about illness and health. We register the material that we have collected in a database, where it is easily accessible. This new work is based on ideas in the Swedish Health Care Law, where stress is laid on the fact that patients have the right to get all the information that they want about their illnesses. The patient has the right to get enough information to be able to decide about his treatment. A necessary condition is then that the patient knows where and how to get this knowledge. We also try to adapt the information to the person who is asking as much as possible.

There are many investigations showing that a patient who is well informed gets less anxious and because of that has greater possibilities to influence his situation. These ideas are also in accordance with the thoughts in the Dala Model, the model according to which health care is organized in our county. The ideas that have inspired us we have got above all from Great Britain, where the Patient's Charter 1992 was a great step in this direction. We have been especially inspired by the work carried out by Sally Knight at Lister Hospital in Stevenage outside London. In Great Britain many other local initiatives have been taken during the last twenty years. We also learnt about similar work in Denmark, especially in Odense where we went to study their work.

We have decided to work together with two other Swedish hospital libraries, Västervik and Karlstad. We think that we all can get great advantages out of such a co-operation. We are going to make our database for patient information available not only in our own library but also to the public libraries of the region, to primary health care and the general practitioners. This means that in fact everybody will be allowed to search in our database. Parts of the material are also going to be available in the public libraries but other parts have to be borrowed from our library. One of the town libraries of the region has already begun to use our new database. When you start this kind of work, it is really very important to make the politicians who grant the money interested in the work. When we went to Odense, for example, to study their library and their methods, we went together with one of our politicians and already when we were on our way home he decided to provide us with one full-time appointment for three months. It is, of course, also very important that you are serious and careful when you select the material for the database. It is also important that we never make diagnoses or give advice concerning a patient's illness. The task of the librarian must always be to search and deliver information. However, we often recommend the patients to discuss the information with their doctor.

The main features of the material in our database will be the following:

The publications that will be found in our database should be of current interest. They should be easy to read and easy to understand. They ought to be, on the whole, written in Swedish and they ought to be available in our library.

The database will above all contain information about different illnesses and diseases but also about preventive medicine and health promotion. We will also put material concerning established branches of alternative medicine into the database, for example concerning acupucture.

What kind of material are we then putting into our database?

1. We have gathered pamphlets from as many patient organizations in Sweden as possible. These organizations produce information material of great quality. These pamphlets will be searchable in our database.

2. There are many books and other publications in our ordinary catalogue that are suitable for this purpose. All these publications will be included also in our database for patient information. It may be books from the medical library that are easy to read. It may also be biographic descriptions, fiction or biographies, wherein patients or their relatives tell about their experiences of a certain illness.

3. We are also indexing suitable articles from different journals and magazines. In addition we can make literature searches in different databases on interesting subjects concerning patient information to get more journal articles on these matters.

4. Pharmacies, drug companies and insurance companies are other institutions that publish material that is of great interest for us in our work with patient information.

5. We have also contacted different clinics in the hospital to find out what pamphlets and other material they use to inform their patients. Several clinics have sent us their material and we have included also this material in our database.

6. In addition we have cassettes with recorded radio programmes dealing with these matters. Video films suitable for patient information will also be available.

7. We also put into our database all information about patient organizations and other associations that may be of interest. You may get, for example, information about contact persons, addresses, telephone numbers and fax numbers. All this material we put into the database and it will be searchable there.

We are going to inform about this work as much as possible in different ways. Among other things we will of course establish contact with all local representatives of the patient organizations. We would also like to arrange days with a certain theme, as has already been done in Odense and to invite experts to make lectures and patients to tell what it is like to live with a certain illness. At last I want to tell you what possibilities you have when you want to search for material in our database. The constructor and designer of the database is Mikael Mikaelsson, who is also a librarian at our library.

There are five different possibilities: you may search for titles, patient organizations, authors and subjects; or you may also use free-text searching. The subject index will probably become the most used index. You just write the name of the disease that you want to know something about, for example DIABETES. Then you notice that we have more than ten documents in the database about diabetes. If you press the enter key you get a list of all publications we have got on this subject. If you press the enter key again you can get complete information about each document and also information about where you may find it in our library. You may also look at EPILEPSY in the same way. When you make a search in the index of the patient organizations you just write, for example, *DIABETESFÖRBUNDET,* which is the Swedish patient organization for those, who have diabetes. You notice that we have more than ten documents in the database from that organization. If you press the enter key you get all information about this organization, for example address, telephone number and fax number. You also get a list of all publications that we have got from that organization. If you press the enter key again you may get full information about each publication. You may also, if you like, get a list of all patient organizations that we have put into the database. The possibility of free-text searching will of course also prove very useful. You may search on any word and you may then be quite sure that you haven't missed anything. You may, for example, make a search on CHILD and DIABETES or on YOUTH and EPILEPSY and in each case you will get a list of all publications that we have got about this in the database. If you press the enter key you may get full information about each publication. Questions from patients and their relatives concerning these matters have always been part of our work but now we make a great effort to extend this work with patient information. We believe that the need for this type of information is very great and we hope to be able to provide people with the information that they need. Hopefully, this will affect their state of health in a positive direction.

THE ATTITUDES OF MEDIA TOWARDS MEDICAL RESEARCH: Are Women's Journals More Receptive Than Medical Journals?

Elisabeth BACON, INSERM 405,Département de Psychiatrie, Hopitaux universitaires de Strasbourg, 1 place de l'Hôpital, BP 426, 67091 Strasbourg CEDEX, France.

Abstract

The aim of the study is to investigate the different levels of the popularization of scientific research and medical information in the written press. The research is based on an attempt to popularize scientific knowledge by a scientific researcher. The information concerns the effects of the anxiolytic drugs on memory. Several articles were written on this subject and submitted to various newspapers addressing different audiences (medical journals, a daily newspaper, women's journals). The research comprises the recordings, progressively, of the events and negociations with the various journals.*

Introduction

The laboratories are the places where the scientific knowledge is elaborated. The background of every scientific activity constructs itself of exchange and communication. Each scientist is handing a role and a responsibility in information. The scientist has the advantage, compared to the journalist, of not being slave to the instant need of delivering information. On the other hand,we can see that, today, there is a growing interest of the public towards science, especially when related to health and medicine : The increasing room attributed to scientific articles or even the existence of science supplements in the general press are revealing this state of mind[19]. But there is not one but several publics, with each his own centers of interests. And the language that their favorite media use also differs. However, in the meantime, one can observe that the effective diffusion of scientific knowledge is very weak. And, concerning the medical domain, it is established that the medical profession is not aware very much of the progresses of their field and that, in the meantime, they supply the consumer with very few information about health and drugs[20].

These statements lead to some questioning : Indeed the researcher should feel interested in the way his research area is popularized. But how is the science transmitted from the researcher to the general public? What is the effective part played by scientists in the diffusion of their research results ? Can they, or must they, popularize their knowledge ? What are the obstacles to this transfer, either voluntary or unintentional ? I tried to find some elements of answer to these questions by studying *the different levels of the popularization of science in the written press.*

Method Used.

I chose to base my research on a concrete experiment of communication of scientific research. In that purpose, I tried to popularize some aspects of *the GABA/benzodiazépine receptor* which was the object of my experimental research at the Center of Neurochemistry in Strasbourg. I am a scientific researcher, PhD, neurochemist, working at INSERM which the french Institute of Research In Health and Medicine. The GABA/benzodiazepine receptor consists of a particular system of nervous transmission. It is the object of study of many research groups throughout the world, either in fundamental research or in clinical research. I have studied the pharmacology of this receptor[21]. Benzodiazepines, for their part, are anxiolytic and hypnotic drugs (The wellknown drugs Valium and Halcion belong to this family). Benzodiazepines constitute a subject of the present day, that interests the layman : they are the worldwide most largerly prescibed anxiolytics, and french people are indeed the biggest consumers of tranquillizers. No wonder that they feel particularly concerned. This also means that french doctors are the biggest prescribers. They should also be interested,

---

Fayard P., Alliage,1993, 1993, 16-17, 226-234.
Medias, santé et information, *La revue Agora*, 1990-91, 16.

for ex. : Bacon E, Girard C. de Barry J. & Gombos G, muscimol and flunitrazepam binding sites in the developing cerebellum of mice treated with methylazoxymethanol, *Neurochem. Res.*, 1992, 7, 707.

therefore, in the progress of the scientific knowledge concerning benzodiazepines and their way of action. This subject is also of great current interest: the European Commitee for Proprietary Medicinal Products (CPMP) recently rendered official recommendations concerning the use and prescription of hypnotics. And the safety of the benzodiazepine Halcion has been the object of a great controversy that lead to the restriction of his delivery in many countries and even his suspension in some others[22].

The first step of my research was "experimental". I wrote several articles on some aspect of the GABA/benzodiazepine receptor (GABA/BZP) and submitted them to different journals adressing different audiences. I tried both to adapt the content and the style of my paper to the nature of the newspaper and to transmit concepts that I consider important in the popularization of science, I mean to diffuse also the questions, unresolved problems and controversies.

Selection of the subject: It was necessary to select an aspect of the GABA/BZP receptor that would interest a large audience. One of them was the effects of benzodiazepines on human memory. Benzodiazepines have this peculiar property that, in some circumstances, they impair memory. Briefly, they affect the acquisition of new information while the recovery of already learned information remain unimpaired. This effect ends when the drug is eliminated from the organism. The amnestic effects of the anxiolytic drugs benzodiazepines are both fascinating and a source of anxiety : how can someone behave normally, but remember absolutely nothing about what they had been doing for a certain lapse of time ? This property has been well known by the anaestetists for the intravenous forms since 1965. But it has been mentioned only since 1993 for the oral forms in the monographies of the french dictionnary of medicine, Le *Vidal*.

The range of the sollicitated newspapers covers :
- an international journal of neurology (*la Revue Neurologique)* in french with an english abstract.
- international pluridisciplinar scientific newspapers (in english : *Nature, Science*)
- international medical journals *(The Lancet, N .E.N.J. Med., Brit. Med. J.)*
  (The above manuscripts have been written in collaboration with François Sellal who is MD, neurologist and has worked on the amnestic effects of BZP at the psychiatric clinic in Strasbourg.)
- the french form of an american popularization magazine(*Pour la Science - Scientific American*)
- a daily french newspaper *(Le Monde)*
- a french medical journal *(Prescrire)*
- feminine magazines *(Vital, Prévention Santé, Santé Magazine, Top Santé)*

This panel of newspapers is enlarged by the submission to some other newspapers of other aspects of the GABA/BZP neurotransmission system. These will not be evoked here.

The second step is analytical and critical. Beyond this direct approach of scientific communication, my research comprises the recordings, progressively, of the negociations and the events with the several newspapers. Each newspaper should react to my proposals according to its specific criteria. Some elements of answear to the important questions previously mentioned shoud emerge from this parallel study.

Results and Discussion

Some articles were published in different media, some are in progress. The submission itself of a paper was always followed by comments that enlight the behaviour of the different editorial staffs. Only the most illustrative results will be pointed out here.

- The article submitted to the neurological journal was a rather classical review of the litterature on the subject of the amnestic effects of benzodiazepines. It was accepted without modification but the title by the two anonymous

---

Cowley G, Springen K, Iarovici D, Hager M, Sweet dreams or nightmares ? *Newsweek,* 19.8.91, 38.

referees[23]. Their comment was that *taking into account the considerable number of prescribers and of users of these drugs in France, it is necessary that doctors are informed of these side-effects. This review brings to light the complexity and the questions that remain today on that subject.* So they entirely understood our purpose and agreed with our point of view. More surprinsingly, the editor commented on the style of our manuscript, saying that is was very exceptional that they do not have to improve it. Indeed they usually observe that scientists, when they address other scientists, consider that it is not necessary to have a good style ! For my study on the diffusion of science this publication constitutes the caution of the competence of the authors on this topic.

- A second step was to submit an article on this subject to an international medical journal. In this second manuscript, we tried to highligt the history and logic of the discovery and the study of the effects of benzodiazepines on human memory. In particular, we wanted to demonstrate how the first observations of this effect were made, why it was unknown by physicians and considered unimportant for such a long time, and how the transformation into an undesirable effect occurred, partially as a consequence of media coverage of a trial. To our point of view, the history of this effect convincingly reflects the complementarity between individual medical observations and strictly fundamental research programs. We thought that this article could stimulate lively discussion in the scientific and medical community on the use of these drug[24].

The manuscript was sent to 3 international english speaking medical journals. As an example of answer, *The Lancet* declined our proposal, arguing that they *receive ten times as many papers as they can find room for, and on this occasion* they said *to be aware of having published rather a lot on the side effects of BZP and related drugs*. Indeed the first derscription of the amnestic effect of BZP was published in the *Lancet*, in 1979, when a dutch Dr, Van der Kroef, described in a *letter to the editor* the strange reactions of some of his patients towards the BZP Halcion. However, since then, the *Lancet* has never published a synthetic article on this theme. I studied their publications on this topic which were done the last 4 years. Most of them were anecdotal and very descriptive *letters to the editor,* along with a few short individual studies. More precisely, I submitted my paper in december 1992. In 1992, one paper about endogenous ligands, a *brief comment* , 3 *news* and 4 *letters to the editor* were published. This is not very much for a weekly newpaper and my impression is that the *Lancet* had no concern of a reflexion on that subject.

- Another step was to submit a paper to a dayly french newspaper. I chose *Le Monde* at the occasion of the limitation of prescription of these drugs which was decided by the french health ministry in the autumn 1991. The reaction of the journalist responsible of the weekly medecine supplement was at first reticent. He was afraid about the readability of a paper written by a scientist. He felt more enthusiastic when he receive the manuscript and published it just as it was[25]. For three main reasons : He was very interested by the "scientific" approach of the subject that scientific journalists have no time to do. He thought that this paper was a good tool for his reader to initiate a personal reflexion on that subject. He also considered the subject as a supplementary opportunity to verify the particular behaviour of the medical community towards information. Indeed he often observed that when doctors popularize medicine, they speak only about benefits and never evoke the risks inherent to the drugs. And this has lead to many health problems in the society, one of the most striking ones being the question of the blood perfusion to haemophils related to AIDS.

- After this article had come out in the columns of *Le Monde*, I asked a french medical journal if they would have published such a paper. The answer was *no* because they considered it as *too theoretical and too fundamental*. After the experience with *The Lancet*, this reinforces my impression that medical journals do not want their readers to have a

---

Sellal F, Bacon E.& Collard M, Mémoire et benzodiazépines, *Rev., Neurol.*, 1994, 150, 5, in press.

Bacon E. and Sellal F., The amnestic effects of benzodiazepines. How an advantageous property becomes an adverse side-effect.

Bacon E, les effets des benzodiazépines sur la mémoire: Dr Jekyll or Mr Hyde? *Le Monde*, 1. 1. 92, 10.

fundamental consideration on their practice. I was told they have to look for that elsewhere. But which media will help them to think it over ?

- In an ultimate step I wrote to 4 french feminine magazines[26]. Only one of them, *Santé Magazine,* gave an answer. They felt surprised and honoured that a scientist is interested by the general public. They appreciated my *care to inform people about the prescription of these drugs which are often improper and thoughtless* . They accepted to present the *essential scientific notions*. They sent me a list of questions that their readers would ask about BZP. These testify to rather concrete concerns, but are also revelative of the imprecision and the anxiety that the classical medical speech generates in the mind of the consumers. (ex : *are anxiolytics and tranquillizers different drugs or the same ? is that true that BZP induce tolerance ? When should one consume them ? are all the anxiolytics BZP ? Is alcool an anxiolytic ?...*). Once again they were surprised that a scientist could be able, they said, *to write a very clear and precise letter* !

Thus, like the specialized neurological journal, like the dayly newspaper, but unlike the medical journals, this feminine magazine felt concerned by some information and reflexion about these drugs. Also, the distrust of the media against the ability of scientists to popularize themselves their knowledge give us an idea of the image of the scientist in their mind. They think that he is able to make himself understandable only by his peers. In turn, the remarks of *Santé Magazine* show that most of the scientists consider that the popularization in such media is a non important activity.

Conclusion

Today, many personalities, either politics, philosophers, sociologists or scientists, have an opinion about scientific research, about his role within the society and about the responsibility of scientists in the popularization. They generally reproach to the scientist not to communicate his knowledge. But my study shows that the media, and particularly the medical journals, also have some responsibility in this state of facts. This original situation that the scientist himself popularizes his knowledge, allows to bring to light, from the inside, which are the real interests ad stakes, and to precise the modalities of the transmission of medical information. It reveals some paradoxes between the need to transmit medical informations and the behaviour of some medical journals. For example, the general physicians, although the biggest prescribers of benzodiazepines, are rather unaware of this adverse side-effect of the anxiolytics. But most of the medical journals would not publish a synthetic review article devoted to the subject.. It questions subsequently which media french physicians employ when looking for scientific information. It seems that they often find them in the scientific supplement of their dayly newspaper (like *Le Monde* or *Le Figaro*) rather than in the medical journals which remain very focused on practice. A french study performed in 1987 reveals even more surprising ascertainements : feminine magazines like *Elle* or *Marie-Claire* have been mentioned as sources of information by medical doctors[1] ! I think that the medical journals should be aware that it is important for the practicians to know more about the progresses of medical research. This knowledge might be helpful for the consideration that the practicians have about their dayly medical practice. And medical journals should feel concerned to be the tool to provide them this information. They should at least feel more concerned than the doctor's wife's newspaper! In a further step, I am intimately convinced that this study will help to improve the dialogue between the researchers, the media, the medical profession and the consumers.

Bacon E., Je n'angoisse plus mais j'ai oublié. D'un effet inattendu des tranquillisants, 1994, in progress for *Santé Magazine*.

SECTION 9

PROFESSIONAL ISSUES

LE RESEAU FRANCAIS DES DOCUMENTALISTES HOSPITALIERS

Françoise Blondel, Centre Hospitalier Universitaire de Rouen, Centre de Documentation Administrative, 1 Rue de Germont, 76031 Rouen Cedex, France

Résumé

Né de la grande diversité de la situation des centres de documentation hospitaliers français ainsi que de l'hétérogénéïté des statuts des documentalistes, le réseau national des documentalistes hospitaliers français a été créé en 1991. Regroupant maintenant 190 adhérents, il se propose de contribuer à leur formation permanente, de faire partager les acquis et les ressources de chacun, de tendre vers la reconnaissance d'un véritable statut de documentaliste, enfin de faire émerger une réelle identité professionnelle.

I - Situation de la documentation hospitaliere Française

A) Les différentes catégories d'etablissements hospitaliers publics. Trois types d'établissements hospitaliers recensent des bibliothèques ou centres de documentation :

- les centres hospitaliers régionaux et universitaires (au nombre de 29) qui se définissent par un plateau technique très élaboré, l'obligation de disposer des services les plus spécialisés et l'apport d'un corps médical hospitalo-universitaire ;

- les centres hospitaliers qui disposent d'un plateau technique destiné à faire face aux besoins généraux et immédiats de la population mais qui n'ont pas vocation à se spécialiser ;

- les centres hospitaliers spécialisés qui comportent une ou plusieurs unités relevant des disciplines concourant au traitement d'une même pathologie comme les hôpitaux psychiatriques par exemple.

B) Les différentes catégories de bibliothèques ou centres de documentation. Trois types de bibliothèques ou centres de documentation prédominent : les bibliothèques médicales, les bibliothèques paramédicales et les bibliothèques administratives. On peut noter que dans les CHRU[27], la tendance serait plutôt à l'éclatement des bibliothèques par spécificité et sites géographiques différents alors que dans les centres hospitaliers la tendance serait plutôt à la centralisation de ces trois catégories sur un même site, bien que des exceptions existent des deux côtés. Il est aussi parfois adjoint à ces centres la gestion des archives médicales. Ce sont en général les bibliothèques médicales et paramédicales qui sont les mieux organisées et pourvues de moyens, les bibliothèques administratives étant plus rares et souvent embryonnaires.

C) Le statut des documentalistes hospitaliers et leur place dans l'organigramme Il n'existe à l'heure actuelle aucun statut "officiel" des documentalistes hospitaliers. La situation de chacun relève donc de dispositions locales dues au bon vouloir des directeurs d'hôpitaux ou parfois prises après délibération du Conseil d'administration. La majorité des documentalistes est rattachée à la grille des personnels administratifs de la fonction publique hospitalière soit dans de très rares cas comme chefs de bureau (catégorie A), soit pour les plus nombreux comme adjoints des cadres (catégorie B), soit malheureusement pour certains comme adjoints administratifs (catégorie C) alors que la plupart d'entre eux ont un niveau minimum bac + 3 en plus de leur diplôme professionnel. Une minorité est rattachée à la grille de la fonction publique territoriale ou au statut des documentalistes de l'Education Nationale.

---

[27]CHRU : Centre hospitalier Régional et Universitaire

Quant à la place du documentaliste dans l'organigramme de l'établissement, elle est aussi très variable et très locale. Les documentalistes médicaux dépendent plutôt du corps médical (président de CME[28] ou médecin-chef de service du DIM[29]). Les documentalistes paramédicaux dépendent plutôt des directrices d'écoles paramédicales (le plus souvent écoles d'infirmières). Quant aux documentalistes administratifs, ils dépendent plutôt du directeur général ou d'un autre directeur administratif (communication ou ressources humaines). Mais là encore, il n'y a pas de règle absolue et tous les cas de figure sont possibles.

D) Les fonds documentaires. Là encore, aucune harmonie. La fourchette du nombre d'ouvrages varie de quelques centaines à plusieurs milliers, les fonds d'ouvrages les plus importants se retrouvant soit dans les bibliothèques paramédicales soit dans les bibliothèques pluridisciplinaires. Quelques centres de documentation ne comprennent que des périodiques. Même inégalité au niveau de ces derniers : la fourchette du nombre d'abonnements va d'une dizaine à plusieurs centaines. Quelques centres, mais ils sont rares, adjoignent à ces documents un fonds audio-visuel, le plus souvent des vidéo-cassettes destinées à l'enseignement médical et paramédical. L'informatisation de ces fonds n'est pas effective pour la majorité des centres de même que l'accès aux banques de données et l'équipement en CD-ROM restent minoritaire.

E) La création du réseau

La conclusion qui vient à l'esprit à l'issue de cette approche est la constatation de l'extrême diversité des situations. On serait presque tenté de dire : à chaque établissement son cas particulier. Diversité dans les statuts, dans la composition des fonds documentaires, dans l'attribution des moyens financiers, dans la reconnaissance de la fonction de documentaliste. Ce constat a entrainé une volonté de regroupement des professionnels de la documentation hospitalière. Né de l'initiative du Directeur Général du CHRU de Rouen (Monsieur Halbout) et de l'une des documentalistes de cet hôpital (F. Blondel), le réseau français des documentalistes hospitaliers est né en 1991 et a vu rapidement le nombre de ses adhérents augmenter de 18 à la première réunion à environ 120 en mai 1994.

II - Le réseau

A) Les objectifs.

- Sortir les documentalistes de leur isolement (car très souvent, ils sont seuls de leur profession dans leur établissement) en leur permettant d'établir des contacts de travail par le biais du réseau.

- Contribuer à leur formation permanente en invitant dans les différentes réunions des personnalités qui apportent connaissances ou expériences.

- Partager les acquis, les ressources diverses de chacun, les expériences positives ou négatives dans le but d'une entraide permanente.

- Faire reconnaître la fonction de documentaliste en tant qu'expert du traitement de l'information afin d'aboutir à la constitution d'un véritable statut.

- Enfin, faire émerger, au travers de ces travaux, le concept d'une réelle identité professionnelle afin que chacun et chacune se sente appartenir à un corps professionnel au service du lecteur.

---

[28]CME : Commission Médicale d'Etablissement

[29]DIM : Département d'Information Médicale

B) Les adherents.

Au nombre exact de 118, ils de décomposent de la manière suivante :

- 57 documentalistes appartiennent à un CHRU (dont 12 de l'Assistance Publique des Hôpitaux de Paris) et représentent 26 des 29 CHRU français ;
- 48 documentalistes proviennent de centre hospitaliers (dont 31 de province et 17 de la région parisienne) ;
- 9 documentalistes travaillent dans des centres hospitaliers spécialisés ;
- 4 documentalistes représentent des instances plus officielles (Direction des Hôpitaux au Ministère de la Santé, Ecole Nationale de la Santé Publique, Centre National de l'Equipement Hospitalier). On notera la parité parfaite entre les documentalistes de CHRU et ceux des autres établissements hospitaliers publics.

De même la répartition géographique des adhérents donne 1/4 de documentalistes parisiens pour 3/4 de provinciaux.

C) Le fonctionnement. Jusqu'en mars 1994, le réseau organisait deux rencontres annuelles d'une journée chacune, toujours à Paris. La Direction des Hôpitaux au Ministère de la Santé, le CNEH[30] ainsi que l'AP-HP[31] ont ainsi accueilli les participants à tour de rôle. La moyenne de membres présents à chaque réunion est de 60 personnes environ (soit 50 % de l'effectif total). Chacune de ces réunions a été l'occasion de recevoir un certain nombre d'intervenants qui ont procédé à la présentation d'outils professionnels : banques de données, CD-ROM, thésaurus en soins infirmiers, Agence de Presse Médicale, Agence d'abonnements internationaux.
Une juriste est venue une fois faire une conférence sur le droit de la reprographie intéressant au plus haut point les membres présents qui voyaient là une réponse concrète à des soucis quotidiens et pragmatiques.

D) Les travaux réalisés. Le premier travail effectué par ce réseau a été la constitution d'un annuaire de la documentation hospitalière inexistant jusqu'alors et répondant ainsi au premier objectif ci-dessus cité. Deux éditions ont été réalisées ; les membres du réseau devenant de plus en plus nombreux chaque mois, une troisième édition est prévue pour la fin de 1994. Une enquête diligentée par la Direction des Hôpitaux a permis de faire le point de l'existant sur les diplômes professionnels des documentalistes, leur place dans leurs établissements, l'informatisation ou non de leur centre, les logiciels éventuellement utilisés... etc. Quelques articles ont été écrits par des membres du réseau dans la presse professionnelle hospitalière afin de faire découvrir la réalité d'un métier.

Des groupes de travail thématiques ont été constitués afin que le réseau avance sa réflexion de façon plus pratique; tous les problèmes ne pouvant être réglés au cours des réunions plénières. Trois thèmes ont été pour l'instant retenus:

Ethique et déontologie de la profession ;
Prêt inter-bibliothèques et fourniture de documents ;
Evaluation économique des centres des de documentation.
D'autres thèmes devraient voir le jour d'ici quelques mois.

III - Prospective et conclusion

A) Consolidation du réseau. Lors de la dernière réunion (mars 1994), un débat de fond riche et passionnant s'est ouvert sur l'avenir de cette structure qui devenait lourde à gérer, vu l'augmentation constante de ses adhérents et qui

[30]CNEH : Centre National De l'Equipement Hospitalier

[31]AP-HP : Assistance Publique-Hopitaux de Paris

n'avait pas de représentant légal mandaté par l'ensemble des collègues pour effectuer des démarches, courriers ou autres activités. La question s'est posée de se constituer en association professionnelle dans le cadre légal de la loi de 1901. Mais la majorité des membres présents s'est opposée à cette transformation qui aurait entrainé des lourdeurs administratives telles que : assemblée générale annuelle, élections annuelles, gestion de trésorerie... etc. La souplesse de fonctionnement d'un réseau informel tel qu'il existait jusqu'à présent a paru à tous, la meilleure des solutions. Cependant afin d'assurer une meilleure organisation et une meilleure coordination dans la répartition des tâches, un bureau de huit membres a été élu dont la présidence a été confiée à Mme Françoise Blondel. La décision a été également prise de ne plus faire qu'une seule rencontre annuelle, mais de deux jours consécutifs, permettant ainsi l'organisation d'une sorte de congrès. D'autre part, ces deux journées permettant des déplacements plus importants, il a été également décidé de "décentraliser" ainsi les réunions de Paris vers la province afin de pourvoir en même temps visiter d'autres centres de documentation et partager encore plus l'expérience des différents centres hospitaliers.

B) Projets.

- Les groupes de travail thématiques cités plus haut, devront trouver une organisation interne propre afin de fonctionner de façon autonome ; les travaux réalisés au sein de chacun de ces groupes devant être restitués de manière synthétique à chaque assemblée plénière.

- La création d'un bulletin de liaison entre les membres du réseau sera discutée lors d'une prochaine réunion.

- Le réseau des documentalistes hospitaliers sera représenté par l'intermédiaire de certains de ses membres au sein de l'Association des Documentalistes et Bibliothécaires Spécialisés (ADBS). Cette association française, forte de 6 000 adhérents, regroupe des documentalistes de tous horizons (public ou privé), toutes disciplines confondues et travaille entre de nombreux thèmes, sur un éventuel projet de statut interministériel des documentalistes de la fonction publique en général. Le réseau apportera donc sa contribution à ces travaux et se tiendra ainsi informé de l'évolution générale de la profession.

C) Conclusion. Ce réseau encore très jeune et donc forcément immature à permis malgré tout depuis presque trois ans, l'émergence d'une identité professionnelle chez les documentalistes hospitaliers français qui ont bien voulu adhérer et qui se sentent ainsi moins solitaires. Beaucoup de travail reste à faire et il faut espérer que d'autres collègues rejoindront encore ce groupe. Le but final reste de faire reconnaître cette profession comme nécessaire et indispensable à la formation continue et à l'information professionnelle des personnels hospitaliers ainsi qu'à l'enrichissement de la pédagogie des écoles paramédicales ou encore à l'aide à la décision des personnels d'encadrement des institutions de soins françaises.

SECTION 10

HISTORY OF MEDICINE

THE PRE-SALERNITAN PERIOD, THE CODICES AND THE ITALIAN LIBRARIES: A Page in the History of Medicine

Brunella Sebastiani & **Giuseppe Salvatori,** Consiglio Nazionale delle Ricerche - Biblioteca Centrale, P.le Aldo Moro, 7 - 00185 Roma, Italia

Abstract
In relation to the history of medicine the 9th, 10th and 11th centuries are called pre-Salernitan period. The analysis of codices dating back to this period and preserved in Italian libraries enables to recreate the medical library of the first Middle Ages when the Greek-Byzantine and Roman models were modified by the introduction of a new element. The personal factor, namely additions due to the hand of unknown writers.

The Middle Ages was a period of crisis and transformation which, as stated by Robertson and later by the great representative of German illuminism Johann Gottfried Herder, represents the coming together of different peoples and nationalities, which somehow managed to merge and join together and give rise to new ethnic and political formations. In this context, it is interesting to recall the separation which occurred between Greek culture, written in Greek and which continued to exist in Byzantium and went on to become the basis for Arab culture in the science - and Latin culture, written in Latin, which survived in the Roman world, preserving only translations and summaries of Greek texts. Thus there were two sources from which the Middle Ages received the classical heritage: Byzantium and the Arab world for Greek culture and Rome, which through the monasteries transmitted what had been saved of the classical Latin texts and what little remained of Greek texts through Latin translations and abridged versions. Medieval medicine therefore has two basic components. The first one is Monastic medicine, which developed before Arab influence reached Europe, and the second one is Arab medicine, which was the heir of Greek tradition, transplanted in Europe in the XII century after revising and reformulating it.

In the period between the fall of the kingdom of the Goths and the rise of the Carolingian empire, what was called monastic medicine arose and developed. It flourished in the monasteries, of which Montecassino represented a major centre. Monastic activity, according to the Benedictine Rule, besides prayer and penitence, also called for dedication to literature, art and science, which included the reading and copying of classical texts. It also called for medical and pharmaceutical practice. Medical activity was carried out initially in infirmaries where only monks were admitted, though subsequently lay people were also admitted. Pharmaceutical activity took place in the pharmacies where the monks processed medicinal plants - the medicines made from officinal herbs - which they grew in the monastery gardens. Another branch of medicine grew out of this monastic medicine, called lay medicine, and at least initially was based on the Latin tradition which was represented by the Salerno School. The reconstruction of the medical codexes in Italian libraries in the IX, X and XI centuries, though limited to the collection of Latin medical texts before 1100, shows the significance of scientific thought during the period.

These three centuries, which range from the flourishing of the Carolingian empire to the first important contacts with the orient and the Arab world, show a calligraphical and cultural standard in which the Carolingian lower-case letter prevails. In this period, these simple, clear forms were the means by which Latin culture in Europe was given new life The development of styles of writing - the basic criteria for assessing the age of a codex - does not, however, allow for highly accurate dating. Changes in writing never take place all at the same time, and vary from place to place. The production of books in various centres undoubtedly shows typical characteristics enabling us to determine the date within a quarter of a century. However, individual scribes often show personal elements which adapt and stabilise their calligraphy throughout much of their lives, thus making dating difficult.

Reference has been made to the cultural reawakening in the Carolingian period, which fostered the reconstruction of scientific knowledge in Western Europe, utilising and expanding classical texts from Gaul, Britain, Italy and Spain. Medicine played an active part in this process, especially in the IX and XI centuries, until the first contacts with the Arab world in the XII century, and the development of the Salerno School. Which works attracted the interest of academics and scribes? A complete answer can only be given by referring to the manuscripts. It should be pointed out that the identification provided in old catalogues is often arbitrary. Then we should add the errors made by the scribes. They often failed to transcribe the whole work, omitting the name of the author, changing the title or the beginning of the work. Other times they mutilated the text or combined different texts, thus modifying the original form, or made extracts and so on. This renewed interest in medicine is shown by numerous codexes dating back to this period. An overall survey shows that there are a number of texts contained in manuscripts which have come down to us. Most of them are in specifically medical texts, and a minority are in the miscellanea, where there is a type of composition which can be defined as minor or for non-specialists.

Medical literature of the period is wholly based on the classical tradition; the original sources are mostly Greek, and Latin authors to a lesser extent. We can also observe a tendency to make practically oriented, short reductions, for example, the Collection on the virtues of herbs and animals of Apuleius the Platonist and Sextus Placitus Papininensis; the one on chronic disease of Liber Aurelii and the Liber Aesculapii; the Therapeutic Manual of Plinius the Younger with the addition of the Liber Dietarum; the Compendium of Muscio; the Chapter on medicine by Isidore of Seville. Together with or inserted in these major works on classical medicine we find fragments and extracts put together by unknown compilers who sometimes signed these works with a famous name. These works state that the text is derived from Greek books, such as in the Gynaecia of Cleopatra. These books are actually just works on popular medicine, rich in superstition and prejudices and with a pratical approach.

In the field of symptoms, texts on the pulse and urine dominate. For specific pathologies, there are works on fevers and diseases of the eye and stomach. The Liber diaetarum diversorum medicorum is a treatise on diet. Pharmacology is represented by a number of extracts and miscellanea with prescriptions inadequately listed by category. Together with medical treatises there are also a number of herbal treatises, sometimes in addition to the one by Apuleius and sometimes separate. Surgery is poorly represented; most of the material is on bleeding. Taking all of this into consideration, we can state that on the whole, the major medical libraries of the early Middle-Ages were influenced by the necessities of life seen almost as a teaching, and this influenced the type of books available at the time. It is reasonable to conclude, that together with tradition, there is also a tendency aimed at renewal taking the first uncertain steps towards preparing a more advanced type of literature. This work involving the manipulation of previous literature, together with initiatives stemming from current needs can be seen clearly, for example, in two Beneventan manuscripts - Montecassino 97 and Vatican Barberini 160 - as shown constantly in the text combinations in the various works. Medical and natural science is often grouped together the Epistles of Hippocrates to Mecaenas + Antonius Musa; or the De Herba vettonica liber + Apuleius the Platonist; Herbarius + Sextus Placitus; Liber medicinae ex animalibus + Dioscorides; Liber medicinae ex herbis feminis + Breves. In Lucca 296, we have the addition of the Curae derived from animals and plants; in Florence Laur. LXXIII a total rearrangement of Apuleius based on a list of diseases from head to foot instead of on a list of herbs In Montecassino 97 (X century) we can see an edition with the original chapters of the Therapeutics added to Glaucus, together with the addition of Compendia of Latin authors. This grouping comes under the name of Galenus in the XI century, circulated in a different form without the abstract of Theodorus Priscianus, together with a note on podagra (Vatican 4417 and Barberini 160). These manuscripts, and others whose contents were manipulated in the same way, clearly form the basis for the early literature of the Salerno School, and form the link between the aformentioned and classical literature. The Antidotarium Nicolai, the official Salerno pharmacopoeia, shows clear evidence of the Prescription Books of the previous centuries, in which the detail and variety of remedies are a clear sign of personal additions to pharmacological sources dating from classical antiquity. Vatican Regin. 1143, No. 4 is entitled "Incipit liber primus medicinalis de multis codicibus ad diversas corporum passiones ordinatus"; another Prescription Book is Vatican Palt. 1088.

The personal touch can be seen in compilers who try to add their own knowledge under a pseudonym to a complete work. To sum up Italy's contribution, we can add a group of manuscripts in Beneventan lower-case letters, a type of calligraphy which developed in Southern Italy and Dalmatia at the same time as the Carolingian style. There are probably only four identifiable codexes at Montecassino: a volume attributed to Abbot Bertarius (d. 833) containing two Prescription Books (Montecassino 69) with an ample collection containing extracts from Galenus, the Commentary on the Aphorisms of Hippocrates, Alexander Trallianus, the grouping of Apuleius, Dioscorides and Sextus Placitus (Montecassino 97), dating back to between the IX and X centuries; another two manuscripts dating to the XI century, under the Abbot Desiderius, containing new translations of Paulus Aeginatae - Greek - and translations from the Arabic by Joannitius including other prescription books (Montecassino 225).

Florence Laur. LXXIII.41, II dates back to the IX century, and has a grouping with Apuleius, Sextus Placitus and Dioscorides, together with two fragments with medical nomenclature and a short treatise on cautery (Florence Laur. LXXIII.41.1), fragments of a prescription book and palimpsests in Rome (Cap. S. Pietro, H. 44). Fragments of palimpsests (Rome, Angelica 1496) and a copy of a grouping of Apuleius (Turin K.IV.3) and a unique example in Beneventan script of the "Bari variety" typical of Apulia and Dalmatia including a medical encyclopaedia with groupings of Apuleius and Galen, the Commentary on the Aphorisms of Hippocrates, Horibasius, Theodorus Priscianus, Quintus Serenus and several prescription books and minor works (Vatican Barberini, 160) date to the XI century.

Together with the tradition based on the text there is also an artistic tradition with miniatures based on Roman or Roman-Byzantine models. From this point of view, a series of miniatures in Florence Laur. LXXIII.41 is highly interesting, with illustrations of cauterization techniques. Another interesting element is the identification of the place of writing, essential for determining which centres had the most advanced medical studies. It is also highly important to identify the pattern of exchange and relationships between the book production centres and the various communities. It should be recalled besides the actual production, each manuscript also has its period of active use. In the pre-Salerno period medicine was already an active discipline. The codexes may have been written in different places, may have been donated, lent or stolen, bound or disbound. Communities and academic centres tried to save the remains of ancient tradition. New works appeared, timidly at first as additions, subsequently gaining confidence from the mid-XI century with the birth of the new medical library, the first step towards modern medicine, and is an essential part of the history of man in nature, as well as being the history of progress; it is the science of man for man and, as Florkin says, not just history but the study of medicine itself.

Citations

Beccaria, A., I codici di medicina (sec. IX, X e XI). Roma, Edizioni di Storia e Letteratura, 1956.
Castellani, C., Un capitolo di storia della medicina: medicazione delle ferite. In Castalia 1963, 19, 3, p. 3-9.
Castiglioni, A., Storia della medicina. v. 1 dalle origini alla fine del seicento. Verona, Mondadori, 1936.
Galeazzi, M.-Trifogli, R., L'Hortulus di Walafrido Strabo. Roma, Cossidente, 1958.
Jandolo, M., Su di uno scritto di Mantica Medica in Codice cassinese del sec. IX e X. Roma, Cossidente, 1958.
Paladini, P., L'arte sanitaria di Montecassino. In La Medicina Internazionale Illustrata 1929, 5, p. 204-207.

SIR WILLIAM OSLER AND MEDICAL LIBRARIES

Frances Groen, McGill University,3459 McTavish Street, Montreal, Quebec H3A 1Y1, Canada

Part I: Introduction

Before discussing Osler's views on medical libraries, I want to review briefly the general chronology of his professional career, and then to present an overview of the place he occupies in medicine. Osler was born in Bond Head, Ontario, Canada in 1849, and following a two year period of study at Trinity College, Toronto, transferred from the clinical program he had been pursuing to the study of medicine at McGill University in Montreal. Following the completion of his medical degree in 1872, he studied elsewhere, returning to the Faculty of Medicine as Professor of Clinical Medicine until 1884. He then accepted the position of Professor of Clinical Medicine at the University of Pennsylvania, leaving there in 1889 to become Professor of Medicine and Physician-in-Chief at Johns Hopkins University and Hospital. In 1905, he accepted his final professional appointment as Regius Professor of Medicine in Oxford where he died in 1919. His career has special significance, resting on the three English language medical traditions of Canada, the United States and Great Britain.

Overview of His Contributions

At this point, more than seventy years after his death, writings and eulogies about Sir William Osler (1849-1919) exceed by far publications by him. Why is it that librarians and physicians alike continue to return to his works for guidance, comfort and insight? Osler's name is not associated with a single great discovery, and it is reasonable to ask to what degree did he augment the medical knowledge base. Today, his writings in the area of medical ethics and the social aspects of medicine, his strong sense of the responsibility of the physician to the profession and to the community served, stand as examples of the continuing value of his ideas. Osler is best remembered as a superb clinician and his casebooks and published case studies provide abundant evidence of his contributions in this area. For librarians, he is most renowned as a bibliophile and a staunch advocate of the importance of medical libraries.

Osler's published writings began in his twentieth year in the field of natural history, documenting his keen powers of observation and use of the microscope, and they continued until the year of his death, 1919. His influence upon his alma mater continues to this day both in his Library and in his influence upon clinical medicine. In the year of his death he was advising the Dean of the Faculty of Medicine of McGill University concerning the importance of full-time clinical professorships:

> "McGill simply cannot afford to fall behind other first class schools in the development of modern clinics in Medicine and Surgery, and Obstetrics and Gynaecology. New conditions have arisen, to meet which it is essential to have sympathetic co-operation of university and hospitals...Medically, Montreal occupies a unique position - a school with a record of splendid work and two of the best equipped hospitals on the continent; but a new departure is needed which will involve change of heart as to methods, etc., and a realization of the full responsibility of the hospitals in this matter. It is their job quite as much as that of the university; and the clinics should be under the control of both bodies jointly."[32]

Five years following Osler's death and this letter, the Rockefeller Foundation gave half a million dollars to McGill University towards the establishment with the Royal Victoria Hospital of a University Clinic, the Director of the Clinic to be Professor of Medicine on a full-time basis. Throughout his career, Osler insisted upon the importance of clinical training and during his years in Baltimore, along with Halstead and Kelly, he reorganized the professional staff of the hospital to provide opportunity for indepth clinical training.

Osler's contribution as a teacher and educator united with his love of learning - his passion to know and his willingness to share his knowledge. He knew the importance of quiet study and, in one of his most memorable sayings commented

---

[32]0. Letter published in *International Association of Medical Museums and Journal of Technical Methods Bulletin*, No. IX. Sir William Osler Memorial Number. Appreciation and Reminiscences. Privately issued in Montreal, Canada, 1926. p. 591.

that "to study the phenomena of disease without books is to sail an uncharted sea, while to study books without patients is not go to sea at all." As early as 1881, Osler noted in a review in the *American Journal of Medical Science* "the paucity of American textbooks of medicine and the modesty of professors who...had left the field in possession of foreign authors."[33]

Osler corrected this situation with the appearance of *The Principles and Practice of Medicine* [34] More than twenty-two editions of this work have appeared since it was first published in 1892. This work was a unique contribution to the field of medical texts, including a systematization of diseases that was to become a standard reference source for librarians and bibliographers and outstanding chapters in the field of contagion, diseases of the heart and circulatory system as well as numerous classical and literary allusions.

Osler's contributions to the corpus of medical writing, extending over 50 years, are overwhelming in number. Golden and Rolland have provided a useful, comprehensive categorization of Osler's writings:

- Natural science, including original research
- Pathology: 1) Comparative (Veterinary Medicine)
  2) Human
- Clinical medicine
- Literary papers, history, biography, bibliography
- Medical education, medical societies, and medical profession
- Public welfare activities (including Tuberculosis and World War I)
- Volumes edited
- Pseudonymous papers - An Egerton Yorrick Davis checklist
- The editions, printings, and translations of The Principles and Practice of Medicine

Bibliographic Research on Osler

The Sir William Osler Memorial Number of the International Association of Medical Museums published in 1926 includes a critical, annotated bibliography of the publications of Sir William Osler. It is based upon a chronological bibliography prepared by Minnie Wright Blogg, Librarian at the Johns Hopkins Hospital during Osler's tenure in Baltimore. Ms. Blogg remembered Osler in reminiscences published in the Bulletin of the Medical Library Association as follows:

> "The present Librarian of the Johns Hopkins Hospital, entering upon her duties twenty years ago...found herself overwhelmed with work and one day arranging books and journals came to a point where she settled herself comfortably on the floor...she was alone in the Library, and was absorbed in arranging the hundreds of journals and reprints which surrounded her. Suddenly, she became aware of a light, rapid step approaching and almost immediately there appeared in the doorway a man who paused and looked at her. Distinguished, keen, slight and wonderfully alert, he stood; he wore a black frock coat, carried a silk hat and gaily swung a slender cane. We looked at each other; neither spoke. Then in a singularly kind and sympathetic voice...he asked, "Is this the new Librarian?" I could not deny it. [35]

Miss Minnie Blogg seems to have been smitten from her first encounter with The Chief and the extensive bibliography she produced for the memorial volume must have been a true labour of love. Other major sources, to help the fledgling Oslerian through the thousands of articles that have appeared about Osler and the frequent reprintings of his writings include An Annotated Checklist of Osleriana by Earl F. Nation, Charles G. Roland and John F. McGovern (1976) and Sir William Osler: An Annotated Bibliography with Illustrations, edited by Richard L. Golden and Charles G. Roland.

---

[33]0. *American Journal of Medical Sciences*, 1880, n.s. p. 175-181

[34]0. Osler, William. *The Principles and Practice of Medicine*, Designed for the Use of Practitioners and Students of Medicine. New York, D. Appleton, 1892

[35]0. Blogg, Minnie W. Osler reminiscences in *Bulletin of the Medical Library Association*, v. 9, n.s. 1919, p. 7-8

(1988). These resources represent the craft of bibliography at its best, Osler valued bibliography very highly, and, in identifying these bibliographies, one recalls Osler's words of praise "there is no better float through prosperity than to be the author of a good bibliography."

Part II: Contributions to Medical Librarianship

His contributions as a clinician and educator are well-known. This paper reviews his thoughts on medical libraries in his own time speculates upon how he might have reacted to some current developments in medical information management. His contributions to medical libraries in general, to professional library associations, and the cultivation of the intellect are also discussed.

Osler's View of Medical Libraries

Few physicians have made a more important impact upon the development of medical libraries than did Sir William Osler.

> "Scores there are and have been that have left an imprint upon one medical library, and there are some whose influence has extended to two or three, but Sir William Osler is the only one whose magic has touched all." [36]

The influence was felt in his gifts of books, his gifts of funds and his support of librarians and their profession. Osler gave generously to any number of libraries including, but not limited to, those of the institutions with whom he was associated. Libraries benefiting from his generosity included the Library of the College of Physicians, the Library of the Medical and Chirurgical Faculty of the University of Maryland, the Library of Johns Hopkins Hospital, the Academy of Medicine of Toronto and, foremost amongst this list that of McGill University, his alma mater. Osler understood that a good library had to be financially healthy and gave generously and encouraged others to do the same.

His most enduring gift, that of his personal library, to the Faculty of Medicine of McGill University, speaks to his thoughtfulness as much as to his generosity. In his own words, he shows himself an early advocate of resource sharing:

> "...I should like to have been able to leave my collection to the [Johns Hopkins] School, but it seems more appropriate to give it to McGill where it is much more needed. After all for the older and rarer books the Hopkins has the Surgeon General's Library at its door..." [37]

Despite his decision on behalf of McGill, Osler continued his interest in other libraries. Just one year before his death, he wrote to Margaret Charlton, at the Academy of Medicine in Toronto:

> "...You should start a special section of the library if you have not already done so, dealing with Ontario medical history - pictures, books, pamphlets, letters, diplomas, etc. I enclose you $100 to be spent by the Library Committee in this work." [38]

Improvements in Access to the Medical Literature

In his systematic writings, Osler rejected mere listings of titles, preferring an approach to bibliography that was selective, critical and annotated. This preferred approach is one indication of how he might have regarded current developments in the control and availability of the medical literature. Certainly he would have welcomed the precision of computer-based bibliographic searching. I suspect he would have been equally enthusiastic when abstracts were added to the MEDLINE database, as an important step towards the annotated bibliography that he espoused. Because of the breadth and scope of his interest and his holistic approach to the treatment of disease, he might well have expressed concern

---

[36]0. Runräh, John, "Osler's influence on medical libraries in America" in *International Association of Medical Museums and Journal of Technical Methods Bulletin*, No. IX. Sir William Osler Memorial Number. Appreciation and Reminiscences. Privately issued in Montreal, Canada, 1926. p. 340.

[37]0. Cushing, Harvey. The Life of Sir William Osler. Oxford, Clarendon Press, 1925. v. 2, p. 557

[38]0. Cushing, *op. cit.* v. 2, p. 625.

regarding a degree of precision that threatened serendipity in creative reading. I believe that he would have been intrigued by developments in artificial intelligence. The model for scanning medical literature, more closely approximating the way the mind works, would have intrigued him, especially the application of "fuzzy" logic searching, with its ability to create more tenuous relationships as well as "hits" in searching the literature.

Bibliographic access and physical access were matters of great concern to Osler. Reading current medical literature was for Osler essential to patient care: "For the teacher and the worker a great library...is indispensable. They must know the world's best work and know it at once. They mint and make current coin the ore so widely scattered in journals, transactions and monographs." [39]

This emphasis on the need to know, to have access to the best and to have it immediately, is a recurring theme in the work of Osler. It is evident in his emphasis on the importance of knowing the current medical literature and the various journal clubs which he established at the institutions where he held positions. In his words, from his essay on "Books and Men", 'it is in utilizing the fresh knowledge of the journals that the young physician may attain quickly to the name and fame he desires' (p. 212). Osler wrote with dramatic effect of the problems created for the library and the user by the rapid obsolescence of medical information:

> "It is sad to think how useless are a majority of the works on our shelves - the old cyclopedias and dictionaries, the files of defunct journals, the endless editions of text-books as dead as their authors. Only a few epoch-making works survive... Now among the colossal mass of rubbish on the shelves there are some precious gems which should be polished and well-set and in every library put out on view." [40]

Cultivation of the Intellect and Lifelong Learning

Osler would have welcomed enhanced access to medical knowledge through the digitization of medical information. But I suspect that he might have regretted the developments in the contemporary medical library that do not allow the student or practitioner to move outside the disciplinary boundaries of medicine, especially in the direction of humanistic studies. Osler instructed his students when he was teaching at McGill University, to develop strong interests in fields outside of medicine:

> "While medicine is to be your vocation, or calling, see to it that you have also an avocation - some intellectual pastime which may serve to keep you in touch with the world of art, of science or of letters. Begin at once the cultivation of some interest other than the purely professional... No matter what that is...but have an outside hobby. For the hardworking medical student, it is perhaps easiest to keep up an interest in literature." [41]

The financing of collections, other than core medical materials has become problematic in all libraries, and librarians and users alike are hard pressed to justify materials outside those that support current research and teaching needs. However, it is well to remember in this context that Osler was attempting to cultivate an interest and an attitude of mind on the part of the medical student, not necessarily a codicil for a collection development policy in a medical library.

Founding an Association for Medical Librarians

In his essay "Osler's Influence on Medical Libraries," Ruhräh remarks that Osler 'did much to do away with the old-fashioned librarian and encouraged the helpful, cheerful variety. He made the librarians feel that their work was of great importance and did much to develop the *esprit de corps* which the Medical Library Association has gone on fostering."

---

[39] 0. Osler, Sir William. "Books and Men." in his Aequanimitas with other Addresses to Medical Students, Nurses and Practitioners of Medicine. 3d ed. Philadelphia, Blakison, 1932

[40] 0. Osler, Sir William. "Some aspects of American Medical Bibliography." In his Aequanimitas. 3rd ed. 1932, p. 299.

[41] 0. Quoted in Thayer, William Sydney. "The Heart of the Library" in OSLER AND OTHER PAPERS. Baltimore, Johns Hopkins Press, 1931, p. 44.

[42] In today's world, Ruhräh's words appear patronizing to the professor of medical librarianship, but there was nothing patronizing in Osler's support of the development of an association for medical librarians.

Osler had experienced in his own work the benefit of professional meetings and the importance of discussion with professional colleagues from a variety of settings. When he was in Baltimore, Osler made it possible for the underpaid librarians to attend regularly the meetings oft he newly formed Association of Medical Librarians, and Cushing refers to these librarian gatherings as "a tonic to them [the librarians] to tide them over another twelve months in their difficult and unremunerative positions... He [Osler] realized the desirability of drawing people with common interests together, but few have been gifted with the genius equal to his of bringing about such combinations and almost wholly through his personal backing the Medical Library Association which has done such important work for the profession was founded..." [43] Sir William Osler, along with Dr. George Gould, of Philadelphia, Marcia Noyes, and Margaret Charlton who had known Osler when he was at McGill University were instrumental in the founding of the Medical Library Association. Sir William served as a President and Margaret Charlton, Assistant Librarian at the Medical Library, McGill University, served intermittently as secretary from 1898 until 1911. [44]

Osler's Library

Today, Osler's love of libraries, reading and learning lives in the Osler Library of McGill University. Osler's 8,000 books left Oxford in 1929 for McGill University, following the completion of the monumental bibliography, *Bibliotheca Osleriana*. [45] Osler's Library consisted of works in the history of medicine and science. It was Osler who planned the structure of the *Bibliotheca*, although it was not published until ten years following his death. It contains eight sections: (1) Bibliotheca prima in which Osler documents the development of science and medicine through a chronological listing of authors of works in the collection; (2) Bibliotheca Secunda containing medical and scientific works of authors Osler did not consider to be of the first importance; (3)Bibliotheca Litteraria, including literature by physicians. Here are listed some of the most precious items of the Library, including Sir Thomas Brocene, Richard Burton and Rabelais, as well as works on spiritualism, immortality and witchcraft.; (4) Bibliotheca Biographica; (5) Bibliotheca Historica; (6) Bibliographica; (7) Bibliotheca Incunabula which itemizes 106 books printed before 1501; (8) Manuscripts.

Osler was a methodical, assiduous and intelligent collector, all virtues still relevant to the development of great libraries. He valued current medical literature, in German and French, as well as in English, and probably would have deplored the increasingly uni-lingual English use in medical literature. He also espoused classical texts in Greek, Latin and Arabic. While at McGill, he was concerned to develop the German collection, helping the Medical Library to acquire complete sets of Virchow's Archiv, the Deutsches Archiv für Klinische Medicin, the Zentralblatt für medicinischen Wissenschaften, Wagner's Archiv, and Max Schultze's Archiv.

He was both generous and slightly forgetful. In 1907, he presented McGill with a 1543 Vesalius, only to have the librarian point out an even better copy on display which Osler had given to the Library some years earlier. Osler determined then that he would give the copy to the Boston Medical Library. On presenting the volume, the Boston librarian showed Osler a book on display in that Library, yet another 1543 Vesalius, which Osler had previously presented to that library. The Vesalius finally found a home in the Library of the New York Academy of Medicine.[46]

---

[42]0. Ruhräh, John. "Osler's Influence on Medical Libraries in America." op. cit. p. 345

[43]0. Cushing. *op. cit*, p. 344

[44]0. Groen, Frances K. Margaret Ridley Charlton, Medical Librarian and Historian." *Fontanus*, 1989. p. 55-63

[45]0. Osler, Sir William. a Catalogue of Books Illustrating the History of Medicine and Science, Collected, Arranged and Annotated by Sir William Osler and Bequeathed to McGill University. First edition published at the Clarendon Press, Oxford, 1929. Reprinted with new prologue, addenda, and corrigenda, by McGill-Queen's University Press, 1969, 1987.

[46]15.. "Introduction: the Collecting of a Library." in *Bibliotheca Osleriana*, 1987, p. xxix

THE PROVISION OF MEDICAL INFORMATION IN A DUBLIN MEDICAL SCHOOL IN 19TH CENTURY

Gabrielle Doyle, St. Luke's Institute of Cancer Research, Highfield Road, Rathgar, Dublin 6, Ireland

Abstract
This paper examines the provision of medical information at the Catholic University School of Medicine. John Henry Newman, Rector of the Catholic University of Ireland founded this School in 1855. The dissemination of medical information through the formal means of communication such as books and journals and through the informal system of communication - the network of scholarly interaction between the School and other similar institutions at home and abroad - is presented.

In 1855 the "Golden Age" of Irish medicine was just declining. A group of Irish doctors in the early nineteenth century brought medical teaching and practice in Dublin to such a level of excellence, that for a brief period during the mid-nineteenth century, Dublin was the leading centre of world medicine. Medical practitioners from Europe and America came to Dublin to listen and learn from Robert Graves (1796 - 1853), William Stokes (1804 - 78) and Dominic Corrigan (1802 - 80), all of whom made important contributions to the study of disease. Their distinguished contemporaries included John Cheyne (1777 - 1836), Robert Adams (1791 - 1875), Sir William Wilde (1815 - 76), Arthur Jacob (1790 - 1874) and Abraham Colles (1773 - 1843). The names of these physicians and surgeons are still associated with clinical conditions that they described, such as Cheyne-Stokes respiration, Colles' fracture, Corrigan's pulse, Graves' disease and Stoke-Adams syndrome. The Irish or Dublin school of medicine, as it was sometimes called, was above all, a clinical school. Its members placed great emphasis on physical signs and the study of pathology. During his career in the Meath Hospital, Robert Graves introduced the system of clinical teaching whereby the student actually examined the patient, as well as writing the clinical history. Slowly his influence on medical education prevailed and this system of clinical education established itself in Dublin.

In the summer of 1854 the Apothecary Hall Medical School in Dublin's Cecilia Street closed down. That same summer it was purchased for the Catholic University of Ireland and in November 1855 it re-opened its doors as a new institution, the Medical Faculty of the Catholic University of Ireland, whose Rector was John Henry Newman. In the years that followed, Newman's small medical faculty, housed in an old building in a back street of Dublin, developed and flourished. Within fifty years it had established itself as the largest medical school in the country. It grew into a centre of excellence in its own right. Its alumni became situated in key positions. It made its impact on Irish medicine. In 1909 the National University of Ireland was established and Newman's Medical School became the Medical Faculty of University College Dublin, one of the constituent Colleges of the National University, which is still flourishing today.

From the available evidence we will look at the informal and formal communication structures in the dissemination of knowledge that we find at work in the institution, the sources of medical information available and accessible to teaching staff and students and the activities associated with the production, dissemination and use of information to, in and from the Catholic University of Medicine.

Library Records
Newman purchased the nucleus of the medical library from Germany. He bought it from Dr. Johann von Ringseis (1785 - 1880), Rector of the University of Munich. It comprised over 5,000 volumes. It represented the select medical literature of the chief schools that flourished in Europe. The languages that it comprised were Greek, Latin, French, German, Dutch, Italian and English. Unfortunately this collection did not survive and there is no trace of it today.

The other evidence to prove that a library existed in the School is a Treasurer's Account Book for the Reading Room from 1874 - 1888. This book has only recently come to light. It records the income and expenditure and provides us with some very interesting data. The main source of income was from yearly subscriptions from the Rector of the University, the professors and students. The expenditure can be divided into three categories:

1) Books
2) Periodicals and Newspapers
3) Miscellaneous - this included book binding, stationery, keys and locks for presses that would indicate that the books were not on ready open access.

The most popular book was Anatomy, Descriptive and Surgical by Henry Gray (1825 - 1861). This book has withstood the test of time. The 37th British edition was published in 1989. Next in popularity came William Senhouse Kirkes' (1823 - 1864) book on physiology. This handbook first appeared in 1848 and ran to several editions. Multiple copies of The Science and Art of Surgery by Sir John Erichsen (1818 - 1896) were also purchased. This was a popular text-book on the subject for many years. One of the best known English text on medical jurisprudence was also in the library. It was Elements of Medical Jurisprudence written by Alfred Taylor (1806 - 1880). It was first published in 1836 and ran to several editions up into this century. Books published in the United States were also represented, for example, A Practical Treatise on Diseases of Women by Theodore Thomas (1831 - 1903) which, in its day was acclaimed as an outstanding work on the subject. The above titles are a few examples that demonstrate the priority attached to relevant curriculum teaching and reference works. This was complemented by the acquisition of innovative works through a subscription to an important contemporary medical publishing society - the New Sydenham Society (1858 - 1907). A subscription to this Society entitled members to a copy of each book published. The objectives of the Society included the reprinting of standard English medical works and the translation of recent foreign works of merit. Thus the works of contemporary foreign physicians and surgeons became accessible to the English speaking world. Some contemporary authors aided the translators in the preparation of the English version of their texts. The teaching staff of the Catholic University School of Medicine helped with the translations. The following is a sample of the authors whose works were published during the years corresponding to the Reading Room Accounts Book: Theodor Billroth, Professor of Surgery in the University of Vienna; Jean Martin Charcot, Professor to the Faculty of Medicine of Paris; Robert Koch, later Professor for Hygiene and Bacteriology at the Humboldt University of Berlin; Peter Mere Latham, Physician to St. Bartholomew's Hospital London. Such works provided the School with an extremely convenient source of international and comparative scientific thought. Thereby this subscription complemented the text-book, multiple copy basic reference function of the Reading Room, which in turn was necessary to complement the learning process at lectures and the practical experience in hospital wards.

Journals

The Reading Room Accounts Book provides us with details of the scientific and medical journals that were purchased specifically for the use of the students and staff. Subscriptions were paid every year for the *Lancet* and *Nature*, two journals that are still core journals in any medical and scientific library today. News of the Irish medical scene came from the *Dublin Journal of Medical Science*. Literary and scientific journals included the *Academy, Saturday Review,* and the *Cornhill Magazine*. The Account Book also reveals that ample provision was made for current affairs material, which reflected different political viewpoints, and for entertainment material. This gave the Reading Room the characteristics of a self-contained club.

In-House Publications

For John Henry Newman, the University was a teaching and a research centre. He wished to demonstrate that the professors and lecturers at the Catholic University were working and engaged in research, each one in their own field. In 1858 he founded the journal *Atlantis: a register of literature and science conducted by the members of the Catholic University of Ireland*. The staff of the School of Medicine wrote articles for the *Atlantis*. Newman also wished to use this publication as a vehicle to establish communication between the University and learned societies and institutions abroad. There was a financial consideration involved here. The University had low financial resources. It could not afford to purchase all the publications that were relevant to its members' interests. At this time, there was a trend for small institutions and societies to publish their own material. Then they could obtain foreign material by institutional exchange or barter. In the *Atlantis,* Number 6, there is an impressive list of journals and other scholarly publications that were sent in exchange for the *Atlantis*. The list comprises general scientific and literary material, and specialised subject publications for medicine, geology, agriculture, astronomy, zoology, botany, meteorology and oriental studies. The publications came from the United States of America, Canada, Austria, Belgium, Denmark, France, Germany, Great Britain, Holland, India, Italy, Norway, Prussia, Russia, Spain and Switzerland.

Institutional exchange based on the *Atlantis* reflected Newman's confidence in the quality of work from his staff. He believed that their contribution to literature and science would be acknowledged and accepted by institutions abroad. It is also worth noting that illustrious academies and institutes were willing to establish bonds and exchange their publications with such a newly founded university.

In 1895, the School of Medicine published an in-house text book for students, entitled Notes on Operative Surgery. The book was designed to be used in class or when attending operations. After each printed page there is blank page on which the students could write in their own notes. The book is well illustrated; it has plates, photographs and many drawings.

The Staff of the School of Medicine

On the subject of the provision of medical information, we cannot forget that the teaching staff of the School played a vital role as information mediaries. These men were extremely active in mobilising the conventions of communication, formal and informal. Within the parameters of the informal communication structure, they lectured, were involved in investigation and research, studied and worked abroad, thus establishing a communication network between the School and centres of learning and research in other countries. Nor did they confine themselves to the informal system, their range of activities was also channelled through the formal system by their publishing activity: textbooks, pamphlets, articles, reports and in some cases by translating overseas books and articles, as shown by the following examples:

R.S.D. Lyons (1826 - 1886) Professor of Medicine and Pathology 1856 - 1886. His medical expertise was called upon to investigate problems in other countries. He investigated the causes of disease among the British Army during the Crimean War. The King of Portugal asked Lyons to come to Lisbon to advise on the problem of containing the outbreak of yellow fever in Lisbon. Reports of these investigations were published. Other publications included a Handbook of Hospital Practice or an Introduction to the Practical Study of Medicine at the Bedside (1859) and A Treatise on Fever (1861). The second edition appeared in 1864.

G. Sigerson (1836 - 1925) Professor of Botany 1865 - 1882, Professor of Botany and Zoology 1882 - 1901 and Professor of Biology 1901 - 1909. During his post-graduate years, he studied in France under Guillaume Benjamin Duchenne, Claude Bernard and Jean Martin Charcot. Sigerson published several original papers on neurology. When he translated the first two volumes of Charcot's Lectures on the Diseases of the Nervous System for the New Sydenham Society, he introduced Charcot to the English world of medicine.

A. Roche (1851 - 1908) Professor of Hygiene and Medical Jurisprudence 1891 - 1907. He translated and edited the Imperial Health Manual. This was the authorised English edition of the official manual issued by the Imperial Health Department of Bismarck's Germany.

Andrew Ellis, Thomas Hayden, Ambrose Birmingham, Sir Christopher Nixon, John McArdle also wrote medical textbooks. They and other staff members contributed papers to the medical journals of their day.

Despite the School's scarce financial resources, we have seen that there was provision for medical reference material, both standard and innovative contemporary works. The dissemination of medical information, through the formal and informal systems of communication, no doubt, contributed to the success of the Catholic University School of Medicine, thus bringing one of Newman's dreams to fruition, as he stated in his Rector's Report of 1856: "As the purchase of the buildings in Cecilia Street was one of the earliest of our successes, so the establishment of the Faculty of Medicine is one of the most important and encouraging. Did our efforts towards the foundation of a Catholic University issue in nothing beyond the establishment of a first-rate Catholic School of Medicine in the metropolis, as it has already done, they would have met with a sufficient reward".

Reference

Doyle, G.M. Information Provision in Dublin Medicine (1855 - 1909) as exemplified by the Catholic University School of Medicine [Dissertation]. Dublin: University College Dublin, 1990. 151pp.

SECTION 11

POSTER SESSIONS

UPGRADING DOCUMENT DELIVERY STANDARDS IN THE HOSPITAL LIBRARY OF ARCISPEDALE S. MARIA NUOVA, U.S.L. n. 9 - REGGIO EMILIA (ITALY)

Laura CAVAZZA & Rita IOR, Iistituto per i Beni Artistici, Culturali e Naturali, Regione Emilia-Romagna, via Farini 28, 40124 Bologna, Italia

Abstract

The poster describes the reorganization of the document delivery service of Arcispedale S. Maria Nuova Library (ASMN) within GIDIF network (Italian Group of Drug Companies and Biomedical Research Institutes Librarians), following staff and budget reductions. After a successful trial run of the new system, the procedures were extended to extra GIDIF libraries.

Introduction

The Arcispedale S. Maria Nuova Library was founded in 1782 and reorganized in 1979. It provides information services to medical staff of USL n. 9, one of the very few Local Health Units actually involved in clinical research. 450 current and 537 ceased journals focus on general clinical medicine. Since 1987, the library participates in the Union Catalogue of GIDIF,RBM devised in order to provide document supply. Active GIDIF Union Catalogue partnership has created a 'double track' situation: on the one hand, the library sees that only members accede to the Union Catalogue, which is the by-product of a private enterprise. On the other hand, the same library supplies services to non members for a fee. So far, 37 libraries are involved and can pool up more than 4,000 titles, annually updated. ASMN Library caters for Emilia-Romagna and Northern Italy, with an interesting - however limited - number of enquiries from Central and Southern Italy.

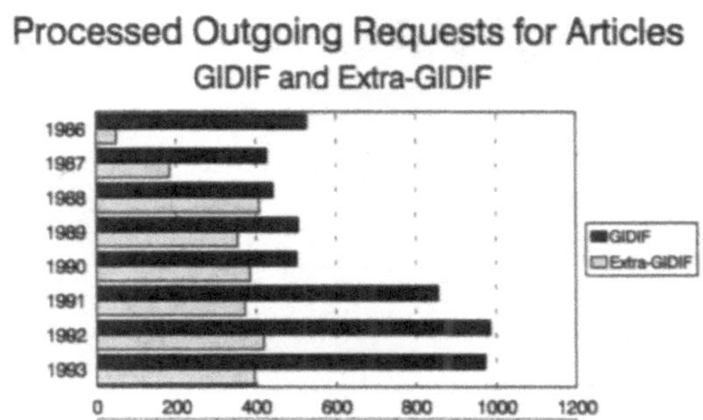

	1986	1987	1988	1989	1990	1991	1992	1993
GIDIF	527	427	443	506	502	855	984	972
Extra-GIDIF	50	184	409	355	385	372	419	396

Table 1

Such a twofold activity can only be explained if set against a national background where no effective medical libraries union catalogue exists or a national medical library either: libraries must rely upon poorly updated or 'local' union catalogues. From 1986 to 1992 the document delivery service was carried out by the same staff who assisted users, one of the four full-time, librarians would process incoming and outgoing requests. The most evident drawback was to be found in the lack of a dedicated fax-line: telephone or mail had to be used instead. As a consequence, information could be imprecise if dealt with orally, or delayed if sent by mail. The standard procedure would be the following: (i) first check of the bibliographical quotations before forwarding them to another library; the same for incoming quotations; (ii) - clearance of the requests within 24 hours; iii) control of the execution of outgoing requests; information to users concerning their requests.

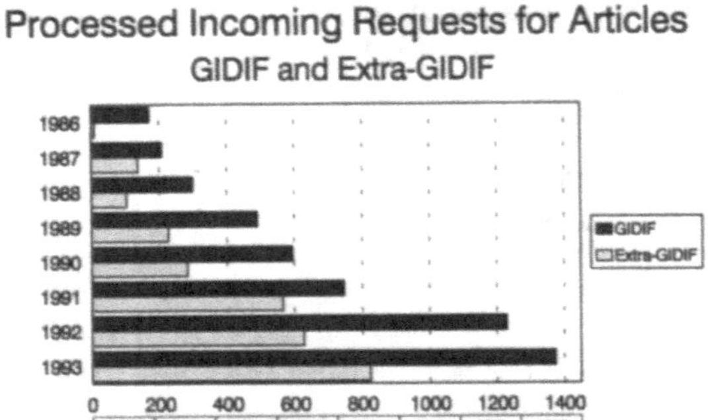

	1986	1987	1988	1989	1990	1991	1992	1993
GIDIF	171	206	299	489	594	747	1229	1374
Extra-GIDIF	10	138	104	227	283	564	627	823

Table 2

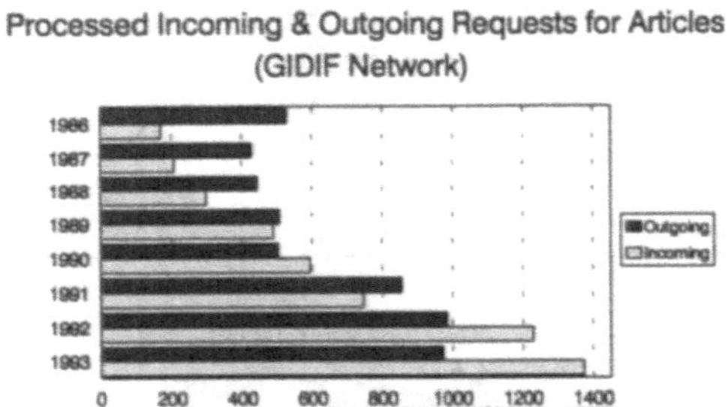

	1986	1987	1988	1989	1990	1991	1992	1993
Outgoing	527	427	443	506	502	866	984	972
Incoming	171	206	299	489	594	747	1229	1374

Table 3

From 1986 to 1992 the number of articles which were asked other libraries for, doubled in volume (see Table 1), while the figure of articles supplied by ASMN Library soared up (see Table 2). Within GIDIF network we can observe an increase of supplies in 1990 which becomes more evident from 1992 (Table 3). ASMN Library qualifies itself as a recipient of the document delivery service until 1990 when its growth to supplier's status is evident, as a result of some important libraries leaving the GIDIF network; their rich collections were similar to those of ASMN and they had shared with ASMN Library a supplier's role within GIDIF. The service came to a turning point in 1992. The incoming requests for articles went up by 30% and, at the same time, the hospital administration decided a staff reduction, while the budget remained unchanged. The quality of document delivery declined as a result of increased demands and workload: (i) operations became hard to control and users often did not receive adequate information concerning the processing of their requests; (ii) processing time for requests/supply would take more than 24 hours; (iii) - monitoring the service became difficult; (iv) time for document supply service was swallowing up the time allocated to other essential library activities. The service was going to collapse and a reorganization plan had to be studied.

Results

Following a first analysis in April 1993, a reorganization plan was launched. It was devised specifically for GIDIF service and applied in a trial run from April to December 1993:

i - all outgoing and incoming requests were to be registered; those addressed to GIDIF libraries were to carry a progressive number;

ii - request slips addressed to GIDIF libraries were to be filed for quick reference in a small filing cabinet on castors;

iii - a dedicated fax line was obtained: telecopies were to be used instead of telephone or mail, for speeding up requests and dispatching urgent articles.

After a few months of trial run, Soprintendenza per i beni librari was contacted and a problem solving methodology was applied in order to check the results. The purpose of the reorganization was studied in detail: upgrading the quality of the GIDIF network document delivery service in a situation of reduced staff, formally unchanged budget and increasing demands. The necessity was felt for an increased control over the processing of the requests, not so much in terms of time, but rather in their flow. As a consequence, ASMN Library quality standards for the service would be enhanced:

i - send or supply articles within 24 hours by fax and record the operations;

ii - inform users immediately about the processing of their requests, both outgoing and incoming;

iii - bird's eye view of service data.

Flow charts of the operations were drawn before and after the introduction of changes in order to analyse the difference between demand and offer. This part was the dark area that had to be investigated to ascertain the most relevant hindering causes. The trial run of 1993 was checked and solutions were selected within the margins actually granted. The experiment was hitting the mark and further adjustments could be devised. Specific attention was paid to negative elicitations as a relevant dark area; the results have been included in the ASMN Library's statistic surveys from 1993 on and a list of causes and solutions is now being drawn.

Conclusions

1. The procedures checked during the problem solving approach hit the mark:

i - the quality of the service is enhanced: fax requests and recording operations are faster and clearer, but not necessarily time saving;

ii - users who enquire about their request, are satisfied immediately;

iii - data can be monitored quickly.

2. Since 1994 ASMN has aimed to control the number of transactions; it was evident that the quality of the document delivery service could not be kept up if the quantity grew. In detail:

i - following further staff reductions in 1994, the service was split into two: document delivery on one side, assistance to users on the other;

ii - a nominal fee would be charged for document supply;

iii - according to new GIDIF guidelines, no more than 5 requests weekly for each member library would be accepted;

iv - all procedures originally meant for GIDIF members were extended to everybody else.

3. ASMN Library will not be in a position to grant the same standard in the future, beyond the maximum height of requests and supplies which has already been touched:

i - if the requests increase, ASMN will have to change the service completely, particularly if the library joins the document delivery project of Italian medical libraries now under way;

ii - negative elicitations ought to be studied in some depth, to find out the reasons why such requests cannot be met notwithstanding preliminary control and rerouting towards other libraries. Criteria should be set in order to select the appropriate library for each request.

References

* L'alternativa si chiama document delivery / Anna Maria Tammaro // In: Biblioteche oggi. - Novembre (1993), p. 34 - 39.
* Document supply in the new information environment / Graham P. Cornish // In: Journal of librarianship and information science. - Vol. 23, n. 3 (1991), p. 125 - 134.
* Interlending and document supply : a review of recent literature: XXIII / Desmond Seaton // In: Interlending & document supply. - Vol. 21, n. 1 (1993), p. 23 - 30.

CURRICULUM INTEGRATION OF HEALTH SCIENCE STUDENTS

Adriana Dracos & Maria Castriotta, Istituto Superiore di Sanità, Viale Regina Elena 299, 00161 Rome Italy

Abstract

University students often meet with some difficulties approaching library resources, because they lack basic bibliographic and information research skills and the scientific faculties, with their dynamic information needs, face this problem with particular frustration. In order to have an overview of educational programs on information retrieval activated in the universities, an analysis was performed utilizing the data derived both from the international literature on the matter and from the results of an "ad hoc" questionnaire sent to the EAHIL members. The screening of the literature was carried out exploiting library-oriented databases, integrated by some multidisciplinary databases, to gain a panorama of the international situation. As to the European reality, the questionnaire had just the aim to collect first-hand data on unpublished experiences ripened in the scientific environment where the European libraries operate. The results show an increasing interest on the matter, even though the organization and structure of the courses are not homogeneous. Finally, the opportunity to plan an organic common program to share experiences and resources appears evident.

1. Introduction

The final scope of University studies is to build up the elements of a specialization that will be acquired later on through the direct experience and the continuous update. The fulfillment of the second objective is achieved integrating the students' curriculum with the essential notions on how, where, when and why the information can be retrieved. This task is nevertheless quite hard to be accomplished, due to the information explosion that creates growing difficulties to academic people searching for specialized literature. Therefore, the need of students' orientation in library research and information management is generally recognized. In such an educational environment, librarians must play their role in the preparation of medical students, proposing themselves as vital partners in medical education.

2. Methods

In order to evaluate the spread of this kind of trainings as curriculum integration of scientific faculties, a double survey was performed: a bibliographic approach and a direct approach. In the first case, a search strategy regarding the topic of the study was verified on six databases, i.e. INSPEC, PASCAL, SIGLE (multidisciplinary files), and LIBRARY LITERATURE, ISA PLUS, LISA PLUS (library-oriented files). Four of them were available online and two of them on CD-ROM. As to the second approach, 108 questionnaires were addressed to the EAHIL members selected among those belonging to the University faculties. First of all, the adressees were asked if their University integrated curricula with literature research skills (item 1), and, in the affirmative case, which scientific faculties were involved (item 2) and which was the academic year of first start (item 3). Finally, some information regarding more precisely the organization of the trainings was required: year/s of the course of study (item 4), number of hours dedicated to the program and subjects taught (item 5).

3. Results

The two different approaches supplied the data to have an overview of the international situation and an updated picture of the European initiatives. The databases exploited through the bibliographic search yielded 96 unique items. The data collected were evaluated considering that the time span of the single files is not homogeneous. Thus, two periods were identified (pre-1985 and post-1985) to assess the geographic spread and the faculty distribution of library science training courses. The results show that the US have always been very active in the organization of such courses, closely followed by Europe, even though the gap between them has increased in the recent period (pre-1985: US 50% and Europe 41%; post-1985: US 59% and Europe 27%). As to the faculties involved in the trainings, Medicine ranks the first all over the years (pre-1985: 31% and post-1985: 62%), while the other scientific faculties share equal positions (10-15% approximately). The results of the questionnaire were divided per item. A total of 43 replies were returned on 108 mailed (39.8 response rate). Among them (item 1), 51.16% answered positively, 37.21% negatively and the remaining 11.63% were planning one more trainings in the academic year 1994-95. As to the scientific faculties involved (item 2), Medicine collected 50%, followed by Life Sciences (13%), Pharmacy (about 11%), Chemistry (8%); the remaining 18% gathered other faculties. The results of item 3 (academic year of first start) were subdivided into segments of five years each. The data show a relatively homogeneous level of interest (10% average) for the segments pre-1976, 1981-85 and 1986-90; whilst an increase in the period 1976-80 (20%) and a meaningfully rising trend in the period 1991-95 (50%) were pointed out. These data include, of course, the faculties that are planning trainings for next academic year. For what concerns the year of the course of study where the training is activated (item 4), the first year (34%) and the third year (about 26%) were the most represented, followed by the second and the fourth year (14% average), while the fifth year (about 4%) was the least involved; the rate of the postgraduate courses was quite low (8%), if we consider the needs and the potentialities of specialized trainings. The results regarding item 5 were divided into two groups: number of hours of training programs of introductory courses and of advanced ones. In the first case, the highest levels were between two hours (about 35%) and three hours (26%), followed by one hour, four hours, and more than ten hours (13% average). On the contrary, advanced courses resulted much longer, with ten hours in most cases (33%), followed by six, four and three hours at the same level (14%); the remaining 25% was variedly shared.

4. Discussion

The panorama emerging from this study suggests a growing interest in the production of bibliographic search courses for university and professional people, due both to the increasing librarians' awareness of their role, and to the great favour expressed by the target persons, who generally evaluate these trainings very positively and profitably. The data collected through the bibliographic approach show a progression of the US for what concerns the quantity of the courses. On the contrary, the European interest has not been constant all over the years: a decrease in the period 1980-90 was indeed pointed out, but the trend is now continuously and definitely rising. The structure and organization of the trainings are anyway very hetergeneous, both considering the number of hours planned, and the deepness of the subjects taught. Moreover, the courses are not always compulsory and regularly integrated in the students' curricula.

5. Conclusions

Actually, the need for an effective, regular information retrieval program is undoubtedly deeply experienced by the scientific faculties' students. The program should be inserted all over the course of study and modulated according to specific local exigencies. At the European level, it is very important to foster a coordinate action among all European librarians and information specialists, so as to take advantage of the existing experiences, optimizing and harmonizing them in a common fruitful effort.

References

Minchow R.L., Pudlock K., Lucas B., Clancy S. (1993) *Breaking new ground in curriculum integrated instruction.* Medical Reference Services Quarterly 12(2):1-18.

Ikeda N.R. (1992) Impact of end-user search training on pharmacy students: a four-year follow-up study. Bulletin of the Medical Library Association 80(2):124-130.

Rankin J.A. (1992) Problem-based medical education: Effect on library use. Bulletin of the Medical Library Association 80(1):36-43.

Le Coadic Y.F., Bretelle-Desmazieres D. (1992) L'enseignement de l'information scientifique et technique en chimie. (La) Vie des Sciences 9(2):137-142.

THE DEVELOPMENT OF A HEALTH EDUCATION RESOURCE SERVICE IN SPAIN

Andrée Manuel Keenoy & Camila Higueras Callejón, Escuela Andaluza de Salud Pública, Campus Universitario de Cartuja, Apdo Correros. 2070, 18080 Granada

Problems

Various organisms in Spain produce material on the same subject and addressed to the same target population. Other areas and target populations are not covered Material available does not respond to users's needs. A research study showed that health promotion workers and producers of educational material lack information on what is available.

Responses

The library of the Andalusian School of Public Health has developed a Health Promotion Resource Service to respond to these needs. A collection of educational material produced in Spain is being compiled and input into a database. Images are scanned and storedin a rewritable optical disk. A printed catalogue has been produced from the image database. Updated versions will be printed regularly.

By-Products

- An image database on an optical disk
- Support material for a network of health promotion
- Exhibitions, workshops, videoviewings, etc.

THE CORE COLLECTION OF MEDICAL BOOKS AND JOURNALS

Maureen Forrest, Cairns Library, The John Radcliffe, Oxford Radcliffe Hospital, Headington, Oxford OX3 9DU, UK; & **Albert Prior**, SWETS

This publication is designed to be an acquisition guide for small or medium-sized libraries in hospitals, postgraduate teaching centres or medical institutions and has a broad-based clinical orientation. The first edition appeared in 1992. The second edition has been completely revised and expanded to include sections on complimentary medicine, medical writing and professions allied to medicine. International Student Editions (ISE) and English Language and Book Society editions (ELBS) are included where appropriate. The selection of material for inclusion was co-ordinated by Howard Hague, the Assistant Librarian at Charing Cross and Westminster Medical School, London who was supported in this task by a panel of booksellers, librarians and publishers under the direction of the production manager Neil Poppmacher, BMJ Books Division Manager. The list has been widely used as both a selection tool and a criterion for the accreditation of UK National Health Service libraries.

The list is published by the Medical Information Working Party, a forum for the exchange of ideas between the UK organizations which form the constituent parts of the information chain. The Working Party was founded in 1984 following informal discussions between representatives of the Library Association Medical Health ad Welfare Libraries Group and the Publishers' Association Medical Group. The participating bodies are; The Booksellers' Association, The Library Association Medical Health and Welfare Libraries Group, The Publishers' Association, The Association of Subscription Agents. The terms of reference include: to liaise on matters of mutual interest and to make recommendations to the parent organizations; to consider problems and topics raised by members and to seek satisfactory solutions to them; to promote better understanding between participating organizations.

MEDLINE PROMOTION

L Locche, A Stanzani & L Loiacono, Biblioteca Centralizzata ,USL 28 - Bologna, Italia

The CD-ROM bibliographic research service of the Library of the USL 28 of Bologna (Italy) is staffed by a full-time librarian (37 hours a week) and is equipped with several SilverPlatter CD-ROM databases (Medline since 1966, ISA Plus, Excerpta Medica Psychiatry, Excer[ta Medica Neurosceinces, Psyclit, and other "try and buy" discs). Its potential users are about 950, subdivided among hospital staff doctors and staff of the Faculty of Medicine. Research is done by the librarian in presence of the doctor on an appointment basis.

The starting point for the investigation was to provide an answer to the question why the service should be utlied only up to one third of its capacit, and to encourage access to the service, as well as to optimize the yield of the librarian's work hours. In order to fulfill this aim, a form was sent to all 950 doctors, through which they were allowed to request by internal mail a certain bibliographic research, which the librarian was supposed to carry out himself, without any need for the doctor to go to the library, nor for the librarian to wait for him, thus allowing a better planning to the latter for his work routine. The form contained 5 simple questions: Title, MESH, Free words, Articles already seen, and Quantitative expectation (Table 1). A table was also set up in order to verify from the correctness in form filling whetreher its formalution was to the point or not (Table 2). The results of the research werre finally transmitted to the doctor along with a questionnaire meant to obtain:

1. Information of the user's attitude toward the service (Table 3);
2. Information on the quality of the research (Table 4);
3. Information as to the future usage of the library (Table 5).

The answers to the questionnare are reported. Three months after the start of the initiative a positibe result is already shown by the 100% increase in the utlization of tyhc service, with respect to the corresponding period of 1992.

TABLE 1: FORM FOR CD-ROM MEDLINE RESEARCH

Fill the following fields:

1. Topic of the research
2. MESH terms
3. Free words
4. Articles already seen
5. Quantitative expectation

Send to the Library

TABLE 2: EVALUATION OF THE EFFICACY OF THE FORM

72 FORMS RETURNED = 100%

1.	Clearness of topic	100.0%
	Fulfilled fields:	
2.	MESH term	50.0%
3.	Free words	87.5%
4.	Already found articles	65.0%
5.	Quantative expectation	64.0%

	How the research was performed	
a.	Directly by the Librarian	94.5%
b.	Need of explanations (telephone call)	4.0%
c.	Need of presence of the User	1.5%

TABLE 3: CUSTOMER'S ATTITUDE TOWARD THE SERVICE

How do you usually find references?		**How the User prefer to access CD-ROM databases?**	
41%	Bibliographic directories	43%	Together with the Librarian
38%	Journal contents	38%	Sending a form to the Librarian
21%	Databases	19%	The User by himself

Have you ever used MEDLINE before?

77% Yes	23% No

TABLE 4: QUALITY OF THE RESEARCH

WELL PLANNED FORM = 97.5%

Outcome of the research	Number of records retrieved
54% OK, pertinent	67% As expected
42% OK, but ... information noise	24% Too few
4% Not pertinent	9% Too many

Comparison between MEDLINE and other sources		
85% Faster	10% Similar	5% Slower

TABLE 5: FUTURE USAGE OF THE LIBRARY

WILL CONSULT A LIBRARY FOR FURTHER INQUIRIES = 90.5%

Which services of the library will be used
50% CD-ROM
40% Consultation of the library journal holding and photocopying
10% Interlibrary loan

MEDICAL DISSERTATIONS - KEEPING OR WEEDING ?

Oliver Obst, University and State Library, Krummer Timpen 3-5, 48043 Münster, Germany

Abstract

Due to a full stack and a beginning retroconversion we decided to weed our medical dissertations acquired by exchange in the seventies. We selected the dissertations by four criteria: actuality, historical outline, deposit copy, and use in the last three years. All other dissertations which did not match these categories were dropped out and pulped. With the help of students (500 hours), only one librarian (190 hours) checked 16.162 medical dissertations. Of these only 4% (i.e. 682) matched our criteria, the remaining dissertations (i.e. 15,480) we threw away. This saved us about 100 running shelf meter and 3,870 hours of retroconversion by a professional librarian.

Introduction

Stack capacities of the University and State Library Münster, an academic library serving as much as 55,000 students, are almost exhausted or will be in the very near future. This is also true for almost every other German library and perhaps even a worldwide problem. In 1986 the Council for Science, the most influential scientific advisory board of the German government, recognized this problem by publishing a report called: "Recommendations to the requirement of stack area of academic libraries." In this report the government was advised not to fund any building of new stacks. On the opposite, the libraries have to throw away unnecessary materials and reduce the exchange to make room for recent accessions. This report has an dramatic impact on academic library management in Germany, and also in Muenster, where we stopped immediately the exchange of medical dissertations. Since that time we have asked ourselves constantly, if we should carefully keep and retroconverse obsolete dissertations but renounced up-to-date ones. Beside better room utilization in virtue of compact shelving and swapping low used volumes like elder newspapers, weeding seems to us a most suitable method for clearing out the shelves in favour of new intakes. Coincidently, the library has started to retroconverse the card catalogue (> 2 mio. entries) in machine readable format. Among them are about 500,000 dissertations with - especially in natural science and medicine - uncertain value to our users. At last, we decided to weed elder medical dissertations (and also dissertations of others subjects like chemistry, mathematics, technical sciences, and agriculture).

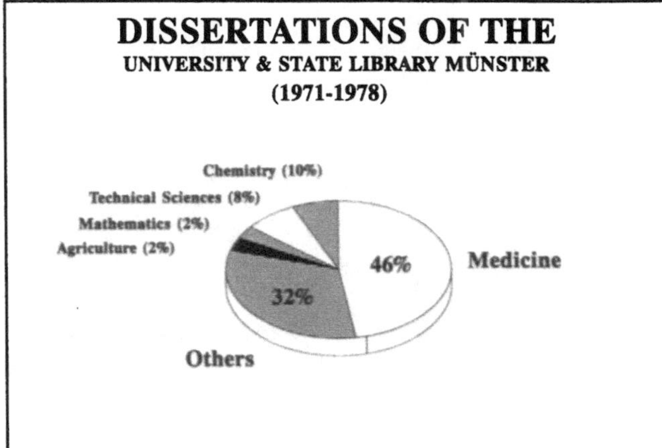

Figure 1

Fig. 1: This graph shows the distribution by subject of acquired dissertations in the University and State Library Muenster from 1971 to midyear 1978. From the total of 35,000 dissertations examined, the major part of 46% (i.e. 16.162) were medical ones. 10% were dissertations in chemistry, 8% in technical sciences, and in mathematics and agriculture 2%, respectively. They were also subject of the selection process. 32% of the dissertations were from biology, physics, or the humanities, which remained untouched. The oversized value of the medical dissertations is due to the fact that at almost every German medical faculty there is a delivery obligation of up to 40 copies.

Usage

In the course of the selection process we detected that more than 99 percent of the medical dissertations has not been used during the past 2 $^1/_2$ years! One main hindrance for utilization might be that only 6% of the dissertations have been subject indexed (decimal classification). The indexed dissertations has been 16 times more often charged out than the not indexed ones, which are only referred in the author catalogue. [Though the use of medical dissertations could possibly elevated by as much as 1,600 % if indexed, there is on the one hand beyond any question no librarian to perform this lengthy task and on the other hand no need for this, because we offer an indexed enduser CD-ROM database including all German dissertations from 1945 to today.]

Criteria for Selection

If the medical dissertations doesn't match at least one of the following criteria, they were pulped:

* at least one use in the last 2 $^1/_2$ years
* historical outline
* deposit copy
* refer to our special collections
* published before the year 1900
* up to date subject

Book Processing

The dissertations were processed in a most pragmatical way:

1. Selection by means of the bibliographic records of the shelf catalogue.
2. Pulling of selected dissertations out of the shelves and pulping.
3. Sorting the cards in alphabetical order.
4. Pulling the cards out of the author catalogue.
5. Deleting the signatures out of the automatic charging system.
6. Printing a list of remaining signatures and pulling not listed signatures out of the subject catalogue.
7. Moving the remaining books closer on the shelf.

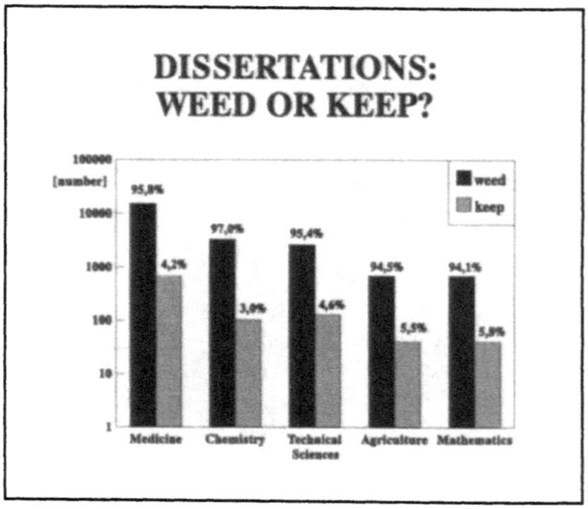

Fig.2: This graph above shows the number of weeded (black columns) as well as kept (hatched columns) dissertations of each subject on a logarithmic scale. The percentage of weeded dissertations ranged from 94.1 to 97.0 % with a mean of 95.4 % .

Conclusion

35,000 dissertations from 1971 to midyear 1978 were examined. 16,162 (46%) were medical ones. 15,480 of them didn't match the criterions for selection and were therefore dropped out and pulped. Only 682 or 4.2% remained in virtue of their supposed necessarity.

<u>This cost us:</u>
* 500 hours of student work
* 190 hours of librarian work
* 120 hours of stack work

<u>This saved us:</u>
* about 100 running shelf meter
* 3,870 hours of retroconversion work

We do not hesitate to keep on weeding ...

LES BIBLIOTHEQUES MEDICALES, LEURS USAGERS POTENTIELS: Besoins et satisfactions dans un contexte non universitaire - L'exemple du Canton du Tessin (Suisse Italienne)

Giuliana Schmid, Manuela Perucchi, & Costanzo Limoni [adresse pour correspondance] Centro documentazione e ricerca, Organizzazione Sociopsichiatrica Cantonale (OSC), ONC, Via Ag. Maspoli, 6850 Mendrisio, Suisse

Objectifs

L'étude concerne le Canton du Tessin (282.181 habitants), région de langue italienne située au sud de la Suisse et ne disposant pas d'université. Les buts de l'enquête sont:

- identifier les besoins d'information et de documentation médico-scientifique des usagers potentiels de deux bibliothèques médicales, l'une specialisée dans le demaine de la psychiatrie et l'autre en santé publique.
- évaluer si les services documentaires du Canton du Tessin répondent d'une façon adéquate aux besoins des usagers, et identifier les éventuels domaines principaux à développer.

Méthodologie

L'enquête a été effectuée au moyen d'un questionnaire mi-structuré envoyé à tous les médecins et les psychologues ayant leur activité au Tessin. Un rappel à tous les médecins a été fait après deux mois. Le questionnaire était anonyme. L'analyse statistique des données a été effectuée avec le logiciel S.A.S. (Statistical Analysis System).

Population

480 personnes (taux de réponse: 50%) ont répondu au questionnaire: 410 médecins (taux de réponse 54,3%) et 70 psychologues (taux de réponse 42,1%) (21% femmes et 79% hommes). 237 travaillent dans le secteur public, 200 dans le secteur privé, 33 dans le secteur public/privé, 11 sans réponse

Questionnaire

Le questionnaire touchait les données suivantes:

a- sources d'information utilisées pour suivre l'évolution des connaissances dans le domaine professionnel et pour la recherche scientifique, types de documents les plus utilisés
b- stratégies développées pour accéder aux documents originaux
c- utilisation des bibliothèques
d- degré de satisfaction des usagers par rapport aux services existant au Tessin: opinions, besoins, propositions
e- services documentaires à développer
f- quelques données concernant les répondants (sexe, âge, profession, spécialisation, demaine de travail)

Résultats*

a- Sources d'information utilisées, types de documents les plus utilisés (fréquence d'utilisation, plusieurs réponse possible)

	chaque semaine (%)	parfois (%)	jamais/presque jamais (%)
bibliothèques	19,4	36,3	35,0
congrès	**32,5**	55,0	8,5
cours de formation	**46,7**	44,8	4,6
relations interpersonnelles	**49,8**	35,4	6,5
industrie pharmaceutique	13,8	37,1	33,1

Les sources d'information des interviewés **les plus utilisées** sont **les relations interpersonnelles, les cours de formation** et **les congrès; les moins utilisées** sont **les bibliothèques** et l'industrie pharmaceutique.

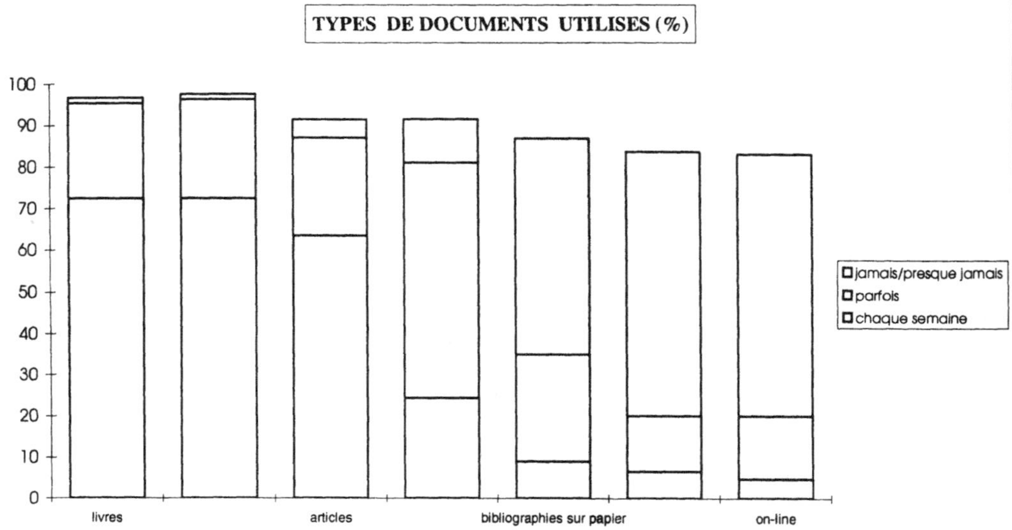

Les types de documents les plus utilisés: livres, périodiques, articles / Les moins utilisés: répertoires bibliographiques sur papier, banques de données on-line et sur CD-ROM

* Il faut considérer qu'il y a un petit pourcentage de non reponse pour chaque question.

b- Stratégies utilisées pour accéder aux documents

	bibliothèques (%)		**achats (%)**		**collègues (%)**		**industrie pharmac. (%)**	
	parfois	souvent	parfois	souvent	parfois	souvent	parfois	souvent
livres	23,8	5	28,8	66,9	41	6,5		
périodiques	25,2	22,1	33,5	43,3	44	11,3	23,3	5,6
articles	22,3	29,8			42,5	22,9		
recherches bibliographiques	18,3	10,4			15	4,4	30,4	5,6

Les bibliothèques sont utilisées surtout pour obtenir des articles et, deuxièmement, pour les périodiques. Le comportement des usagers varie beaucoup selon le type de document. Pour ce qui concerne les livres, la majorité les achète, mais presque la moitié s'adresse aussi "parfois" aux collègues. On remarque donc qu'il existe une circulation d'information assez importante entre collègues, surtout pour les articles et les périodiques. Pour la recherche bibliographique les services et les instruments sont utilisés plus "parfois" que "souvent". En faisant la somme des "parfois" et des "souvent" on peut établir la liste des services et des instruments les plus utilisés: industrie pharmaceutique le 36%, bibliothèque le 28,3%, base de données on-line le 22,9%, répertoires bibliographiques sur papier le 22,7%, dodki le 22,6%, base de données sur cd-rom le 20,8 %, les collegues le 19,4%. Il y a des différences entre les médecins publics et les médecins privés pour ce qui concerne le parcour suivi pour se documenter. Les médecins publics utilisent plus les bibliothèques pour accéder à la documentation; les médecins privés s'abonnent plus "souvent" aux périodiques et utilisent davantage la commande des articles directement à l'auteur.

c- Utilisation des bibliothèques selon le secteur d'activité, l'activité de recherche et la profession

	N tot*	**OUI %**	**N**	**NON %**	**N**
médecins	410	42,9	176	55,4	227
psychologues	70	**65,7**	46	32,9	23
secteur public	200	**69**	139	30,5	61
secteur privé	237	27	64	70	166
chercheurs	166	**68,7**	114	30,1	50
non-chercheurs	314	34,4	108	63,7	200
total	480	46,3	222	52,1	250

* comprend aussi les non répondants

Les chercheurs, les personnes qui travaillent dans le secteur public et les psychologues utilisent plus les bibliothèques que les médecins du secteur privé.

d- Bibliothèques du Tessin: degré de satisfaction et besoins

Opinions (Nombre de réponses N=222, taux de réponse: 46,25%):

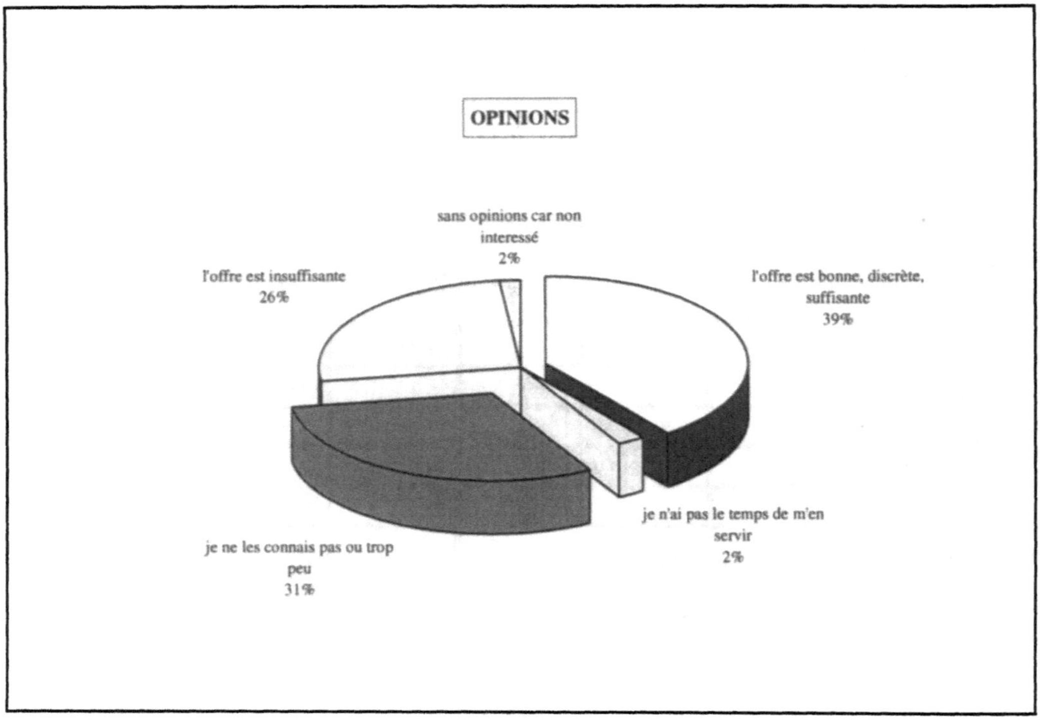

Besoins prioritaires des potentiels usagers:
A la question, à savoir quels sont les services que les interviewés utiliseraient s'ils avaient la possibilité de s'adresser à une bibliothèque médico-scientifique, les comportements parus à propos de l'utilisation actuelle des bibliothèques (voir question b) se confirment, avec comme besoins prioritaires la consultation de revues et d'articles (souvent: revues 44,2%, articles 38,3%, livres 30,6%, recherches bibliografiques 30%).

Propositions exprimées par les interviewés pour améliorer l'acces à l'information scientifique N = 136, taux de réponse = 28% (valeurs absolues, plusieurs réponses possibles, question ouverte):

-. centraliser les services ou du moins une partie (33)
-. miser sur l'informatique (on-line, cd-rom) (28)
-. améliorer et coordonner les services existants (22)
-. plus d'information sur les services existants (14)
-. créer des bibliothèques dans les hôpitaux (12)
-. plus de personnel qualifié dans les bibliothèques (11)
-. ouvrir les bibliothèques des hôpitaux aux usagers externes (8)
- faire circuler l'information concernant la documentation (5)
- pas besoin de nouveaux services (3)

Conclusions

La méthodologie appliquée à l'enquête a permis d'évaluer les besoins des usagers potentiels des deux bibliothèques et de disposer de données pour identifier des solutions adéquates et ciblées pour y répondre. En ce qui concerne les résultats on pourrait dire que: les personnes qui travaillent dans un contexte public consultent plus les bibliothèques, ainsi que qui fait de la recherche; dans le cas où l'on devrait renforcer l'offre existante, les services les plus requis concerneraient la demande d'articles et de revues; au niveau cantonal, il sera souhaitable que la coordination/centralisation, l'informatisation et l'information soient améliorées.

OLD POSSIBILITIES BUT NEW FEATURES: European Online-Database HECLINET

Rüdiger Schneemann, Technische Universität Berlin, Institut für Gesundheitswissenschaften/Public Health, Dokumentation Krankenhauswesen, Straße des 17.Juni 135, D-10623 Berlin, Germany

Abstract

1. **Bibliographic Database** To solve the growing information problems in the field of hospital care, in 1969 two German hospital institutes started the *Dokumentation Krankenhauswesen*. The task was to collect all kind of hospital related litera-ture, to index it and to put it in a retrieval system, and to give as far as possible support to the users.

2. **Old Possibilities** The main traditional tools have been: Indexing and citating the national and international literature; using EDP to collect the data and build up a database; publishing bimonthly the *Informationsdienst Krankenhauswesen*; editing the *Thesaurus Krankenhauswesen* to organize the search terms.

3. **The International Cooperation HECLINET** Based on that system, in 1974 several European hospital institutes started the *Health Care Literature Information Network (HECLINET)* to combine their activities, to optimize data collections with their limited resources, to solve information problems with existing technics. Since 1980, lead by the *Institut für Krankenhausbau (IFK)* of the Technical University Berlin, *HECLINET* has been offered worldwide by the host *DIMDI*, Cologne, as a database.

4. **New Features** The database HECLINET is completely bilingual German/English searchable. All documents are indexed and easy accessible stored. Nearly 90% of the originals are microfiched. The documents are not only indexed by descriptors but also described by abstracts and classified by qualifiers. DIMDI supports HECLINET - as well as any other offered database - with *Duplication Check*, *Superbase* function for cluster seaching, *Online Ordering*, *Statistics* tools, *Synonym* search aids, and *Menu*-Driven user surface.

5. **Further Developments** The scope of literature will dramatically widen: In 1993 the *Institut für Krankenhausbau* changed its name into *Institut für Gesundheitswissenschaften/Public Health* (similar to the Swiss Hospital Institute) and the covered field of research will expand into that area; there are additional cooperations in discussion to round off the documented field of health care, with numerical data producers; the production of a CD-ROM version of HECLINET is to be expected as well as more highly sophisticated search tools by DIMDI.

UK UNIVERSITY MEDICAL SCHOOL LIBRARIANS GROUP (UMSLG)

Peter Morgan & John van Loo [Correspondance to] Cambridge University Medical Library, Addenbrooke's Hospital, Cambridge CB2 2SP, UK

The Group

The University Medical School Librarians Group (UMSLG) is the representative group for the librarians of undergraduate and postgraduate medical schools in the United Kingdom and the Republic of Ireland. Membership of the Group is *ex officio*, being restricted to the librarian in charge of each library. There are currently 45 members. The Group held its first meeting in 1983, to raise the political profile of medical school libraries at a time when the UK's universities and the National Health Service were both undergoing periods of substantial change. Its main objectives are:

- to improve communication and co-operation among medical school libraries
- to represent its members' interests at national level
- to develop links with other library organisations
- to organise meetings on topics of interest to members and others.

There is a programme of regular meetings and other activities. The Group holds a minimum of two full meetings a year: these provide members with the opportunity to discuss topics of mutual concern and to share their experience with others, and most meetings will also include a seminar devoted to a selective theme. The Group also organises an annual national one-day forum to which representatives of other health-care library organisations are invited, in order to review and debate major topical issues. Open seminars and workshops are held on specific subjects, such as the use of bibliographical databases and developments in networked information services for health-care.

An important aspect of UMSLG's work lies in its dealings with various governmental and other national bodies that are concerned in some respect with library policy-making and funding. A number of statements have been issued by the Group, either on its own behalf or as joint submissions prepared in collaboration with other organisations. There is close liaision with the Standing Conference of National and University Libraries (SCONUL) and particularly with SCONUL's Advisory Committee on Health Services. There is also an established working relationship with the NHS Regional Librarians Group, and new links are emerging with the recently-constituted Health Sciences Group. Until 1992 UMSLG was administered by a single officer, the Group Secretary. Since then, following the adoption of a new constitution, its affairs have been directed by an executive committee headed by a chairman and secretary. The Group's current executive committee is:

Mr Peter Morgan *(Chairman)* (Cambridge University)
Miss Lindsay Curtis *(Secretary)* (Royal Postgraduate Medical School, London University)
Dr Felicity Grainger (Glasgow University)
Mr John Lancaster (University of Wales College of Medicine)
Mr Martin Lewis (Sheffield University)
Mr John van Loo (United Medical and Dental Schools, London University)

Contacts

UMSLG members use electronic mail (email) and discussion lists extensively to communicate with one another via the UK's JANET (Joint Academic NETwork) system. The discussion lists allow any registered user to send a message to all the other registered users, either to pass on useful information, to seek help, or to provoke debate. UMSLG maintains three electronic mail discussion lists. Two are closed, and available only to members of the Group. The third is an open list called LIS-MEDICAL, and anyone interested in health-care libraries, and who has access to the Internet, may join it. If you wish to join, send a message to the email address

mailbase@mailbase.ac.uk

leaving the subject line blank. The message text should say

join lis-medical <your first name> <your last name> (for example, "join lis-medical jacques delors").

You will receive an automatic reply with more information on LIS-MEDICAL. The Group is interested in developing links with other European groups that share similar interests. Please contact the Chairman (Peter Morgan, Cambridge University Medical Library - address above; tel: +44 223 336757, fax: +44 223 336709, email: pbm2@cus.cam.ac.uk) or Secretary (Lindsay Curtis, Royal Postgraduate Medical School Library, Ducane Road, London W12 0NN, UK; tel: +44 81 740 3246, fax: +44 81 740 3203, email: lcurtis@rpms.ac.uk) to discuss this.

Medical Education in the UK and the Republic of Ireland

Medical education follows broadly the same pattern in the United Kingdom and the Republic of Ireland. Teaching is centred on the university undergraduate medical schools. Students pursue a course lasting 5-6 years, depending on the university, before obtaining their degree. The curriculum must meet the requirements of the statutory body that licences doctors to practise: in the UK this is the General Medical Council (GMC). The traditional undergraduate course consists of two phases, each lasting for about half of the total course length. First, students study "pre-clinical" subjects, covering the basic medical sciences. After completing this phase successfully, they move to the second, "clinical", phase. either at the same medical school or at another university. In the clinical phase, students are usually based at teaching hospitals, but community-based teaching is becoming more common. The undergraduate medical curriculum is currently being revised, and in future pre-clinical and clinical instruction will be more closely integrated. Each medical school has at least one library, which usually also serves medical and other staff employed by the National Health Service.

After graduating, doctors must serve for a year in approved training posts before becoming licensed medical practitioners. Further training and qualifications may be obtained both through postgraduate degrees awarded by the universities, and by passing the examinations of professional bodies like the Royal College of Physicians and the Royal College of Surgeons.

UMSLG Member Institutions

United Kingdom

London University:

- Charing Cross & Westminster Medical School
- Hunterian Institute
- Institute of Cancer Research
- Institute of Child Health
- Institute of Dental Surgery
- Institute of Neurology
- Institute of Psychiatry
- King's College School of Medicine & Dentistry
- London Hospital Medical College
- London School of Hygiene & Tropical Medicine
- National Heart & Lung Institute
- Royal Free Hospital School of Medicine
- Royal Postgraduate Medical School
- St Bartholomew's Hospital Medical College
- St George's Hospital Medical School
- St Mary's Hospital Medical School
- University College (3 sites)
- United Medical & Dental Schools

Aberdeen University
Bath University
Belfast - Queen's University
Birmingham University
Bristol University
Cambridge University
Cardiff - University of Wales College of Medicine
Dundee University
Edinburgh University
Glasgow University
Leeds University
Leicester University
Liverpool - School of Tropical Medicine
Liverpool University
Manchester University
Newcastle University
Nottingham University
Oxford University
Sheffield University
Southampton University

Republic of Ireland

Cork - University College
Dublin - Royal College of Surgeons in Ireland
Dublin - Trinity College
Dublin - University College
Galway - University College

EDUCATION OF POTENTIAL HEALTH-CARE INFORMATION END-USERS BY PHARMACEUTICAL SPECIAL LIBRARY

Nada Trzan-Herman, Lek d.d., R&D, Verovskova 57, 61000 Ljubljana, Slovenia

Abstract
Educational objectives of Lek's special library are presented and we find it very important that we move our information resources closer to health care professionals who work on various working areas - not only in Lek.

Introduction
Lek d.d. is a pharmaceutical and chemical company which serves as a rotation site for young graduated pharmacists - before their licence exams. Lek's special library (later on: Lek's library) enables young professionals to become well acquainted with information sources and modern information technology. The objective of such training is to distribute scientific information for pharmacists and other medical professionals and contribute to personal career development and to the effectiveness in a professional's everyday work.

1. Lek's Library Fonds
Lek d.d. is ranked on the 100th position among the world's pharmaceutical firms (Scrip Report BS 509,1992, Table I: Leading Companies By Pharmaceutical Sales). Lek's library is a part of the Department for Industrial Property and Informatics which is situated in R&D. USD 250.000,00 was spent on sources of scientific information last year. Modern information technology is used for gathering and distributing information. The most frequently used information sources are the following:

- monographs (cca 500 new titles per year)
- periodicals (cca 350 titles per year)
- CD-ROM data bases (14 different titles - introduced in 1987)
- on line data bases (DIALOG, STN)
- specialised data bases (e.g. Lek's bibliography)

Information resources are as important as production, finance, or humans for business results and Lek follows the intensive development of information technology and new information sources. Lek's library has developed also a good relationship with libraries like Central Medical Library, Central Technical Library, libraries of scientific institutes in Slovenia etc. and there is a good interlending exchange. Many articles and patents are ordered from British Library.

2. User Education in Lek's Library
We find it very important that our end users are well informed about the use of Lek's special library. They are not only the Lek's professionals but also the students of the Faculty for Natural Sciences and Technology - most of all the students of the Department of Pharmacy, graduated pharmacists and our professional partners in institutes, faculties, laboratories, pharmacies etc., who can obtain copies of articles and some on-disc searches free of charge. Lectures given in the Lek's library aim at two different end user's group: lectures for new professionals; for new Lek's employees; lectures for young graduated pharmacists to whom Lek serves as a rotation site. We would like to point out that every year more than twenty freshly graduated pharmacists attend a one month education program in pharmaceutical industry (e.g. Lek) which is a part of one year training before a final licence exam. Lek's library serves to inform them about modern information technology and information sources and this is an opportunity to present to our future professional partners the use of Lek's library whenever professional questions arise in their everyday work.

3. Our Findings
We realise, however, that pharmacists from various working areas use Lek's library mostly when they do their master or doctoral theses or specialisations. The second type of requests include simple questions about brand names and medicinal products. After five years of giving lectures we can find these young professionals satisfied with our free of charge information sources. Each year we provide the following items for various health-care information end users: articles from our journals (300 per year); - on disc searches (60 per year); - value added information (40 per year).

The essential quality of educational objectives is their relevance to the health needs of society.

4. Discussion

High quality of information is an essential part of any successful work. We believe that the existing Lek's information sources can help young health care professionals with their personal career development and with their everyday professional work. Another considerable advantage worth underlining is that our information sources are free of charge what might be stimulating as far as the use is concerned. We move our information resources closer to health care professionals who work on various working areas (hospitals, pharmacies etc.) (1) and mostly to pharmacists whom pharmaceutical industry sometimes does not pay as much attention as to physicians (2,3,4,5,6). A short comment (7) can illustrate a distance between pharmaceutical firms and students of pharmacy: a group of students was put a question what they would do to advance pharmacy if they were presidents of a pharmaceutical factory. Several interesting answers were obtained:

pharmaceutical industry should:

- support pharmaceutical education at all levels
- encourage education of pharmacists and patients
- improve communications between pharmacy and industry

Conclusion

However, according to our findings and consideration of young professionals' remarks, it is clear that our free of charge information sources for pharmacists and other health-care professionals can contribute to good health care information environment in our society.

Literature

1. Roser M. (1993) New-Age Pharma Companies. Pharmaceutical Technology Europe vol.5 No.6 p.8
2. Canadian Medical Association (1994) Physicians and the pharmaceutical industry (update 1994). Canadian Medical Association Journal vol.150 No.2 256A - 256F
3. Lexchin J. (1993) Interactions between physicians and the pharmaceutical industry: what does the literature say ? Canadian Medical Associaton Journal vol.149 No.10 1401-7
4. Robbins J. (1994) How Schering won pharmacist loyalty.Medical Marketing&Media vol.29 No.3 58-61
5. Sagar G.V. (1992) Pharmaceutical Industry Interaction with Pharmaceutical Schools. Pharmatimes vol.24 Sep. p.15,17
6. Caliendo G.C. & Danyluk A.P (1993) Drug information education in the pharmaceutical industry. ASHP-Midyear Clinical-Meeting vol.28 No.12 P-147(R)
7. Essay Contents Winners (1994) Out of the mouths of students: Bright ideas for industry. Drug Topics April 25 p.12

STUDY ON SERVICES OF MEDICAL SCHOOL LIBRARIES: Comparison of Japan and China

Kazuo Urata & Zhang Haiqi, [Correspondance] Medical Information Centre for Education and Research, Jikei University School of Medicine, Tokyo 105, Japan

Abstract

The objective of this study was to tell the differences from services of medical school libraries between China and Japan. It was concluded that resource sharing in Japan were generally well - employed as compared to China. The common problem encountered was to strengthen the information and education link between users and the information resources.

Background

In 1993, there were 99 schools of Western medicine and 23 traditional medical schools in China according to the annual statistics by the Ministry of Health. 13 of these were funded by the Ministry of Health, 4 by the People's Liberation Army and the remainder by provincial or municipal governments[1]. In 1992, there were 105 medical libraries according to the 63rd annual statistics by the Japan Medical Library Association. 42 of these were funded by the national university or colleges. 10 by the prefectural university or colleges, 53 by the private university or colleges[2]. The majority of medical schools in China, unlike most of those in North American, are not part of a larger university so that the libraries are somewhat analogous to a faculty. The Japanese medical school libraries (MSL) belong to the administrative offices of their schools, on the other hand, Chinese MSL belong to their faculties, and have a librarian with faculty status.

Key Medical Libraries

In China and Japan, the formal medical information servicing facility are the medical libraries of the university or colleges. There are hundred libraries specializing in medical sciences which are located around the both countries. However, only some of the libraries have relatively large expenditures to deal with ever increasing expenses in Japan and, only one library, Peking Union Medical College, has relative large expenditures to deal with ever increasing expenses in China. Table 1 indicates the statistical information of the key MSL in both respective countries.

Table 1:

Statistical information of Key MSL in China and Japan

Medical School Libraries	Personnel	Expenditure	Study Seats	Square Meters	Number of Volume
Peking Union Med. College	66	3,700,000	150	3,600	410,000
Beijing Med. University	62	861,000	1564	10,200	404,541
Sun Yat-sen Univ. of Med. Sci.	56	768,000	496	7,348	544,422
West China Univ. of Med. Sci.	74	940,000	1100	8,840	545,104
Tongji Medical University	73	870,000	417	6,458	448,648
China Medical University	52	535,000	800	3,300	460,000
N. Bethune Univ. of Med. Sci.	64	587,000	570	8,400	450,000
Xian Medical University	42	360,000*	500	5,600	550,000
Sapporo Medical College	18	161,893**	101	1,275	159,535
Jichi Medical School	18	244,028	240	3,828	190,569
University of Tokyo	35	176,722	174	5,226	258,975
Keio University	33	442,505	90	30,695	230,869

Tokyo Medical College	22	231,708	152	1,301	158,620
Jikei Univ. School Medicine	20	147,394	206	2,420	209,479
Kyoto Prefectural Univ. Med.	14	1,185,994	253	2,567	214,731
Osaka Univ. Life Sci. Library	26	422,914	327	6,481	366,903
Kyushu University	21	245,543	251	4,216	280,130
* Chinese ¥ 360,000 yuan ** Japanese ¥ 161,893,000 yen					

Personnel of Medical School Libraries

There are five national ranks for librarians in China: research librarian, assistant research librarian, librarian, assistant librarian and assistant. The first three are equivalent to the academic ranks of professor, assistant professor, and lecturer and, assistant librarians are equivalent to the residents[3]. Table 2 shows the personnel of 90 MSL in China[4].

Table 2:

Statistical Personnel of Ninety MSL in China

Personnel	Male	Female	Total	
	1056	1836	2892	
Professional	top level	middle level	low level	not decide
	176	726	1300	680
Experienced years	under 30	30 - 50	51 - 60	up 61
	910	1431	391	27
Special fields	medical	information	languages	others
	535	889	183	1202

There are three types of staff in MSL in Japan: curator and vice curator, professional (670 full-time, 7 concurrent, 69 temporary) and others. Table 3 shows the personnel of 105 MSL in Japan.

Table 3:

Full - Time Staff Experiences

	Professional				Non-Professional			
	1 year under	5 years under	10 years under	10 years or more	1 year under	5 years under	10 years under	10 years or more
Total number	34	136	117	485	156	251	81	111
of libraries	105	105	105	105	105	105	105	105
average	0.4	1.3	1.1	4.6	1.5	2.4	0.8	1.1

All key personnel in MSL management play an important role in the library developments and in keeping good services with the information technologies.

Medical School Library Services

The function of MSL are to serve the teaching and research needs of both staff and students in China and Japan. Although traditional ways of running library services are still as much in China, the services provided in both respective countries are: answering reference queries; preparing subject bibliographies; preparing index for medical journals; providing photocopies; teaching users on the use of the library's resources; current awareness services; selective dissemination of information; online search services; CD-ROM service and interlibrary loans.

The Medical Library Associations play a very important part in the MSL services in the both respective countries. The Japan Medical Library Association was founded in 1927 and engaged in the coordination and organization of exchange and supply of materials, interlibrary loans and photocopying and, promotion of mutually advantageous relation with other related organizations[5]. With leadership and funding the Ministry of Education and Culture, the Osaka University Nakanoshima Branch Library was developed as a national biomedical center library in order to satisfy interlibrary loan requests in 1977 and the two sub-centres were established in the medical libraries of the Tohoku University and Kyushu University[6]. The Association of Libraries of Chinese Medical and Medicinal Colleges and Universities was set up in 1985, which marked the formal establishing of the MSL network and had taken a decisive step to turn the loose coordination among libraries into a formal close well organised common body of libraries[7]. The MSL in Beijing, Shanghai, Shenyang, Xian, Wuhan and Guangzhou had set up CD-ROM medline computerized retrieval system and. some had link to the National Library of Medicine in U.S.

Evaluations and Conclusion

Based on the information that has been collected. MSL in both respective countries revealed some differences: A major difference was clearly demonstrated by the fact that a major function of the reference services was to produce and edit abstracts and index the medical literature. Network were to be carried out in both countries, however, there was tend to be weak on interlibrary loans and photocopy services due to the slow communication systems in China. CD-ROM service was not largely used for improving information dissemination as compared to Japan. Although online information retrieval service is available to some MSL in China, there were found that it impossible to subscribe to large numbers of journals because of the critical shortage of the budgets. It was concluded that resource sharing in Japan were generally well-employed as compared to China. The common problem encountered was to strengthen the information and education link between users and the information resources.

References

1. The annual public health of China. People Health Publishing House. Beijing, 1993.
2. 63rd annual statistics the Japan medical Association, JMLA. Tokyo. 1992.
3. Crawford DS & Xiong DZ, Report of a cooperative venture between the China Medical University Library and the Medical Library of McGill University. Bull Med Libr Asso. 76(1), 64-72.
4. Huang SQ & Wang FS. Investigation of information services of libraries in medical schools. Medical information Services. 1991 (6) 12-19.
5. Suga T & Urata. Medical library cooperation: asian countries and the Japan Medical Library Association. J Interlibrary Loan & Info Supply. 1993. 3(4) 25-30.
6. Yamada S & Yamazaki S. A recent trend of interlibrary loan activities in the member libraries of Japan Medical Library Association. Procs of the 5th ICML. Tokyo, JMLA, 1985, 808-12.
7. Zheng XQ. The network development and resource sharing of medical libraries in China. Medical libraries: keys to information: Procs of the 6th ICML, Delhi. Medical Library Association in India. Regd 1990. 487-490.

THE IMPLEMENTATION AND DEVELOPMENT OF PHARMACY INFORMATION NETWORK

Linda Lisgarten & Lesley Downs [For correspondance] School of Phamacy, Univ. of London, 29-39 Brunswick Square, London WC1N 1AX, UK

Pharmacy information provision in the UK is currently supplied to a variety of sectors through a wide number of disparate groups. By creating a dialogue between those engaged in this area at a variety of levels the authors believe that the potential benefits to pharmacy information specialists and their client-base will be considerable. At the current time there is no existing body which fulfils the needs of librarians interested in pharmacy information. Consequently the Pharmacy Information LibrarianS (PILS) network has been introduced and developed under the leadership of 2 major pharmacy libraries within the UK (the Royal Pharmaceutical Society of Great Britain, and the School of Pharmacy, University of London). The group has taken the form of an informal network and is initially aimed at those pharmacy librarians working within the university sector. Emphasis has been placed on attaining a better knowledge of the material, personal expertise, needs and requirements of the disparate institutions involved in an attempt to create direct and easy access to the various collections. Membership to the Group will ensure a better awareness of those specialists working within the area, with emphasis placed upon ensuring that entry to the network at any point will result in the most applicable and relevant information source being provided by those best equipped to deal with the enquiry.

The group's first meeting was held at the Royal Pharmaceutical Society of Great Britain's London headquarters on 5th May 1994. Many of the initiatives suggested will be developed to help provide a more fully comprehensive service at this level with the intention of extending the Group's membership to include those working in hospital and industrial information centres. Further plans include specialist training days and seminars designed to cover a wide variety of the different aspects of pharmacy information retrieval. Owing to the success of this first meeting the group will be looking to extend its membership and to form more distinct links with such bodies as the Association of Information Officers in the Pharmaceutical Industry (AIOPI) and the various hospital pharmacy drug information groups based throughout the UK.

Although the network was initially developed with the UK pharmacy subject specialist in mind, its activities and in particular its training courses will be designed to be of wider interest to those working within related fields of information provision. It is also hoped that it will be possible to extend the network further on an informal basis to encourage a more European input based on an assessment of the network's success in the UK.

SHARING RESOURCES - CIRCUIT LIBRARIANSHIP

Hanne Christensen & Lise N. Christensen [For correspondance] Medical library, Aalborg Hospital, DK 9000 Aalborg, Denmark

Many libraries now experience severe cut-backs in their budgets. The skyrocketing prices of books and especially medical journals have further aggravated the situation. As librarians we know the importance of access to the medical literature for the quality of health care, education, and research. It becomes essential to find ways of exploiting and sharing resources. In the United States a "Circuit Librarian Program" was first established in Cleveland, Ohio 1973. The idea was for smaller hospitals and institutions in a certain area to share expenses. The circuit librarian had a base in the resource library and would visit the institutions on a regular basis providing database searches, document delivery, and other library services.

In Denmark **Viborg** County offers similar services. The medical library at Viborg Hospital (a 400 bed hospital) has a travelling librarian who visits 4 smaller hospitals in the region. In the Northern part of Jutland the hospital library in **Aalborg** extends its services to all physicians (including general practitioners and specialists) in the county. Hopefully this poster can inspire librarians to set up programs that enable them to extend services and make the most out of their resources.

A MEDICAL LIBRARY AND ITS NEW USERS: A 3-Year Experience with the Nursing Staff

Rosamaria Rotolo & Aris Zonta, Biblioteca del Dipartimento di Chirurgia, c/o Patologia Chirurgica 1, Policlinico San Matteo, 27100 Pavia, Italia.

Summary

From January 1991 through December 1993, the University library of the Department of Surgery of Pavia, which is mainly dedicated to oncology literature, has also been used by an increasing number of employed nurses and student nurses of the Hospital Nursing School. The first group had specific interests in advancing methods for post-operative care of surgical patients. The others asked for literature concerning medical and surgical treatment of diseases and basic nursing techniques. The Authors highlight the importance of access to up-to-date information for employed and student nurses. Their experience confirms that nursing staff needs to get technical knowledge from libraries, and that, at present, most of Italian University libraries are not prepared to provide such information for nurses and to solve their specific needs.

Introduction

In this work the Authors review the problems which arose due to the nurses' requests in a Medical University library which is primarily attended by physicians and medical students. They describe the solutions offered and discuss the advantages and limits of the service provided.

Results

From January 1991 through December 1993, we received a total of 35 requests, 10 (30%) from employed nurses and 25 (70%) from student nurses. We observed a trend of increasing requests during the 3-year of the study period (Tab. 1). The majority of the requests from student nurses occurred during the training period in surgical wards or in specific months (January-May) corresponding to the time of school examinations. We have been able to satisfy requests in all cases, most of the time with our in-house material, in the remaining cases providing information or referring the users to other libraries. Fig. 1 shows that 85% of the requests were covered using the listed sources while in the remaining 15% additional sources were needed. Most of the users (85%) were not familiar with the use of bibliographical instruments and computers and they needed help to retrieve information. Nurses preferred textbooks and journals written in Italian because of the limited comprehension of foreign languages. For the same reason a very few users asked directly for MEDLINE searches on CD-ROM and other repertories available. Unfortunately, it was difficult to get documents from elsewhere because nursing libraries are not numerous in Italy and because in most medical libraries there is a lack of literature devoted to nursing. Furthermore, our users required quick, essential information and swift delivery of documents. For these reasons we chose to acquire such literature with a preference for texts written in Italian (Fig. 2) and also suggested searching for these texts (Fig. 3) in the Nursing School's library and to their teachers.

Discussion

This work highlights the importance of up-to-date information for employed nurses and student nurses. Our experience confirms that there is an increasing use of the medical library from nursing staff and student nurses. They ask for information related to medical basic and clinical science and to specific instruments and equipment. Unfortunately, there is a lack of nursing libraries in Italy. Furthermore, most of Italian medical libraries are not equipped for nurses' specific needs since they are usually attended by researchers, physicians and medical students.

We have been able to satisfy the requests for the following reasons:

- The wide and updated collection of scientific journals and books already present in our medical library.
- The acquisition of specific literature dedicated to nursing during the 3-year period of the study.
- The possibility to have access to computerized systems for bibliographic search.

The role of the librarian to retrieve information has been essential because he provided:

- suggestions for the specific bibliographical sources;
- assistance for the use of computerized systems;
- contacts and exchange of documents with other libraries.

Nurses appreciated the availability of literature offered by our library also because it was found concise, easy to read and significant for their educational and professional development.
For the future, we expect improvements in our service because of a better cooperation with other Italian medical libraries for a literature exchange and because of a higher level of autonomy reached by the users within the service provided.

Fig. 1. Sources of information available in the library

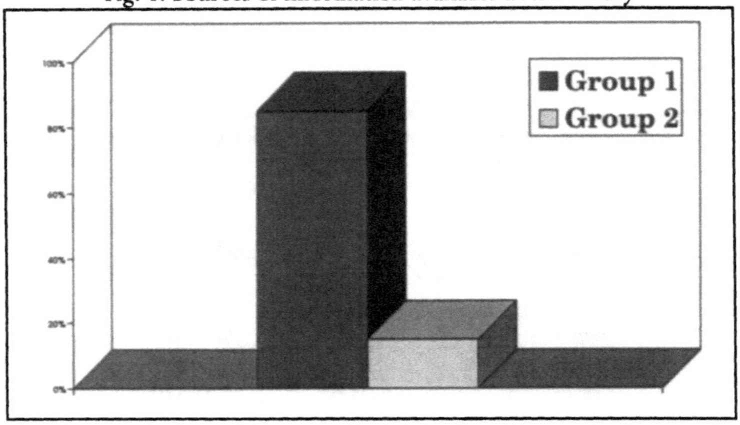

Group 1 (85%)

- Textbooks for physicians and medical students
- Textbooks for nurses
- Other publications related to nursing
  (Proceedings of congresses, meetings and education courses; guidelines from Hospital Management Office and National Department of Health)
- Medical journals and bulletins in Italian

Group 2 (15%)

- MEDLINE on CD-ROM
- Medical journals in foreign languages
  (French, English)
- Others
  (Medical dictionaries, Excerpta Medica...)

Fig. 2. Acquisition of literature devoted to nursing

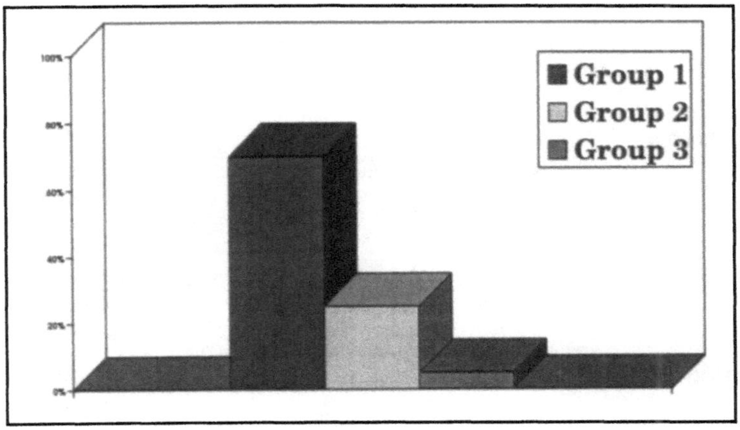

Group 1 (70%)	Exchange of duplicate issues or gifts
Group 2 (25%)	Purchase of books for nurses written in Italian
Group 3 (5%)	Document delivery from other libraries

Fig. 3. Other sources of information for nurses

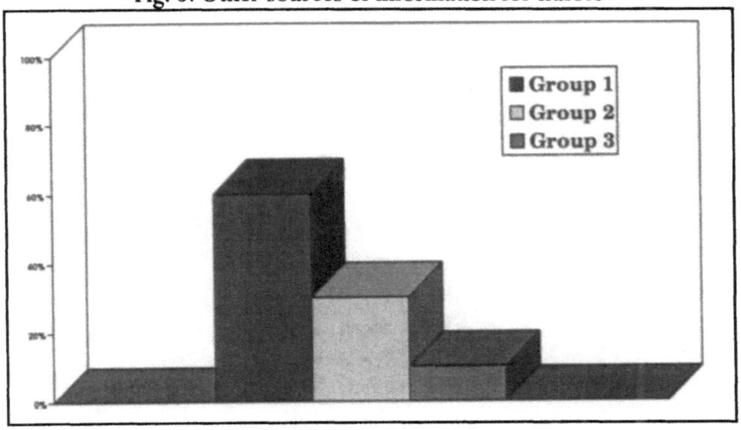

Group 1 (60%)	The Nursing School's library
Group 2 (30%)	Teachers at the Nursing School
Group 3 (10%)	Other medical libraries

	1991	1992	1993
Employed nurses	2	4	4
Student nurses	5	8	12
Total	***7***	***12***	***16***

Tab. 1. Distribution of nurses' requests

Acknowledgements

The Authors thank Dr. Rubina Ruggiero and Dr. Carletto Genovese for their technical assistance, and Dr. Mario Alessiani and Dr. Hugo MacManus for their suggestions and comments.

References

1. BRANDON AN, HILL DR. Selected list of books and journals for the small medical library. Bull Med Libr Assoc 1991 Apr;79(2):195-222
2. BUNJAN LE, LUTZ EM. Marketing the hospital library to nurses. Bull Med Libr Assoc 1991 Apr;79(2):223-5
3. CARPENTER KH. Evaluating library resources for accreditation: results of a study. Bull Med Libr Assoc 1992 Apr;80(2):131-9
4. COGNETTI G. Scuola di biblioteca per infermieri: due passi avanti e uno indietro. Bibliotime 1991;Suppl. 2:21-4
5. CURTIS KL, WELLER AC, HURD JM. Information-seeking behavior: a survey of health sciences faculty use of indexes and databases. Bull Med Libr Assoc 1993 Oct;81(4):383-92
6. FISHER WW, REEL LB. Total quality management (TQM) in a hospital library: identifying service benchmarks. Bull Libr Med Assoc 1992 Oct;80(4):347-52
7. HOLST R. Hospital libraries in perspective. Bull Med Libr Assoc 1991 Jan;79(1):1-9
8. LOVAS I, GRAHAM E, FLACK V. Health professionals' use of documents obtained through the Regional Medical Library Network. Bull Med Libr Assoc 1991 Jan;79(1):28-35
9. OKUMA E. Selecting CD-ROM databases for nursing students: a comparison of MEDLINE and the Cumulative Index to Nursing and Allied Health Literature (CINAHL). Bull Med Libr Assoc 1994 Jan;82(1):25-9
10. OLSON K. Strengthening the link between research and practice. Can Nurse 1992 Jan;88(1):42-4
11. WATSON MM, PERRIN R. A comparison of CINAHL and MEDLINE CD-ROM in four allied health areas. Bull Med Libr Assoc 1994 Apr;82(2):214-6

GIDIF, RBM 1983-1993: Ten Years of Activities

Gruppo Italiano Documentalisti dell'Industria Farmaceutica e degliIstituti di Ricerca Biomedica Piazza S. Agostino, 24, 20123 Milano, Italia

GIDIF, RBM, the Italian Association of Information Professionals in the Pharmaceutical Industry and Biomedical Research Centers, started up informally in 1983, like a meeting of colleagues. These club-like arrangements went on for three years but in 1985 the leading group realized that a formal association would improve the quality and quantity of meetings. The aims of GIDIF,RBM are to promote and defend the documentalist's professional image; to promote training and continuing education courses for all members; to contribute to the study and development of tools and methods useful in the information professional's work. The decision to group together people from the pharmaceutical industry and biomedical institutes arose from the basic "dualism" of the medical world and reflects the association's aim to combine different experiences and points of view in order to help members solve everyday problems and extend their professional skills. Members of the Association are people working as information professionals in the biomedical field or similar disciplines; in public or private institutes, firms or associations working in the field; in public or private institutes, firms or associations not working in the field but interested in supporting the association's aims and initiatives Ten years of the Association work are summarized.

Members

At present the Association has 156 members from:

- Universities, Hospitals, Research Institutions (43)
- The Pharmaceutical Industry (96)
- Others- freelance, brokers, etc.- (13)
- Associate members (Elsevier Science, RadioSuisse, Swets & Zeitlinger, Derwent Publications, Lange & Springer)

Meetings and Workshops

Since its informal birth in 1983, GIDIF,RBM has organized annual conferences and workshops. The former generally deal with questions of policy and managerial aspects of documentation, the latter with technical points related to updating. These meetings are open to non-members. GIDIF,RBM members are often invited to speak to other associations'.Speakers from all over Europe have made valuable contributions to the conferences, attended by approximately 1000 partecipants.

Newsletter

A newsletter "Notizie" is published every three months and mailed to all members. It keeps members informed of what is going on in the information field in Italy and elsewhere. The newsletter includes editorials, reports from national and international congresses, seminars and conferences, surveys on new products, alerting on courses, meetings and new books, recommended reading, and a "forum" on the profession.

Working Groups

The working groups are set up by the members to look closely into topics such as education, new products,techniques and tools, which could be of interest for the profession.The findings of three such groups have been published in Italian and international journals. The fourth working group is presenting its preliminary results as a poster at this meeting.These working groups have tackled several specific themes:

Adonis: A Feasibility Study

After a workshop on Adonis in Milan in May 1990, a working group was set up to assess whether a subscription to Adonis would be of advantage to small to medium sized libraries and information centers.Over a period of three months using specific software, 68 libraries were asked to keep a record of the articles retrieved outside. Then the working group examined how many requests could not be met using the GIDF,RBM union catalogue. At that time Adonis covered 441 titles, 339 of them overlapping with the GIDIF,RBM catalogue.However, since the Adonis collection was a life span of only one year, less than 10% of the requests could have been satisfied by a subscription to this product. "ADONIS: Valutazioni preliminari di un nuovo prodotto per il recupero di fonti primarie", Bibliotime 1991; 2, suppl.2: 33-35 . Documentation services and the documentalist's job in Italy in the nineties In 1992 a working group conducted a survey to identify various professional features of the people who work with scientific documentation

in Italy in public and private research institutes and companies. The results highlight the knowledge, innovative and managerial spirit this people put into their job in order to achieve institutional objectives.
The history and structure of documentation centres and libraries were analyzed and their services and products, technologies and resources examined. "Documentando - Profilo dei Professionisti del settore della informazione scientifica in Italia. Risultati di una inchiesta" -Cronache Farmaceutiche 1993;32(5):199-206 -"Documentation Services and the Documentalist's Job in Italy in the Nineties" - Drug Information Journal 1994;28(2).

Quality Assurance in Drug Information Centres

A study was set to define a suitable procedure of quality assurance for documentation centres.The aim was to define quality measurements and develop assessment questionaires.The first step was to identify the products and services offered by individual centres. Objectives for a hypothetical drug information centre were drawn. Essential common quality indicators adequate to the full range of products were identified. Specific quality indicators have also been produced. Overall assessment of the service was not tackled as resources were considered important.The understanding of needs and queries of customers emerged as crucial to the achievement of quality. "Quality Assurance in Drug Information Centres" - Online & CDROM Review, 1993;17(5):279-283. - "Documentando - Qualita' nei Centri di Informazione" - Cronache Farmaceutiche 1994; in press. Potential interactions of of biomedical information centres with marketing agencies and biomedical public media: a search of new customers/suppliers. Poster at this Meetings

Union Catalogue

One of the Association's first initiatives was to create a union catalogue to facilitate the retrieval of journals.A reference committee studied the formal and technical aspects of the catalogue management and prepared a list of rules for cooperation among participants. In 1990 the catalogue was computerized and an electronic edition is now available.The catalogue is updated annually. So far about 35 libraries from companies and institutions have joined the project, and the catalogue collects more than 4,500 titles.

Future Activities and Projects

In the last few months GIDIF,RBM has started cooperating with the leading Italian journal on librarianship "Biblioteche Oggi".Every two months two pages of the journal are devoted to the voice of the Association. A fellowship has been established in cooperation with The British Council in Rome. One member of GIDIF,RBM will have the opportunity of spending two weeks working in the United Kingdom. He/she will spend this period visiting public and private information centers to share experience and gain further knowledge in this field.

MONOTHEMATIC OR TRADITIONAL DATABASES?

Mt. Pesenti & M. Colombi [For correspondance] via Paleocapa 8, 24122 Bergamo Italia

Introduction

To approach the Italian market of neurology, epilepsy in particular, we had to collect published scientific literature on that topic and to make it available in an easily accessible, and economical form for inhouse end users. We therefore built an inhouse database on our new antiepileptic drug and on the main topics of epilepsy. Our aim was to provide support for medical (researchers, monitors, and physicians) and for the marketing users (product managers, trainers, etc.). For the process of evaluation that led to the decision to build this database, reference is made to D.Smith-Cohen's article (Special Libraries, 1993;84:9-17).

Methods

First of all we selected and evaluated the primary sources and the most easily accessible secondary sources. Primary sources were the journals and books already available in our library. As secondary sources we considered the main biomedical databases supplied by DataStar and BRS. We took as an exhaustive source the database EPIL, produced by the National Epilepsy Library of the Epilepsy Foundation of America, one of the most important and bestknown research institutions in the field. We collected information and the thesaurus about this database by getting in touch with the Epilepsy Foundation.

Then, according to our experience we selected the following "unspecialized" medical databases: Medline, Embase, Biosis, International Pharmaceutical Abstracts, whose thesauruses and structures we knew quite well.
Our search strategy considered:

a) all the possible names, trade names and synonyms of our product
b) the main clinical and epidemiological aspects of the disease.

We ran the strategy a) in all the above databases and strategy b) in EPIL and Medline.

Results

Surprisingly enough, the information available in EPIL was fewer and less up-to-date than the "unspecialized" databases. Thus, EPIL could not be contemplated for use as the sole or even the main source of data about epilepsy.
We retrieved some hundreds of records from all the above sources and reindexed them using an in-house established thesaurus. The EPIL thesaurus was very useful in helping us build this inhouse indexing system because it is almost complete but at the same time simple. Finally we organised the material using an information retrieval software (Inmagic).

Conclusions and Comments

The study's most interesting finding came from the evaluation of the secondary sources, particularly the ones which were basically supposed to be specialized and exhaustive. We are sufficiently experienced to know that we have always to consult a number of databases in order to obtain as complete information as possible, but we had hoped that a database prepared by a specialized institution would be reliable and would shorten or at least simplify our work. This was not the case, so the authors' suggestion in case of highly specialized searches is to refer to both specialized and more general databases to ensure reliable results and broad coverage.

STRATEGIC PLANNING FOR A PROFESSIONAL JOURNAL: a Case Study of *Health Libraries Review*

Shane Godbolt & Susan Crawford, British Postgraduate Medical Federation,
33 Millman Street, London WC1N 3EJ , UK

At a recent psychiatric conference, the speaker told a rather bemused audience: "If you trained before the 1960s, your orientation would be heavily psychoanalytic; during the 1970s it would be sociological - community mental health centres and all that. If you trained in the 1980s, it would be psychopharmacological - you would prescribe drugs, and today, if you choose psychiatry, you would be trained in all three directions - and be simply confused".

So it is with information professionals who:

* Are challenged with the pace and scale of change
* Must recognise paradigmatic shifts and keep abreast of issues and trends
* Need to respond appropriately by developing programs and forming alliances
* Must continue professional development over their entire careers

An important means for finding our evolving identity and for keeping up with changes in the technological and socio-economic environment is through scientific and technical journals. But journals, as their readers, need also to evolve and to change with time. This paper addresses the evolution and the strategic plan of a health information journal, the *Health Libraries Review*. HLR began as a short newsletter for the Health, Welfare and Medical Group of the British Library Association. By 1984 it was evident that the health library sector needed a professional journal for more lengthy contributions reflecting the spectrum of activity and research of in health care librarianship. In consequence, HLR was established and has since grown into an internationally recognised journals. With increasing readership and importance of the European ideal, we felt that active involvement of colleagues across the continent would give the Review a more broadly based dimension and focus. We began a strategic plan for broadening the scope of HLR which articulates a vision; identifies and sets goals; defines a reader base; develops an action plan; and implements the programme.

The Strategic Planning Process

Vision and Goals: The vision is to support health care and its delivery through improved communication and co-operation among health information professionals. Selected goals are:

* Respond to interests and needs of the readership
* Keep in touch with the readership
* Support at practitioner level by sharing and reporting best practice
* Support at research level by reporting innovation and change
* Draw on experience across national boundaries
* Consider issues concerned with the identity of the journal
  - Editorial Board Structure
  - Expansion of scope
  - Title
* Redefine objectives to meet existing and identified new needs of the readership
* Seek comparative studies to share experience and good practice across boundaries

Environmental Analysis: Where are we? What are our strengths and weaknesses? The objectives are:

* Identify strengths and weaknesses of the journal relative to its statement of aims
* Look at environmental trends to determine whether objectives need to be modified

* Assess opportunities presented
* Assess impediments posed

Participatory Planning: Who are the key players in the appropriate sectors? How can we ensure interactive participation in the planning process?

* Across sectoral boundaries
* Across national boundaries
* Investing in strategic alliances between sectors:
  - Education
  - Industry (particularly pharmaceutical)
  - Government (national and local)
  - Voluntary

Action Plans and Implementation

* Plan that future issues include a series of articles on themes of current interest
* Always seek to develop European perspectives
* Provide up-to-date coverage on information technology applications
* Organise and synthesise information to make it meaningful to the readership
* Ensure financial and human resources to accomplish objectives
* Monitor and evaluate achievement of objectives regularly

The plan is to make the ***Health Libraries Review*** relevant and attractive. It must stimulate new approaches, share experience across national boundaries and be a journal that must be read to enhance professional development.

LOGOS: Literature on Gastroenterology on Diskette Supply

Manuela Colombi, Documentation Service Manager, Schering -Plough S.p.A., Via Ripamonti, 89- 20141 Milano, Italia

Summary

One of the main tasks a pharmaceutical company has to accomplish, is to encourage the cultural updating of the medical doctors who are addressed for advertising. Our first interest was towards Gastroenterologists, working in medium-sized hospitals, who rarely have the possibility to widely consult world literature on topics related to their specialization. Urged by the marketing department to study a new way to approach the distribution of information to doctors, we combined the scientific data from Current Contents, by The Institute for Scientific Information Inc. and the flexibility of Headfast, by the Head International Software Ltd., to realize **LOGOS** (Literature On Gastroenterology On Diskette Supply). Copyrights have been asked and granted from both Companies. Details of the selection operated on Current Contents and of the characteristics of the software choosen will be given. **LOGOS** itself will be described in order to point out its peculiarities and the advantages over Current Contents as far as the selected end-users are concerned.

Introduction

Since many years Schering-Plough considers medical information one of the strengths of a pharmaceutical company. Therefore a dedicated library and a documentation service have been available since the Seventies for internal staff. Starting in the late Eighties with the spread of online databases, the service opened its doors to the field force and to the medical doctors and pharmacists they visited. At the early beginning all information was distributed on demand as photocopy or printed matter and a real activity of updating was not feasible. With the strong wish to start a pro-active service to involve a certain number of gastroenterologists in an initiative of professional update, we have been engage in finding the topics and the best technology to achieve the goal. It was January 1993.

The Topics

We evaluated all the in-house available texts, serials and databases, online and offline, to find the most complete and up-to-date scientific literature. *Current Contents* by The Institute for Scientific Information (ISI) Inc. Philadelphia was identified as one of the best-known and up-to-date secondary sources, available in house on diskette with abstract in the two editions Life Science and Clinical Medicine. Out of the more than 1500 journals considered we prepared a selection of 25 titles covering the main aspects of Gastroenterology (see table 1). Table 1

LOGOS

Literature on Gastroenterology on Diskette Supply
List of Selected Journals

Acta gastro-enterologica belgica
Alimentary pharmacology and therapeutics
American Journal of clinical nutrition
American journal of gastroenterology
Digestion
Digestive diseases
Digestive diseases and sciences
Endoscopy
European journal of gastroenterology and hepatology
Gastroenterologie clinique et biologique
Gastroenterology
Gastroenterology clinics of North America
Gastrointestinal endoscopy
Gut
Hepato-gastroenterology
Journal of clinical gastroenterology
Journal of gastroenterology and hepatology
Journal of hepatology
Journal of parenteral and enteral nutrition
Journal of pediatric gastroenterology and nutrition
Liver
Pancreas
Revista espanola de enfermedades digestivas
Scandinavian journal of gastroenterology
Zeitschrift fuer Gastroenterologie

The Technology

Electronic is nowadays heavily adopted and is well integrated in each reality. Consequently we decided to use these means to approach the problem. The amount of data to be distributed was high (about 700,000 byte or more per issue and 8 issues per year) and a software was necessary to group the information and make it easily retrivable. HEADFAST, from Head Software International, was choosen. Its strenghs are:

- its peculiar characteristics of information retrieval system
- ease of use, speed and flexibility
- it could be personalized
- search screens could be translated into Italian
- the availability of a separated search and update module for end-users
- the acceptable price
- the possibility to use it in the future for optical archives

The Application

The application was designed in cooperation with Winch (a Milan based consultancy and dealer of the software), translating the search screens into Italian, selecting relevant information for the database and preparing output formats for display, printer and file. A brief manual in Italian was prepared to help in the installation of the program, in the upload of the data and in the use of the two search modules

Quick Search (one field at a time)

Form Search (field combination)

The results are shown in the following 'screens'

Copyrights

The software was bought in the correct amount of copies. The Institute for Scientific Information (ISI) Inc., Philadelphia Pennsylvania USA was asked for permission of downloading and re-distributing their data and the permission was granted.

Conclusions

On March 12, 1993 the training to the Product Specialists of the field force took place. Even those who were not confident with computers accepted the initiative. We assured them a continuous support on the phone for solving all possible problems which could arise during the installation and running of the program. As a matter of fact we did not receive more than 15-20 requests of help, and the Gastroenterologists accepted **LOGOS** very well, as they had finally a huge amount of classified information on their specific subjects of interest. The initiative is still running, other specialisations have been approached and we now distribute data to more than 1,000 doctors and are planning to convert our magnetic files into optical files with the introduction of CD-roms.

PARTICIPATION OF THE MEDICAL FACULTY LIBRARY IN GRADUATE AND POSTGRADUATE MEDICAL EDUCATION

Milan R. Spála and Frantisek Choc [For correspondance] Institute for Scientific Information, First medical faculty, Charles University, Salmovská 3, CZ-12108, Praha 2, Czech Republic

Abstract

A comparison of two studies (1986/1987 and 1992/93) shows that the change of political and social atmosphere itself stimulated the students (e.g. knowledge of English raised from 48 to 78 %). Librarian and information literacy requires a continuous comprehensive training before graduation (92 resp. 89%). That is why the Medical Faculty Library (a section of ISI) participates in pregraduate (M.D.) and postgraduate (Ph.D.) programmes since 1992 (Medical informatics, Social medicine, Introduction to biomedical research).

Introduction

It is generally supposed that in the course of university studies students will get acquainted with basic methods of searching and retrieving scientific information, during the studies for seminars, problem-oriented education and examinations, and at the end for their theses. In the Czech Republic (and similarly in former Czechoslovakia) medical students/doctors, however, who do not have to submit a thesis to get the degree, have insufficient theoretical as well as practical experience how to utilize libraries and information services. After World War II, this librarian and information literacy had not received a due attention, neither in high-school nor in postgraduate studies. In the period 1948-1989 the totalitarian system contributed to this situation by its endeavour to restrict access to scientific information, especially to non-soviet/non-russian sources. This situation, in addition to restricted travels abroad , led to a general decline of foreign language studies which - besides the ideologic and economic restrictions - resulted in creation of language barriers for utilization of scientific information.

However, for responsible academic teachers or librarians it is necessary, if not interesting at least, to know the students'/information users' capability of searching and utilizing medical literature. That's why we decided to compare two studies [1,2] from the time before the 1989 "velvet revolution" with results from the years 1992/93 when an influence of free contact with other countries, including the influence of market-economy, can be expected.

Material and Methods

In the first study [2] from 1986/87 a questionnaire containing 14 questions with 27 items was presented to 164 medical students (67% of the total) in the fourth pre-clinical year. The present results (1992/93) were obtained by a similar method: 12 questions with 23 items, 220 students (61%). Since 1991, the Institute of Medical Information (ISI) has been participating in pregraduate teaching (M.D.) in the subject "Medical informatics" and "Social medicine" at the First Medical Faculty and since 1992 also in postgraduate (Ph.D.) "Interdisciplinary biomedical studies" at the Charles University in Prague. The teaching team consists of four M.L.S.'s and one M.D.,Ph.D.

Results and Discussion

Table 1. Survey of answers to selected questions

Questions/Answers (yes)	1986/7 (n=164)[1]	1992/3 (n=134)[1]
1. Do you prepare for exams from obligatory or recommended literature only?	34%	25%
2. Which libraries do you use?		
Med. Fac. Central Library	34%	40%
National Med. Library	17%	9%
National Library	18%	12%
Academic Library	9%	4%

Other Libraries[4]	12%	25%[4]
None	13%	10%
3. Do you know any medical journal?	66%[2]	73%[2]
Cas.Lék.Ces.(J.Czech Physicians)	35%	40%
Prakt.Lék. (The Practitioner)	13%	12%
Vesmír (similar to "Nature")	7%	5%
Other Czech journals	27%	15%
Foreign journals	18%	28%
4. Can you speak any foreign language?	55%[2]	72%[2]
English	48%	87%
Russian	28%	4%
German	16%	4%
French	8%	3%
Other	-[3]	1%
None	-[3]	1%
5. Do you work as volunteer at any department or clinic?	43%	11%
6. Have you ever delivered a paper at the student scientific conference?	21%	4%
7. Do you know the correct meaning of the term:		
a - informatics	66%	50%
b - search	21%	25%
c - abstract journal	9%	5%
d - data base	-[3]	40%
8. Would it be useful to obtain comprehensive training in this field before	92%	9%

Notes: [1] - number of respondents (100%), [2] - represents 100% for further calculations, [3] - this question was not included in the questionnaire, [4] - since 1990 mainly the library of the Czech Medical Students Association supported by foreign sponsors.

The results (see *Table 1,* questions No. **1** - **8**) show an increased number of students who make use of other literature for their study, too, not only of the obligatory and recommended titles (**1**). This was obviously enabled by the services of the renewed library of the Czech Medical Students Association (**2**). The students also use foreign journals in greater measure than before (**3**) which is undoubtedly enabled by a better knowledge of foreign languages, especially English (87%) (**4**). Then we can suppose that *the change of political and social atmosphere itself stimulated the medical students in their study.* Recent comparative studies (1991) of knowledge of German and English with adults and high schools students (2,790 resp. 2,300 persons) made by the Faculty of Social Sciences of the Charles University showed that the students with whom English prevails have better knowledge of both languages [3]. On the other hand, the financial restriction of faculty budget for research, as *a result of general restructuralization of national economy and still evolving schemes of research funding,* have reduced the number of students interested in research (**5**) as well as their publication activity (**6**). The librarian and information literacy (**7**) is the same, i.e. equally insufficient, and the students themselves feel they should complete their practical skills in this field (**8**). After two years of the graduate programmes iniciated by ISI ("Bibliographical and literature search systems" in "Medical informatics" and "Fundamentals of scientific communication in medical sciences: lecture, poster, article" in "Social medicine") the number of students in noncompulsory lectures and seminars increased by three fourths. In the postgraduate programme (Medicine, Biology, Bioengineering) the ISI ensures the above mentioned themes directly with individual fellows for their concrete theses as well as in the programme "Introduction to biomedical research". For this purpose the bibliography of recent titles covering nine chapters was compiled (see *Table 2*). After first year of this programme the number of base users (MEDLINE and SCISEARCH) in postgraduate study doubled. Such engagement of libraries in graduate and/or postgraduate medical education is usual in other countries now [4].

Table 2. "Introduction to Biomedical Research" - A bibliography

Chapters
1. Introduction to Biomedical Research
2. Introduction to Clinical Research and Clinical Trials
3. Philosophy of Science
4. Science Education and Teaching
5. Scientific Literacy
6. Ethics and Rights in Biomedical Research
7. Science Funding
8. Communication of Scientific Information
9. Animals in Biomedical Research

References

[1] Brdicková E., Spála M.: Investigation of librarian and information literacy of medical students during their studies of pathophysiology *(In Czech)*. Cs. Fysiol., 37 (4) :435, 1988.

[2] Brdicková E., Spála M.: Are medical students prepared to use libraries and information centres? In: Days of Scientific Information in Medicine. Vrábelová R. *(ed)*, Bratislava, 1988, pp. 141-142.

[3] Prucha J.: Study of foreign languages at the schools in the Czech Republic *(In Czech)*. Aula, (3) : 15-23, 1991.

[4] Fourth European Conference of Medical and Health Libraries (EAHIL) - Abstracts. Oslo, 1994, p.17: Brazier H. - *Ireland*; p.17: Barker J.M. - *Wales*; p.18: Rabow I., Akerblom H. - *Sweden*; p.25: Bawden D. - *England*; p.40: Atton C. - *Scotland*; p.42: Petrak J. - *Croatia*; p.43: Fridén K., Oker-Blom T. - *Sweden*; p.58: Iivonen R., Suckcharoen S. - *Finland*; p.78: Dracos A., Castriotta M. - *Italy*; p.98: Spála M.R., Choc F. - *Czechia*. (For full texts of these papers see these proceedings.)

INFORMATION SYSTEMS FOR NURSING SPECIALITIES

David Bawden & Kay Robinson, Department of Information Science' City University, London EC1V 0HB

Summary
A study of the information needs and information seeking behaviour of midwives is reported, based on interviewing of practitioners and information providers.

Acknowledgements
We are grateful to the British Library, Research and Development Department for providing financial support for this project. All opinions expressed are those of the authors, and do not necessarily represent the views of the sponsors. We are also grateful to those healthcare workers and information providers who have taken the time to help us in this research.

Aims
The aim of this project was to investigate the information needs and information seeking behaviour of healthcare workers in specialist branches of nursing, and In particular, to compare them with general nurses, whose information needs have already been the subject of British Library sponsored research. The study focused on two groups: midwives and psychiatric nurses. Some preliminary results for midwives are outlined here.

Methods
This study was based on semi-structured interviewing of

- practitioners
- librarians
- database producers
- professional associations

together with examination of systems and sources. This qualitative approach allows for a full appreciation of the place of information access and use within professional practice. The study examined all aspects of library and information services, and also more general computer-use, within the context of the emerging discipline of nursing informatics. The study was carried out among practitioners (midwives, psychiatric nurses, managers, tutors, and computer project staff) working in the National Health Service, in a variety of locations, in London and South-East England, among local librarians in this geographical area, and other information providers nationally. The in-depth interview / examination of sources and systems approach has allowed detailed contextual information to be gathered.

Some Preliminary Findings
A wide range of sources are available and used, both general and specialised, printed and computerised. Knowledge and use of sources is variable, and dependent more on individual situation and inclination, than on location, grade or job. Usage is determined more by convenience and simplicity than by perceived quality or utility. Computer-awareness is similarly very varied, and seems linked to more general information awareness. The role of the local librarian in supplying information should be crucial, but is in fact carried out with variable effectiveness. Midwife tutors, in particular, seem to play an important " gatekeeper" role. Reorganisation within the British National Health Service is having a significant impact on information provision, as is the move towards a more community-based role. Reorganisation of the educational structure, with nurses and midwives receiving formal training in higher education institutions rather than hospitals, is having a considerable effect on information provision.

Some of the specialised information systems and services available (e.g. MIDIRS, MIRIAD, and Cochrane) are of a high degree of sophistication and quality. They are not widely enough known, nor their particular values appreciated, among the library community as well as among practitioners.

Some Preliminary Conclusions

The nursing specialities represent an interestingly differently group of professionals from general nurses, in information terms. Although "typical practitioners" in their need for convenient and relevant information, they seem more "information conscious" than most practitioner groups. In their adoption of specialised information tools, in addition to general ones, and in their increasing requirement for community-related multidisciplinary information, they are taking a leading role in information service development, which will be followed by other professional groups. Recommendations for information service improvement will relate, *inter alia*, to publicity and promotion of library services, links between "traditional" library/ information services and health informatics, and networking.

Full Results

The results of the study will be reported in full as a British Library Research Report. They will be available towards the end of 1994.

WIDE USE OF MEDLINE ON CD-ROM BY STAFF MEMBERS AT THE FACULTY OF MEDICINE LIBRARY OF THE UNIVERSITY OF LIEGE, BELGIUM

Françoise Noel-Lambot, Bibliothèque de la Faculté de Médecine - Université de Liège, Centre Hospitalier Universitaire du Sart Tilman - Bât B35 - B4000 Liège, Belgique

Abstract

Taking advantage of a particular context (large availability of networked CD-ROM stations, existence of regular training sessions), the entire staff of the library of the Faculty of Medicine of Liege (mainly composed of individuals without professional background in library science) has been trained to use some data bases on CD-ROM. Results are clearly positive : these powerful reference tools can be used for various library activities with the consequences of improved services and augmented job satisfaction.

1. Special Context At the Library

1a. Staff requiring particularly library training: In our library, as in many academic libraries throughout Belgium, the staff is largely composed of individuals who do not possess a vocational or professional background in library sciences. When the library of the Faculty of Medicine was created in 1987, staff members were mainly recruited inside the university from laboratories and secretariats. The actual staff is made up of 3 "reconverted" scientists, 2 librarians, 8 "reconverted" technicians or secretaries. The importance of the library can be precised by the following figures : 1000 current subscriptions, 40000 monographs, 4000 users, 2000 sq.mt. in self-access. In spite of their status, the responsability of these people to fulfil the sundry traditional library functions as well as the everevolving, electronic medium data demands resides within their daily routine as representatives of the library. The existing gap between employee preparedness and the job at hand is being addressed at the Faculty of Medicine library of Liege through supplementary in-house training provided to each staff member. Such continuing education is assumed on a weekly basis by our professional staff. Each Tuesday, the library is only accessible to the public from 10 h a.m. so the entire staff can participate to these activities.

1b. Existence of an intralibrary network linking the endusers CD-ROM stations and the "administrative" stations. Our LANtastic network links 4 public CD-ROM stations as well as 4 "administrative" stations (used mainly by staff for library management but also available as auxiliary CD-ROM stations). By this way a large access to CD-ROM is offered to all staff members.

2. CD-ROM Training and its Consequences

In this particular context, the challenge to acclimatize the personnel to electronic retrieval systems was greatly assisted. Via our training sessions, the entire staff (12 people) was taught the general principles and practical applications in the use of Medline (first Compact Cambridge, now CD Plus) and other data bases on CD-ROM which are currently available to the reader population accessing our facility (Cambridge Life Sciences Collection, IPA ...).

2a. Staff members can take advantage of their new skills for various activities. First they are able to advise the endusers, most particularly for software features (limits, printing, saving ...) but also for performing simple searches. Moreover they have at their disposal powerful reference tools useful for various library tasks :

- Bibliographic controls in the activities of interlibrary loan (correction of inexact references of journal articles requested in photocopy)
- Various controls related to serials management (publication of volumes, title changes...)
- MeSH indexing guidance in the process of monographs cataloguing : Medline consultation on a specific subject can provide help for this difficult task.
- Use of the data base as a medical dictionary (ex : what is the meaning of an abbreviation such as COPD ?)

2b.Very positive experience Result of our effort to upgrade skills have shown themselves to be clearly positive.

- Nearly all staff members are able to perform simple searches.

- These performing bibliographic tools provide the means to deliver improved services and to enhance the employee's range of daily responsabilities.
- More difficult to measure, yet clearly evident among the members of our staff, is the increased value added to their work and subsequent augmented job satisfaction that is derived from the understanding and competence of CD-ROM data bases.

3. Conclusion

It is well established that CD-ROM constitute an attractive and useful tool for library endusers. We are firmly convinced that they also represent a means by which staff members can upgrade existing skills and also maintain contact with the evolution of their "tools of the trade".

ORGANISATION OF AUTOMATED ARCHIVES FOR HANDLING CURRENT AWARENESS BULLETINS AND BIBLIOGRAPHIC SEARCHES

Nadia Baroni & Alberto Bottacini, GLAXO S.p.A., Via Fleming 4, VERONA - ITALY.

Introduction

The aim of R&D Scientific Services (SSR) at Glaxo Research Italy - one of the main pharmaceutical research centres of the Glaxo Group is to provide appropriate scientific information support to R&D projects and other scientific disciplines. This support is ensured by the periodic publication of the "CURRENT AWARENESS BULLETINS", thus providing regular updates on several topics such as information on competitors , monitoring of published scientific literature and patent alerting. "CHEMICAL NOVELTY and BIOMEDICAL SEARCHES" are also provided to support specific queries from researchers. The functional organisation of the above mentioned SSR activities has made it necessary to place this information on an automated system, so as to have the following available in real time:

a) specific front cover for each type of document produced by SSR;
b) retrieval of previous Current Awareness Bulletins and Searches;
c) statistical analysis of SSR activities.

This gave us the opportunity to create a "CONSULTATION FILE", periodically updated and available to researchers and which contains all the information about services developed by SSR. To achieve this, automated archives have been created by Glaxo Italy, using the RDBMS "ORACLE" on a Digital Vax platform (VMS operating system).

Methods

1 - AUTOMATED ARCHIVE FOR HANDLING BIBLIOGRAPHIC SEARCHES

1.1- handling of salient data specifying details of the bibliographic search/structure, with a printed "COVER" to be attached to the search before it is forwarded to the client.
Front cover example:

FROM **BARONI N**	Planning and Scientific Services	02 May 1994
TO **BRAGA A**	Pharmacology Directorate	

TITLE: **CALCIUM ANTAGONIST PHARMACOLOGY**
Project: CARDIOVASCULAR

Number of references: 50 Search code: 94/B/125
Search carried out of the following data banks: **EMBASE, MEDLINE.**
Please contact me for any further details.

1.2 - handling of the information keyed in by the operator, to produce lists for different **statistical** needs. The information handled by Oracle is as follows:

search code (a single, personalised code for each operator)
applicant(s) & directorate
title of search
research project
number of bibliographic references obtained
number of structures
data banks consulted
confidential or not

Oracle example:

BIBLIOGRAPHIC SEARCHES ARCHIVE

94/B/125	**Date processed**: 02 May 1994
Applicant	BRAGA A
Directorate	PHARMACOLOGY
Title:	CALCIUM ANTAGONIST PHARMACOLOGY
Project:	CARDIOVASCULAR

Number of references: 37 Confidential (N/Y)
Data banks consulted: EMBASE MEDLINE

1.3 - automatic management by the system of the monthly list specifying searches completed, with two possibilities:
- an E-mail through the Glaxo Holdings network (to be sent to any client)
- an on-line FILE which researchers (Glaxo Italy) can consult directly on their PCs.

2 - AUTOMATED ARCHIVE FOR HANDLING CURRENT AWARENESS BULLETINS

2.1 - handling of salient data specifying details of the bulletin, with a printed "COVER" and distribution list to be forwarded to the client.

Front cover example:

PLANNING AND SCIENTIFIC SERVICES
Research and Development Directorate

Current Contents
ANTIBACTERIALS n. 18

Person i/c: BARONI N.

DISTRIBUTION LIST Date 02 May 1994

1 Braga, A.
2 Cracco, M.
3 Rigo, B.
4 Venturini, A.

Please contact the person named above for any comments or suggestions.

2.2 - handling of information to produce lists by different **statistical** procedures.
The following information is handled by Oracle:

BULLETINS:	*code*	ISSUES: *year*
	description of bulletin	*volume*
	person i/c	*date acquired*
	research project	
	frequency	
	type (sdi, current awareness ...)	

READERS:	*copy number (if for consultation or copy for user)*
	client
	order of distribution

Oracle example:

CURRENT AWARENESS BULLETINS ARCHIVE

Title	ANTIBACTERIALS.		
Description	Current contents awareness E-mail distributed. Selection of reference and abstracts on biochemistry and physiology of bacteria. Antibacterial projects.		
Person i/c	BARONI N.	**Area**	R&D
Frequency	weekly	**Category**	Current Contents
Year	1994	**Volume**	18
Date acquired	02 May 1994		

MANAGEMENT OF BULLETIN DISTRIBUTION

Copy number	**User**
1	Braga, A
2	Cracco, M
3	Rigo, B
4	Venturini, A

2.3 -automatic handling by ORACLE of an on-line FILE which researchers (Glaxo Italy) can consult directly on their PCs.

Conclusions

The ORACLE system, already used in the Company for a number of activities, has made it possible to set up automated archives to meet the operational requirements of Scientific Services. The system has also been used to set up FILES, which Glaxo Italy researchers can readily consult by direct access on their PCs. This hardware-software configuration, offers considerable further advantages, including:

- password-controlled access
- automatic back-up to data
- use independent to peripheral hardware
- concomitant accesses.

READER FRIENDLY: Maximising the Availability and Use of Library Stock

Penelope Bonnett, BMA Library, Tavistock Square, London WC1H 9JP

The BMA library (BMAL) is one of the largest medical libraries in the United Kingdom, operating from a single site in central London. It exists to provide library services to its 100,270 personal members and 590 library members. It also serves its own staff at headquarters and in the 16 Local Offices throughout the UK. Our readers are very scattered - 95443 personal members in the United Kingdom and 4827 overseas. Similarly, 550 library members in the UK and 40 overseas. Fast document delivery is one of the services provided by BMAL, currently sending, on average, 280 articles per day. It is therefore essential, given the nature of BMAL and the services provided, to develop strategies for speeding and easing access for those applying directly to the central base, and also to take the library out to members in their own locations. It is also necessary to ensure that the stock is reflecting members' needs. This was done by carrying out a bibliometric study over five months. From this, much valuable information on the use of the collection was obtained and the journal collection was re-shaped to reflect current demands.(1) This paper deals with the subsequent steps taken to maximise use of the collection.

Firstly, it became apparent that the physical arrangement of the journal collection did not match up well to the demands of readers and staff. At that time there were 220 titles held on open access. These were arranged by subject and runs spanned the last 30 years. Our initial reaction was to cut the runs to the last five years, previous studies having shown that a journal is used most heavily in the first five years after publication(2). After analysis of journal usage from our bibliometric study we found, to our surprise, that our journal runs are used heavily for a longer period. We put this down to the fact that BMAL is used as a library of second resort by our member libraries, who have copies of many of the more recent journals, but come to us for the older titles. Therefore our collection remains active for longer than would normally be the case. This being so we decided to keep runs on open access for the last 15 years. This would still enable us to bring a substantial number of heavily used titles up from closed access. Figures from the bibliometric study were used to identify the heavily used titles, and two lists were compiled. One list of all the heavily used closed access titles for possible move, and secondly a list of all titles on open access at that time.

Our next stage was to obtain measurements for all these titles. During the Easter holiday eight students were employed to carry out initial work prior to the move. Each student was armed with a measuring tape and lists of titles and year spans to be measured. This information enabled us to start planning in detail the procedure for the move. Starting with the most heavily used, closed access titles were fitted into the space made available by cutting runs to 15 years, this enabled the transfer of 200 titles to open access. Finally a complete list of all the titles to be on open access was drawn up This was in alphabetical order and the footage to be taken for each title allowing for one year's growth. Next we had to work out a strategy for the move. It was very important that planning was as detailed as possible, as normal library services had to continue throughout the move. Many of the journals on closed access had to be moved to make room for the older journals coming down and of course all titles on open access had to be moved to accommodate the new alphabetical sequence. Many lists were drawn up showing the sequence of moves, as space became available. It was also necessary to establish holding bays to accommodate titles which were waiting to be slotted into their correct place. So the first move to take place was to relocate some material to establish holding bays, one set of holding bays in the Reading Room, and one set in the basement.

The actual move took place during the Summer, and was undertaken by the same eight students. Apart from the initial planning, library staff only had minimal involvement with the actual move. The students worked in pairs, two pairs in the closed access area and two in the open access. Those in the open access area had a complete list of the alphabetical sequence and worked steadily through that bringing titles from either open or closed access as required. Those in the closed access area were given lists each day of the titles to be moved, this was to make room for 15 years coming from open access. Each title moved was given a waybill giving the title, where it had come from and where it had gone to. At the end of each day these were all collected and all the library records were changed. A list was also made each day of titles in the holding bays. This list was displayed at various points in the library. In this way all titles were available for use throughout the whole move. This method worked extremely well, in all approximately 600 of the 3000 titles were relocated and the whole operation was completed in four weeks.

Fig 1: BMA LIBRARY 1990 MOVE - WAYBILL

Details of Journal

Details of relocation
From: To:

The results were evident. Readers visiting the library were able to find the required titles more easily and overall a greater percentage of titles used. 67% were now on open access. There was also considerable benefit for the library assistants involved with the photocopying process. Previously two library assistants had been spending most of the day in the closed access area getting out and photocopying articles. After the move they only needed to spend two to three hours each day below ground!

The second step concerned BMAL's 38,000 book stock which we felt was not being fully utilised. It is important to provide a good level of service to our members wherever they live, and although known items are sent to members and member libraries all over the UK and sometimes books are sent in response to topic requests, for members unable to visit the library, personal "browsing" access is not available. There was a need to circulate the book stock more widely and this could be done through our close links with member libraries throughout the United Kingdom, to ensure that the fullest use possible is made of our book stock.

The BMA's mobile library service was started in August 1992. The new service places "sample" selections on specific, requested, topics on member libraries throughout the United Kingdom. Display panels and a range of supporting hand-outs are sent with the books. During the three months loan the selections are displayed by the member library, and are available for loan to BMA members. Each library can ask for books on three or four topics. This may be to fit in with particular courses, where the books stock is weak, or just special interest of their readers. In two cases libraries preferred to have a selection of recent books covering all topics. In retrospect this has been found to be less successful. To avoid duplicating a library's stock a list of books which have been selected is sent or faxed. Very often one or two titles are changed at the request of the receiving library. The books are then processed, an explanatory notice is put in the front of each book, so that they can be clearly identified. The books and other material are then posted out to the member library.

To ensure that the greatest possible use is made of the collections whilst on loan, notices are sent out in various ways. Notices are prepared by the BMA's News Information Unit. These are distributed to Regional Offices and 300 BMA members who have agreed to post notices on hospital, health centre and postgraduate medical centre notice boards. In addition extra notices are sent with the books which can be posted up around the hospital at the librarian's discretion. The service has been well received. Already 22 libraries have made use of this facility and some are coming back for a second time. Some libraries, who advertised the service throughout the hospital felt that it made medical staff more aware of, not only the library facilities the BMA offers, but also its own library. One library sent a list of the books with a covering letter to all consultants, registrars, senior house officers and house officers, in the subject areas chosen. They found, to their delight, that the entire ophthalmology department arrived on the first day and were delighted with the selection. Other libraries have also said it has brought new members and stimulated greater interest in the library. Many librarians have said it has helped to boost their collection and have found it invaluable for book selection.

IT WORKS ! A NEW HOSPITAL LIBRARY AND ITS SERVICES.

Valentina Comba, Elisabetta Gandini, Laura Rolando. [For correspondance]. USSL 70, Ospedale di Alessandria, Alessandria, Italia.

Summary

The Alessandria General Hospital opened its new library In March 1992: the available periodicals were collected from the wards, an information service based on Medline CD-ROM was offered, a photocoping service and, at least, one librarian were ready for the users. Two years later data about the use of the library and its services can be gathered. The number of users increased, as have Medline searches. The Authors discuss whether the library helped medical doctors write their scientific papers and reports. A short questionnaire was designed to investigate the impact of the new services on their research and clinical problems; one of the goal of the questionnaire was to gather data about all kinds of scientific communication (reports, papers, posters, ecc.) presented or published by the respondents in the past four years.

Introduction

In the 1989 a number of medical doctors and managers of the Alessandria General Hospital established a Library Committee whose aim was to create a library ; two years later a consultant was appointed to draft a project and train the future librarian. The Committee's most difficult task was to find premises for the library since previously two library rooms had been used by administrative staff. Training was quite intensive . The librarian, Mrs. Elisabetta Gandini, learnt to order, check issues and catalogue journals and to search Medline on a Cd-ROM. The heaviest job , before opening the new service, was to carry all the back issues of 500 periodicals from the wards to the library. The opening of the libray was marked by a conference , where the hospital history was explained and the new services illustrated.

Users and Services

Library service use and Medline searches were monitored in the April-December 1992/January-September 1993 periods and compared. Data show an increase of the number of users and searches, both on in-house and external demand. In the period April-December 1992 the highest number of users per month reached 92 , but in the period January-September 1993 the highest number was 182, with an average of 129 users per month. The number of Medline searches for internal users increased from 118 to 352 in the same monitored periods (from an average of 13 searches per month to 39, with a maximum of 61 searches on the September 1993). For the external users the increase was form 16 searches in the first 9 months to 60 in the second period observed. This is considered a good result, as the Hospital is located in a huge building and the library is not so easily accessed from some wards. Moreover, during the Spring 1993 all the journal collections at the Paediatric Hospital (a smaller building 700 m. from the main hospital) were moved to the library ; paediatricians had to come to the library to read their journals. Wards were supplied with a very efficient service of Table of Contents copies . The number of photocopies requested to the library (copies and Medline searches are free for the Hospital medical staff and nursing staff) increased. The library provides 40,000 photocopies a year on average.

Questionnaire

A user opinion survey on the new library services was carried out with a questionnaire. There were 50 respondents, that is 1/7 of hospital medical staff. A future survey of the nurse users will be held in the future, as there are still a very few nurse users and the library still does not offer services suited to their special needs (there are only 7 subscriptions to journals for nurses). The questions are about :

1) when did they visit the library for the first time.
2) What are the main areas in which they consider the services had improved :
    - opening time
    - document delivery
    - journals access and availability
    - Medline searches
    - photocopying services
3) The new services were of use for the patient care/for research and publications
4) How many publications (papers, case reports, short communications, posters) were written in the 1990-1992 period and how many in the 1992-1994 period (with the help of the library services).

The users greatly appreciated the opening hours, the Medline search service, and the availability of journals in the library; the answers to the others questions listed above where also quite positive.

Papers and other publications deserve a special mention. There has been a marked increase in the number of papers published since the opening of the library service. In the years 1990-1991 242 papers, short communications and posters were published in journals and conference proceedings; since the library opening (1992-1993) the number of the published papers increased to 334. We decided ask respondents about the number of papers, posters etc. because the Medline records do not indicate the Hospital scientific production. In fact, many medical doctors partecipated to conferences with short communications or posters, which are not indexed in Medline. Moreover, about half of these papers were written in Italian . As many Italian librarians know, the indexing process of Italian journals in Medline takes about 6-9 months ; for instance, at the beginning of June 1994 there are some Italian articles dated October-November 1993. It was therefore important to compare the data supplied by the users. It is also important to note that in Medline there are about 70 articles from 1990 to 1993 with "Alessandria" in the ADDRESS field.

Conclusions

It works ! The new library services are increasingly successful. The centralization of the journals in the library might dissatisfy those medical staff used to browse issues while on duty . The library does not lend journals, as some hospital libraries in Italy do, and therefore results on centralization were uncertain. Users appreciate the new services and, in the questionnaire, aknowledge thework library staff: this proves that changes have given good results.

Now the new goals are :

* to increase the library staff (one librarian with temporary staff is not enough !)
* to improve the document delivery service
* to establish the library interconnections to the Internet (in Italy : GARR network)
* to merge the journal catalogue into the Italian Union Catalogue of Periodicals.

DOCUMENT DELIVERY IN ITALIAN BIOMEDICAL LIBRARIES

Gabriella Poppi & **Maurella Della Seta**[1] Istituto Superiore di Sanità Biblioteca,
Viale Regina Elena, 299 00161 Roma, Italia

Abstract
This study aims at presenting a short picture of the Italian situation concerning document delivery with particular regard to the utilization of the national resources such as union catalogues, directories and cooperative projects. An outline is given of the different information structures existing in the country which all converge to make document delivery effective.

Introduction
The scope of this survey is to look at the Italian situation regarding document delivery from a specific point of view. This investigation is concentrated on the efforts to create an Italian document delivery service by using the tools produced by single biomedical libraries, coordinated in a collective effort. Libraries have indeed access to a variety of information through traditional reference tools but it is not an easy task to translate the bibliographic information into the factual access to the document of its intellectual contents and this is rather frustrating for the end-user. This paper aims at underlining possibilities and limits of document delivery in Italian biomedical libraries.

Methods, Analysis and Results
Through data emerged from a questionnaire sent to Italian biomedical libraries to produce the first Italian directory or existing informative structures which has been published in 1993 (1), typologies an dimensions of the libraries involved, classification schemes and thesauri adopted, as well as services offered to users, were pointed out. Before examining the problems related to document access, it must be remarked that biomedical libraries, for geographical and historical reasons have not developed all in the same way. An unbalanced growth emerges, due to a lack of a coordinated policy for the integration of different situations. It is interesting to underline that about 50% of the libraries considered are small, holding between 1000 and 5000 monographs and between 100 and 500 periodicals. Aside from their dimensions, 60% of the libraries participates in local or national periodicals union catalogues and uses them as the most common way for localizing a periodical. Another widely diffused practice is the exchange and cooperation with other libraries, as a consequence of the fact that Italian biomedical libraries usually have small dimensions; they normally employ 1-5 persons, not always qualified and this is especially true for University libraries which own very specialized collections (it may happen that a periodical is held by one library in the country). In addition, small libraries usually have limited budgets and availability of financial resources is essential for a fast service and for a real-time information.

How can these small-sized libraries face the problem of document delivery? Mostly through an efficient photocopy service, but it must be remarked that only 177 libraries of the over 300 that answered the questionnaire, offer photocopy services. If we consider the chronic shortage of personnel, efforts undertaken to achieve this goal must be appreciated. However photocopy service should be improved at any rate: the original documents in a biomedical library must not be removed, or at least, should have a limited circulation. Assuming that the document delivery process is made easier and faster by the applications of library automation, it seems suitable to examine achievements, projects and national professional literature in order to evaluate the initiatives in progress in our country on this matter.

It appears that the level of automation is improving. Over 41% of biomedical libraries have computer-based procedures, but only 27% has some online connections to databases, or takes part in a network. Also the use of CD-ROM is increasing: 20% of Italian biomedical libraries interrogates databases on CD-ROM, integrating the online reference service. Noteworthy is the initiative recently promoted by the medical library V. Pinali in Padua. Italian users have access to all library catalogues which have been integrated with periodicals titles of ADONIS CD-ROM. Document delivery service is fulfilled upon payment within 24 hours from the request. Copies of articles are sent by mail or by fax. To be a number of a national or regional network is extremely important for the future of document delivery services and many efforts have been made in Italy to achieve this goal. The network of Italian libraries (SBN), which became operative about two years ago, links at present 150 libraries and the connection of a further 300 is in progress. Among these, about 30 are biomedical libraries, mostly belonging to university departments (2).

The small percentage of scientific and biomedical libraries in the Italian library network is due to a lot of different factors. In this respect we may mention, for example the different classification schemes adopted: SBN uses Decimal Dewey Classification, whereas biomedical libraries usually prefer the NLM classification scheme. The problems derived from the use of different standard services and functions in the single biomedical libraries suggested the opportunity to produce suitable interfaces that could allow the integration of various systems. A further possible step for the harmonization of the existing informative structures is the integration of SBN and GARR through the well known network INTERNET. GARR (Gruppo armonizzazione reti di ricerca) is the Italian academic network which involves the majority of biomedical libraries with great benefit either for the localization of documents, or for their delivery. GARR network makes possible, in fact, the access to the catalogues of the libraries not involved in SBN. Of course, this is not a solution for those informative structures with limited resources which will forcedly remain isolated and excluded from the network. It seems that SBN will be able to offer those libraries access to data through offline supports (magnetic or optical memories).

Access to online catalogues, offered by SBN, which has historical merit but collects only a minimal part of biomedical libraries, does not represent the only way to support document delivery in Italy. One of the oldest and most interesting realizations is ACNP (Archivio Collettivo Nazionale dei Periodici) (3), a serials online database produced by Istituto di Studi Sulla Ricerca e Documentazione scientifica (ISRDS) of the National Research Council (CNR) on three different supports: this is the first important Italian project of union catalogue in the serials field, and it has been published in its last printed version in 1990, on CD-ROM and at present also on diskette. The catalogue is also available online and it may be searched at CNUCE Centre (Pisa) and at Bologna University through ALMATEL network (both poles accessible via INTERNET). ACNP represents a daily working tool for Italian librarians because of its remarkable dimensions (it incudes 2,000 Italian libraries for a total of about 85,000 bibliographic records). It's not fully comprehensive, since it does not include all Italian libraries, owing to the absence of institutional agreements at a central level which would force the libraries to contribute with their holdings and to update their data.

ACNP may be considered the basis of an interesting experience developed subsequently and independently by the Italian Group of documentalists of pharmaceutical industries and of biomedical research institutes (GIDIF/RBM): the union catalogue of serial owned by biomedical libraries taking part in this group (4). Forty libraries participate in this catalogue which has been produced with the explicit aim of supporting document delivery between the associated libraries and is updated annually.

Strict and precise rules allow a satisfactory document delivery service to libraries which are part of this consortium. Various catalogues have also been produced by libraries using DOBIS/LIBIS system (5) and some of the twelve installations in Italy give access to their catalogues (OPAC) through INTERNET to accelerate localization of documents. The most common way to acquire documents is still the local lending arrangements between libraries or the information establishment of exchanging documents on a reciprocity basis that does not require financial management. This voluntary type of agreement is due to end because it is not able to create an efficient document delivery service. A general experimental agreement (named BDD, Biomedical Document Delivery), has been tentatively established this year, by initiative of the librarians operating in the most different typologies of biomedical libraries. This agreement was reached to evaluate the real possibility of exchanging document at a national level. Two meetings on this matter were held in Bologna in February and in June 1994. Terms for exchange of documents between libraries were discussed according to the possibilities offered by technology developments and the integration of new media with traditional procedures.

This kind of experimental project is important also in view of a European policy of document exchange. Some Italian biomedical libraries are taking part in AIDA project (Alternatives for International Document Availability) which was presented to DGXIII CEE in 1993, in order to develop a network among Italian, French and Portuguese libraries, for an efficient and fast document delivery service. This network will be interconnected with other infrastructures already existing in the countries involved (GARR in Italy; RCCN - Rede de Calculo Cientifico Nacional in Portugal and the French network) and in the future access will be granted to other countries.

Conclusion

There is a growing need to integrate international projects for international document delivery with an Italian solution to the problem. Many attempts and initiatives are oriented in achieving a centralised solution, even if in the present situation local initiatives suggested by specific situations still prevail. In effect all biomedical libraries, whatever their dimensions and resources, are fully engaged in attempting to fulfil the scientists greatest expectation: to get the document on their desks.

References

(1) Associazione Italiana Biblioteche. *Guida alle biblioteche biomediche italiane.* Milano: Vita e Pensiero, 1993.

(2) FOGLIENI, O. *La rete SBN e le biblioteche biomediche*, II Jornadas APDIS. Documentacao e informacao de saude, 1994. (in print).

(3) CNR/ISRDS, *Catalogo collettivo delle pubblicazioni periodiche.* Roma, ISRDS, 1990.

(4) *Catalogo collettivo dei periodici delle biblioteche biomediche del GIDIF/RBM.* Gruppo italiano documentalisti industrie farmaceutiche e istituti di ricerche biomediche. Milano: GIDIF/RBM, 1993.

(5) - *Catalogo collettivo dei periodici.* Università degli studi di Perugia. Ufficio per l'automazione delle biblioteche. Perugia, 1991.

- *Catalogo dei periodici correnti delle biblioteche di Parma e provincia.* Amministrazione provinciale di Parma. Parma, 1988.

- *Catalogo dei periodici.* Università degli studi di Modena. Modena, 1988.

ROLE OF RESEARCH LIBRARIES IN SCIENTIFIC INVESTIGATIONS OF MEDICAL AFTER-EFFECTS OF CHERNOBYL DISASTER

E P Ivanov, V S Lazarev[47], D Yunusova, L Velkovich, G Laysha, Research Institute of Hematology and Blood Transfusion, 160 Dolginovsky Tract, Minsk 223059, Republic of Belaruz

The reasons for the increasing role and responsibility of research libraries in the fulfilment of biomedical investigations of Chernobyl health hazards are pointed out. Some sights have been found of a special "out-burst" of information, devoted to Chernobyl related medical problems. At the same time, the medical library stocks in Belarus are not sufficient.

Introduction

The unique character of radiation exposure, caused by Chernobyl, and, therefore, the shortage of knowledge possessed by researchers as well as, generally, the shortage of knowledge in radiobiology possessed by clinical medicine scientists and vice versa seem to be the main general reasons for the unique role of research libraries in scientific investigations of Chernobyl medical after-effects. Among the specific political reasons of this even more important role in the post Chernobyl Republic of Belarus the absence of reliable data on immediate dosage exposure that requires now more special knowledge for reconstructing the missed notions; scientific and mass media censorship till 1989, stimulating still shorter knowledge of Belarussian scientific findings in 1986-1989 and the absence of epidemiological research sufficient backgrounds should be mentioned. It is important to know in this context if the thematic scattering of world's Chernobyl related (ie, relevant for the fulfilment of the various studies of medical after-effects of Chernobyl) scientific documentary information flows (DIFs) is really so vast or it is just seems to be so because of the above reasons; if there are any other specific features of world's Chernobyl related DIFs and if the Belarussian library stocks of scientific biomedical journals are sufficient.

Methods

By sorting *de visu* the relevant abstracts, disseminated during 7 months, 1990-1991, by a computerized scientific information service system that processed *all* the All-Union Institute of Scientific and Technical Information databases, disciplinary, as well as geographical, language and species structure of DIFs in 3 case to-pics, viz, assessment of incorporated radiation doses (A), leukemia treatment and prognostication of leukemia development (L) and morphological and functional state of haematopietic system under radiation exposure (M), were studied, alongside with the estimation of the "quotas" of references in journal papers per an average paper of each collection [1:2] and counting the number of journals, which papers were abstracted. The disciplinary orientation of the abstracts was determined according to the name of a database containing them and the thematic scattering of DIF was estimated according to the number of disciplinary-orientated databases, reflecting a concrete DIF. The number of cited references was taken from the abstracts.

Since the Republican Scientific Medical Library (RSML) is the largest one in Belarus, its stocks are available to any researcher, physician, medical student, etc ... and no other institution in Belarus has currency for subscribing foreign journals, it was enough to consider the RSML foreign periodicals stocks and to compare the value of *impact factors* (IF) of available journals (that reflects their general scientific value, viz, recent relative impact of an assessed journal in scientific development in general) with the IF values of the same number of journals in the same disciplines that have the highest value of IF and correspond to the specific features of the development of a discipline (represented by a journal) in Belarus. The journals in the following disciplines were chosen for the analysis: Hematology, Oncology, Immunology, Cardiovascular System, Genetics and Surgery. Since we have no JCR in Belarus since 1988 we were to use 1988 data.

Results and discussion

The results of the studies of Chernobyl-related DIFs (A, L and M) structure are plotted in Table 1.

---

47 To whom all correspondence should be sent.

Table 1: Characteristics of world's DIFs structure in topics A, L & M

Topic	DS	GS	LS	SS	JN	RQ
A	27	36	14	51.68/17.20	121	13.61/56.68
L	19	33	19	92.3/0	305	16.97/45.35
M	21	20	7	80/12	52	13.61/49.11

DS Disciplinary structure in terms of number of disciplinary-orientated databases;
GS Geographical structure in terms of number of countries
LS Language structure in terms of number of languages
SS Species structure in terms of parts of journal papers/conference abstract (%)
JN Number of source journals
RQ References quotas in an average non-review/review paper

We consider the DIFs thematic scattering as rather *too much high*, especially and undoubtedly for the topic A. Such a large number of related disciplines is more natural, when the scattering of CITED literature is under study because the processes of information usage seems to be inevitably more interdisciplinary in its nature than the process of "classification scattering" itself. Therefore, WE THINK THAT RESEARCH LIBRARIES INFORMATION SERVICE SHOULD REALLY PAY SPECIAL ATTENTION TO THIS PROBLEM, TRYING TO DELIVER AS MUCH AS POSSIBLE COMPLETE INFORMATION RETRIEVAL IN ALL IMAGINABLE SOURCES and not concentrating only on *specialised* databases. This conclusion is of a special importance in the content of a greatest special responsibility of Chernobyl-related medical scientific research.

At the same time, nothing very special is found about the geographical and language structure of DIFs (though, the number of countries where the research work on topic A is being fulfilled seems to be a bit more than trivial). Yet, the species structure is rather noticeable. On one hand, The unusually large part of conferences abstracts on the assessment of incorporated radiation doses might evidence about the research activity "burst-out" In this area since the first results are normally being published in this form immediately; on the other hand, the species structure of the DIF on leukemia treatment and prognostication of leukemia development with the enormous prevalence of journal articles is characteristic for a very stable development of a scientific branch not influenced by any urgent problems. (Our epidemiological findings of post Chernobyl childhood leukemia proves that no expected increase of radiation-induced leukemia appeared so far, so it might be possible that we put too much "Chernobyl status" to the topic L). As for the reference "quotas", taking into account the results of Price's studies [1:2], we came to a conclusion that the best grounded recent studies (out of the taken into account) are the ones for L, the best grounded review are on A. It is known, concerning non-humanities, that the greater number of references (within the range of 15.22 references in an average non-review paper from a collection) evidences about a potentially higher scientific value of the collection under study.

Table 2: Journals in selected disciplines in the RSLM stocks - their IF values vs. IF of "top quality" journals

DISCIPLINE	JOURNAL TITLE	"IF"	Rank of The Journal According Its "if" in the Disciplinary List	Average "if" Of the Available Journals	Average "if" for The same Number of top Journals of the Same discipline

Haematology	Blood	6.849	1	3.660	6.255
	American Journal of Pediatric Hematology and Oncology	0.671	25		
Genetics	Cytogenetics & Cell Genetics	3.753	7	2.305	10.908
	Journal of Medical Genetics	1.857	27		
Surgery	Laser in surgery & Medicine	1.421	12	0.727	2.512
	American Journal of Surgery	1.303	13		
	Plastic & Reconstruction Surgery	1.242	14		
	Transplantation Proceedings	1.096	17		
	The European Surgical Research	0.892	22		
	Journal of Bone & Joint Surgery	0.748	26		
	Der Unfallchirurg	0.101	68		
	Der Chirurg	absent in JCR			
Cardiovascular System	Circulation	6.676	1	3.699	5.617
	American Journal of Cardiology	2.619	10		
	American Heart Journal	1.801	18		

At the same time, it is known that a number of 40 references in a paper gives it a status of a review automatically, though there are also reviews with much less quantity of references. Again, it supports indirectly the opinion that the studies on L are oF a very stable character (possibly alongside with not so good realised cumulative function of reviews), whereas there is a kind of a "burst-out" of reviewing activity in the field of A. The results of the studies of the sufficiency of world's biomedical journals library stocks in Belarus are plotted in Table 2 except the ones in oncology (despite the fact that there is very powerful Research Institute of Oncology in Belarus. RSML has only one journal, whereas oncology is the field of medical science with the highest information scattering that has about 100 only *specialised* journals!) and immunology (RSML has 2 journals referring (not devoted!) to this field that a are not in JCR list of immunological journals and there is no heading "immunology" in the RSML international journals list! At the same time, the Republic of Belarus has a specialised immunological institute and several powerful departments and laboratories of immunology in other institutes).

So, the world's biomedical periodicals library stocks in Belarus are absolutely insufficient. Having 2-3 journals in a discipline is nothing, especially if these journals are not of a top value. Being very important parts of medical sciences, immunology (it's a leader!) and oncology (the biomedical discipline of the most documentary information scattering!) are ridiculously bad presented in the stocks. This is especially dramatic in Chernobyl context, in which these disciplines plays still even more important role.

So, there are some sights of a special "burst-out" of information devoted to Chernobyl-related medical problems. Tremendous thematic scattering could be traced at least for some of them. At the same time, the medical science in belarus is suffering from the "information hunger". After the break-up of the Soviet Union, when the state system of scientific and technical information became russia's property and due to some other economical reasons there is no possibility to obtain information from neighbouring russia. The Belarussian library stocks are not sufficient.

What could be kindly done for Belarus?

In fact, two Amercian programs of corresponding assistance are put into action. However, the problems remained, since no bibliometric criteria were applied to the journals selection for searching the appropriate ones, no specific features of Belarussian medical science and organizational structure of it (and, also scientist poverty) were taken into account.

Our idea of sufficient help supposes that a structure of biomedical post chernobyl belarussian science as well as the specific information needs ought to be taken into account and the "top quality" bibliometrically selected journals *themselves* should be generously provided. Also, the idea of giving such an assistance in reality to the research institutes seems to be fruitful.

References

1. D.J. de S. Price: Network of scientific papers: SCIENCE, 14 (1965) N3638: 510-515
2. D.S, Price: Citation quotas of hard science and soft-sceinces technology and non-science: VOPROSY FILOSOFIJ (1971) N3: 149-155 (in Russian)

CURRENCY ON CD-ROM OF ARTICLES FROM MEDLINE

Vincent Maes, Pfizer SA, 102, rue Léon Theodor, B-1090 Brussels, Belgium

Summary

On the 1993 CD-ROM disks of Medline, 371,010 descriptions were found over 3,271 serials. The overall average currency of information was 6.92 months. Values ranged from a minimum of -2 to 329 months. The mean journal currency ranged from 2 to 324 months, with an average of 9.18 months. Priority level, periodicity and prior database were found to have a highly significant influence on mean journal currency. The 10 most important serials (regarding ISI's impact factor for general medicine) are shown as examples of the secondary result database.

Introduction

The objectives were to:

- quantify the currency of the general average articles from Medline on CD-ROM
- quantify the mean currency for each serial
- establish influence of the priority level
- establish influence of the periodicity
- establish influence of the prior database : (Abridged) Index Medicus, Index to Dental Literature, and International Nursing Index
- obtain, as a secondary result, a database that summarizes for each serial characteristics and currency values

Graph 2 : Serial mean currency

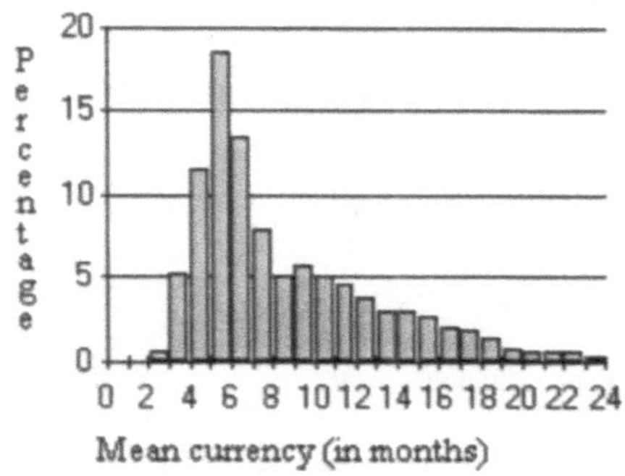

Graph 1 : Article currency

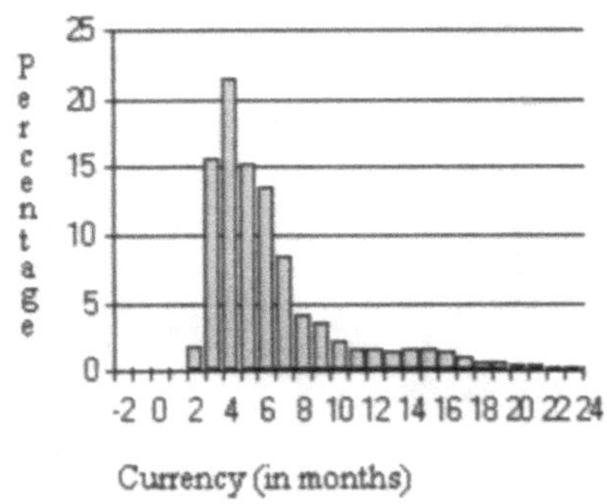

Methods

Appropriate fields were downloaded from the1993 disks of SilverPlatter Medline, and from Serline. Some adjustments had to be made to publication date and dates of receipt of the disks in order to make them complete. Periodicity was divided into 14 categories. All statistical tests were two-tailed and performed with SPSS.

Results

Graph 1 summarizes the distribution of the article currency. A total of 371,010 descriptions appeared in the

Graph 3 : Serial mean currency by priority level

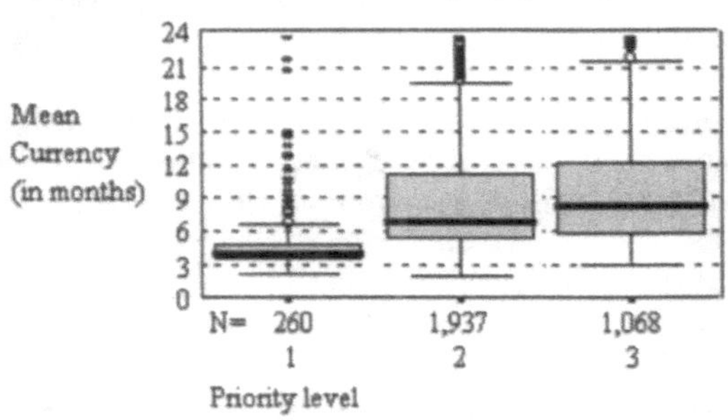

1993 disks. The overall average currency was 6.92 months with a standard deviation of 8.72. Values ranged from a minimum of -2 to 329 months. Negative values were checked with the NLM and this concluded to description errors from indexers. True minimum is 1 month. Such errors being possible, we had kept data from Medline. Graph 2 summarizes the distribution of serial mean currency. The mean journal currency of the 3,271 serials ranged from 2 to 324 months, with an average of 9.18 months and a standard deviation of 9.72.The priority level is an internal processing code to the National Library of Medicine as a means of control-ling workflow. It induces differences in indexing process : priority 1 and 2 journals are the journals indexed at NLM, respectively more or less in demand by users, and indexed in depth. Attempts are made to complete them respectively within 30 days and 60 days of receipt. Priority 3 journals are primarily regional interest journals, or others for which indexing is performed by the American Dental Association or the American Journal of Nursing Company. Articles are indexed less in depth and within 60 days of receipt.

Priority level was found to have a highly significant influence on serial mean journal currency. High priority journals tended to appear earlier on CD-ROM ($p<0.0001$). Verification with partial correlation controlled for periodicity test confirms influence.

Graph 3 shows the distribution of serial mean currency by priority level. We decided to detail the study of priority 1 journals mean currency.

Graph 4 shows the distribution of this. They had a median currency of 3.92 months. Only 5% of such journals appeared on CD-ROM within 3 months of publication, but 53.8% appeared within 4 months. First and last were respectively 2.2 and 23.75 months after publication. Although overlap is noted, priority 1 journals appeared 1 or 2 months earlier on CD-ROM.

Graph 4 : Serial mean currency for priority 1 journals

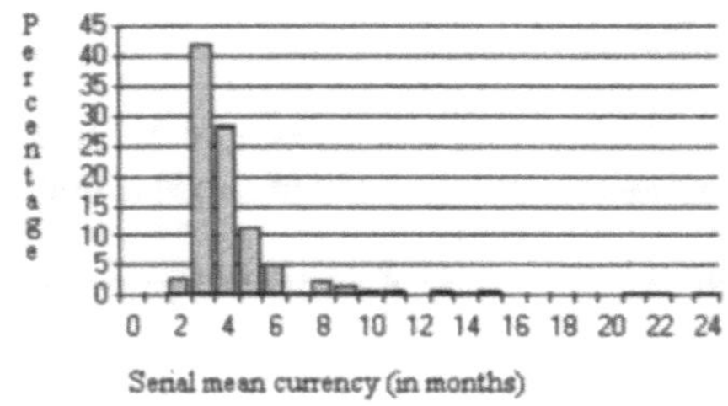

Graph 5 : Serial mean currency by periodicity category

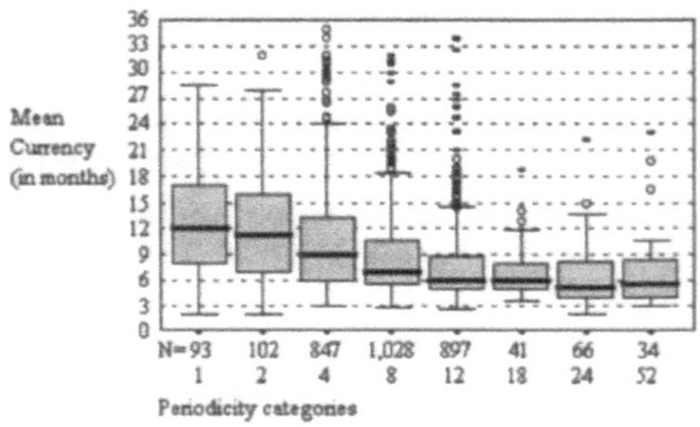

Graph 6 : Serial mean currency by prior database

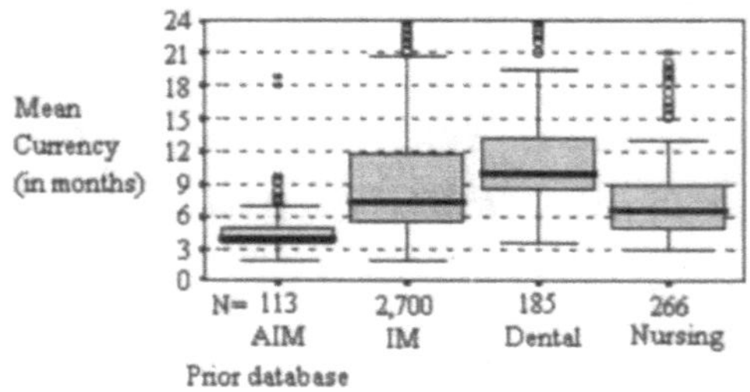

Periodicity categories reflects average number of issues per year. Serial mean journal currency was found to be highly significantly influenced by periodicity. As Graph 5 clearly shows, frequent periodicity tended to appear earlier on CD-ROM ($p<0.0001$)

Medline is the sum of the references appaering in Index Medicus (IM), Index to Dental Literature (Dental) and International Nursing Index (Nursing). Abridged Index Medicus (AIM) is a subset of IM containing a huge core of 115 biomedical English-language journals. These journals are mainly indexed as priority 1 journals. There was a significant difference in mean journal currency with regard to the prior database. Titles from the AIM database tended to appear earlier on CD-ROM than others.

A database was obtained as secondary product of the analysis. For each serial, it gives abbreviated title, type of date description in Medline (T), ISSN, periodicity (P), currency - mean (av), minimum (m), maximum (Mx) and standard deviation (std) - the number of articles (Nb), priority level (P), and prior database (Db). The 10 most important serials by ISI impact factor for general and internal medicine are shown in Table 1 as example of the built database.

Table 1 : Serial database : the 10 most important serials

Title	T	ISSN	P	Currency (in months)				Nb	P	Db
				av.	M	Mx	std			
N.Engl.J.Med.	1	0028-4793	W	21.85	2	320	76.27	1,427	1	AIM
Lancet.	1	0023-7507	W	6.60	2	187	25.66	2,977	1	AIM
Ann.Intern.Med.	1	0003-4819	SM	2.20	1	3	0.65	645	1	AIM
JAMA.	1	0098-7484	W	2.57	2	15	0.63	1,447	1	AIM
Diabetes.	2	0012-1797	M	3.14	3	4	0.35	273	1	AIM
Medicine.Baltimore.	2	0025-7974	BM	4.67	4	5	0.48	27	1	AIM
Diabetologia.	2	0012-186X	M	5.08	4	6	0.65	203	2	IM
BMJ.	1	0959-8138	W	4.48	3	6	0.58	2,071	1	AIM
Diabetes.Care.	2	0149-5992	M	4.08	3	6	0.84	404	2	IM
Arch.Intern.Med.	1	0003-9926	SM	3.02	2	4	0.69	324	1	AIM

Discussion

Currency of information in a database, although being an important part of coverage, seems to interest information scientists mainly for on-line databases. Other media, such as Diskettes or CD-ROMs are not very much studied, and the only information widely available and used is frequency of updates. The results of this study show that frequency of updates is not a very useful information on currency of the information. It is at most an indication of the evolution of coverage (whether coverage grows every week, or every month, etc.) and of a minimum possible with respect to its currency. Adjustments made to the publication date from Medline demonstrates that periodicity, period covered and publication date should better be given as three clearly different data. Another preoccupation is the sometimes great difference between the publication date and the actual date of receipt of a serial. Imbrication of characteristics studied - Abridged Index Medicus contains almost only priority 1 journals, which have at least a quarterly periodicity to qualify for sufficient importance - made it uneasy to show the correlations of each of them with currency, but partial correlation tests confirmed this with important significance level ($p < 0.0001$). The spread of the distribution is very wide : from 1 month to 27 years (!), and such large values are dedicated to at least one issue. These are certainly the result of completion of old collections, or addition of new titles. This is confirmed by the large standard deviations of serial mean currency, and relatively low median article currency compared with maximum.

Is the shown time-lag acceptable with regard to the time-consuming processing needed from publication to availability on CD-ROM ? If we look at the indexing process, 2 months seems to be the time needed, instead of the one-month attempt. Compared with time lags between submission and publication of an article, it seems quite low. Comparing with on-line, the production and the mailing of the disks are the two only supplementary processes of CD-ROM media. Thus, theoretically, on-line can only be 1 or 2 months more current than CD-ROM, which represents nevertheless 8% or 16% of the information of one year! And, as Re'em says, "*even if it is economically possible to update CD-ROM weekly, CD-ROMs can't be updated in real time instead of on-line*" A comparable study of Medline on-line would give precise information on the differences specifically induced by the CD-ROM medium. We hope this study has made information scientists aware of currency, and not only on CD-ROM.

Acknowledgements

My thanks are due to Dr K. Blot for his invaluable statistical help, to Mr P.J. Lottefier & Mrs M.-L. Chantraine for reviewing the manuscript, to Mr P. Chantraine for the layout of the poster, and to all people who send me information.

THE DATABASE NORINA: a Norwegian Inventory of Audiovisuals

Adrian Smith, Karina Smith & Richard Fosse [For correspondence] Laboratory Animal Unit, Norwegian College of Veterinary Medicine, P O Box 8146 Dep., N-0033 Oslo, Norway

Objectives

The debate on the ethics of using laboratory animals has led to discussions at many institutions on the necessity of using animals in routine teaching. The problem of finding suitable material has been tackled by the development of a database called NORINA (A Norwegian Inventory of Audiovisuals) containing information on approximately 1400 audiovisual teaching aids.

Methods

The Laboratory Animal Unit at the Norwegian College of Veterinary Medicine, Oslo, has compiled an English-language database of audiovisuals for use in the biological sciences. The primary purpose of this non-profit venture is to offer an overview of possible alternatives or supplements to the use of animals in student teaching, at all levels from schools to university. The database consists at present of around 1400 entries, including computer programs, interactive video, films and more traditional teaching aids such as slide series, 3-D models and classroom charts. There is also a section for Contact Persons who are developing and/or using audiovisual at their institution, and for suppliers of audiovisuals. Users, developers and suppliers of audiovisual are invited to send in details for future upgrades of the database. NORINA is available as a "stand-alone" version that will run on any IBM-compatible PC with harddisc, with no additional software. It is also available as a Filemaker Pro file, that will run on a Macintosh or IBM Windows machine where the database program Filemaker Pro is already installed. The price is US$150 (for networks with up to 30 workstations: US$750). Demonstration floppy discs and a set of sample printouts are available.

Further details are available from Professor Adrian Smith at the address above or by fax (+47 22 96 45 35), telephone (+47 22 96 45 74) or email (adrian.smith@veths.no).

INTERACTIONS OF BIOMEDICAL CENTRES WITH MARKETING AGENCIES AND TECHNICAL-MEDICAL MEDIA: New Customers/Suppliers?

L Vercellesi , GF Miranda , A Beretta [For correspondence] Zeneca S.p.A., Medical Department, Via F. Sforza, I-20080 Basiglio MI

Summary

Through questionnaires and structured interviews, present and potential relations between Biomedical Information Centres and Technical Medical Media (TM) or Pharmaceuticals Marketing Agencies (A) were investigated in Italy. Information Professional (IP) show attention to material produced by TM and A, recognising them as major source of information for prescribers. Their present role as suppliers is mainly mediated and for primary documentation and searches. TM and A have expressed needs which could be solved by IP, and the possibility of closer relations emerged, even as regards value-added information. The authors consistute a working group of GIDIF, RBM.

Introduction

Common perceptions in our association are:

- a sporadic use of information sources, other than scientific biomedical publications.
- a too-limited role of our professionals in support to technical-medical media and marketing agencies.

Aims of this study were to ascertain these perceptions in Italy. Responders were allowed to express more options; accordingly percentages can be higher than 100.

Information Professionals

Two-part questionnaires were addressed to all GIDIF, RBM members interviewing them about their role as costumers and suppliers.Results are evenly distributed between pharmaceutical industries and research institutes/hospitals, except for:

- Document delivery, which is mainly secured by research institutes/hospitals (41% vs 19% of pharmaceutical industries)
- Pharmaceutical literature, which is almost not collected by research institutes/hospitals, in spite being the main information source for prescribers. Only 17 IP answer queries directly; further 14 through intermediaries (scientists, medical, marketing functions); 23 neither receive queries nor know which is the point of contact in the institution.

Table 1. Demography

58/150 IP answered		PHARMACEUTICALS INDUSTRIES (n)	RESEARCH INST/HOSPITAL (n)	TOTAL (n)
54 questionnaires were evaluable	DOCUMENTALISTS LIBRARIANS	32 5	10 10	42 15
	TOTAL	37	20	57

Table 2. Activity as suppliers

		INFORMATION SUPPLIED	
		DOCUMENT DELIVERY (n)	SEARCHES & INFORMATION (n)
Activity as suppliers is mainly for primary documentation	MARKETING AGENCIES	12	5
	TECHNICAL MEDICAL MEDIA	12	2
	PRESS AGENCIES	5	1

Table 3. Activity as customers

		PRESENT USE OF SOURCES (n)
Acquisition and retrieval are occasional. Further 40% IP show a potential interest.	TECHNICAL MEDICAL MEDIA	29
	PHARMACEUTICAL LITERATURE	21
	PRESS AGENCIES	13

Technical Medical Media

Technical medical media (TM) are overall secondary, non-indexed journals. Their contents are abstracted, reviewed or commented scientific papers, general comments, news, over-views of congresses. 15 TM corresponding to this definition were identified through two Italian official directories: CSST (Consorzio Stampa Specializzata Tecnica) and USPI (Unione Stampa Periodici Italiani). 14/15 editors answered a structured interview.

Table 4. Selection of news

		MAIN PARAMETER (% of respondents)	SECONDARY PARAMETER (% of respondents)
Core journals are the main source	SOURCES	100% scientific literature (inhouse scanning or through consultants)	78% press agencies
	CRITERIA	86% relevance	17% originality
	APPROVAL	100% reliability	36% originality

Table 5. Sourced used

		SOURCES INVOLVED IN MEDICAL WRITING (% of respondents)
Editors process news without referring to originating researcher	PRIMARY LITERATURE DATABASES CONSULTANTS ORIGINATING RESEARCHER	71% 57% 21% rare

Table 6. Feedback received

		FEEDBACK TO NEWS (% of respondents)
Feedback is common: never received from IP	PUBLICATION AUDIENCE LAY PRESS CONSULTANTS ORIGINATING RESEARCHER	43% 36% 14% 7%

Table 7. Perceived needs

		POTENTIAL SERVICES (% of respondents)
Only 29% TM refer to IP 93% express a need for a continuing support.	LITERATURE SEARCHES DOCUMENT DELIVERY CURRENT AWARENESS CHECKS: CONSISTENCY, RELIABILITY, ORIGINALITY COPYRIGHT CLEARANCE	93% 86% 43% 43% 36%

Marketing Agencies

No specific association federates pharmaceutical marketing agencies (a) in Italy. The commonest estimated number is 20. The most known agencies were contacted: 10/13 answered a structured interview, through directors, copies and accounts.

Table 8. Sources used

		ACCESS TO INFORMATION (% of respondents)
Three scenarios were identified as regards information facilities	CUSTOMERS' CENTRES EXTERNAL CONSULTANTS INHOUSE INFO CENTRE	60% 60% 40%

Table 9. Selection of information

		MAIN PARAMETER (% of respondents)	SECONDARY PARAMETER (% of respondents)
Legal requirements for approval of literature demand the use of scientific source and criteria	SOURCES	90% inhouse literature	10% consultants
	CRITERIA	90% core journals and first line papers	10% minor or local publications (best available)
	CHECK	100% strictly scientific criteria	

Table 10. Processing of information

		PROCESSING OF INFORMATION (n)
Mixed modalities are followed in provision of information for medical writing. Criteria followed are as above.	INHOUSE RESOURCES	6
	CUSTOMERS	4
	EXTERNAL CONSULTANTS	2

Table 11. Perceived needs

		POTENTIAL SERVICES FROM IP (n)
The potential request of services by A is limited (*activities considered copywriters' responsibility) The four A with inhouse info centres receive the full range of services.	SEARCHES	4
	DOCUMENT DELIVERY	4
	CURRENT AWARENESS	4
	COPYRIGHT CLEARANCE	3*
	CHECKS: RELIABILITY. ORIGINALITY, CONSISTENCY	3*

10/10 A refer to IP for primary documentation or searches (often 50%; sporadically 40%).

At least Medline on CD-Rom is available in all A.

2/10 A still consider possible referencing literature after copy-writing.

Discussion and Conclusion

In spite of difficult retrieval, due to lack of indexing, IP show an attention to enlarge the typical sources of information to technical-medical media and pharmaceutical literature. This reflects an understanding of the common sources of information for presribers. Routine acquisition is envisaged in particular from public centres. Mediated contacts with technical-medical media and pharmaceutical marketing agencies confine the role of IP mainly to suppliers of primary documentation. No TM has a formal information centre; few search literature databases. All perceive a need for a support from IP, in particular for document delivery and literature searches, confirming a traditional view of librarian services. In addition to the four A with an information centre, further 4 would appreciate the support from IP for primary, secondary and value-added information. None plans to create an inhouse structure to avoid fixed costs. In our opinion needs emerging from this study could be satisfied by IP, whose potential is underestimated by TM and A due to mediated contacts (scientists, marketing. medical functions). In return IP could experience a qualitative expansion of their role in favour of value-added information. Direct integration with enduser and better knowledge of their institutions will help IP in this direction.

MAINTAINING QUALITY IN A MEDICAL INFORMATION GROUP

Luisa Vercellesi, Medical Department, ZENECA S.p.A., Via F. Sforza, I-20080 BASIGLIO Milano, Italia

Summary
A project to improve quality was decided and started with mapping of the group situation and promotion to customers. Assessment was carried out yearly, with feedback to users, and remedial actions planned. Restart of the quality cycle was foreseen. Improvement in one area showed a carry-over effect on the whole production. Feedback to customers made them more realistic and satisfied enquirers.

1990 - Introduction
An internal mission statement requiring to supply professional services at a level exceeding the average originated a local quality project (1). Aims were:

- to improve quality of services/products
- to define suitable methods and carry out assessments.

1991 - Material and Methods

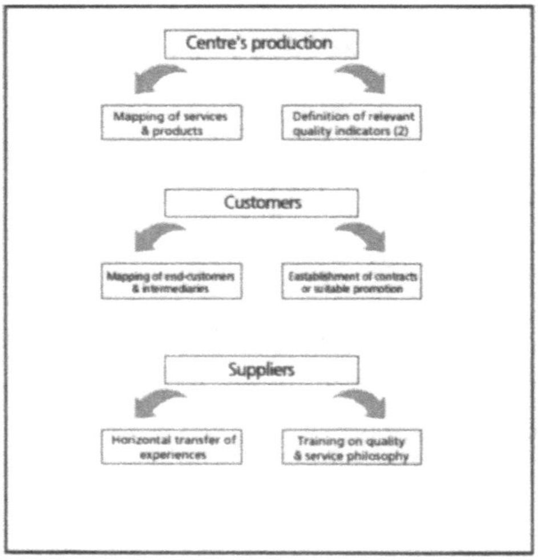

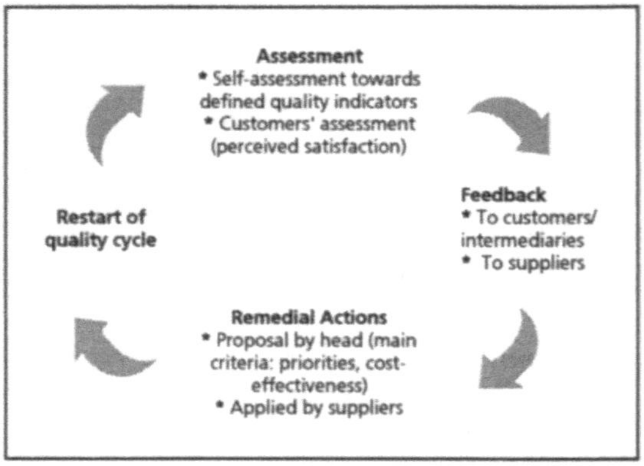

1992/1993 - Results
In 1992 all products/services were assessed by all customers/intermediaries and internally. Production was considered for remedial action if global assessment scored < good in > 20% of answers. After implementation of remedial actions, in 1993 a streamlined procedure was adopted.

	1992		1993	
Group of products Assessors	remedial > good critical issues actions > good			
Reactive service/Document delivery				
Health profession	91%	language	no	n.a.
Reps	92%	time/language	yes/no	95%
Internal customers	69%	timeliness	yes	>80%*
Self-assessment	75%	timeliness	yes	75%
Alerting service (Ref + Abs)/Dissemination of information				
Investigators	95%	n.a.		
Internal customers	9%	full paper	>80%*	
Self-assessment	78%	advisable	yes	85%
Periodicals circulation				
Internal customers	69%	timeliness	yes	>80%*
Self-assessment	85%	85%		
n.a. = not available; * = informal feedback				

1994 - Discussion and Conclusions

Internal customers appeared to be more severe and closer to self-assessment; stressing a strong company perception of information potentials. Some critical issues could find a reasonable remedy (eg, duplicate subscriptions to main circulating journals with consultation copy in the library) others legally debatable (eg, full papers distributed with alerting); in some other cases technical solutions could be possible, but not feasible for budget constraints (eg, timeliness in paper ordering). The critical issue "language" could not find technical solutions due to lack of Italian literature databases, and paucity of publications in Italian. Assessment is a time-consuming activity still deserving attention. A quality improvement in an individual product showed a "carry over" effect on the whole production. Explanations to customers made them to be more realistic enquirers, even if more demanding.

1. Vercellesi L., Enhancing quality in a medical information group. Bakker S. & Cleland M.C.: Information transfer: new age - new ways. Kluwer Academic Publishers, Dordrecht, 1992, pp347-350..

2. Vercellesi L., Colombi M., Pesenti M.T. etal, Quality Assurance in Drug Information Centres. Online & CDRom Review Vol. 17, 279-283, 1993.

SUBJECT INDEX

Index to Authors

FSC
www.fsc.org
MIX
Papier | Fördert
gute Waldnutzung
FSC® C083411

Kolibri 360 GmbH
Ferdinand-Jühlke-Straße 7
99095 Erfurt, Deutschland
produktsicherheit@kolibri360.de